BLUEPRINTS
NEUROLOGY

Third Edition

BLUEPRINTS
NEUROLOGY

Third Edition

Frank W. Drislane, MD
Associate Professor of Neurology
Harvard Medical School
Comprehensive Epilepsy Center
Beth Israel Deaconess Medical Center
Boston, Massachusetts

Michael Benatar, MBChB, DPhil
Associate Professor of Neurology and
Epidemiology
Director, Electromyography Laboratory
Emory University
Atlanta, Georgia

Bernard S. Chang, MD
Assistant Professor of Neurology
Harvard Medical School
Comprehensive Epilepsy Center
Beth Israel Deaconess Medical Center
Boston, Massachusetts

Juan Acosta, MD
Neurologist, Clinical
Neurophysiologist
European Medical Doctor
Best Doctors
Madrid, Spain

Andrew Tarulli, MD
Instructor in Neurology
Harvard Medical School
Division of Neuromuscular Disease
Beth Israel Deaconess Medical Center
Boston, Massachusetts

Louis R. Caplan, MD
Professor of Neurology
Harvard Medical School
Cerebrovascular Service
Beth Israel Deaconess Medical Center
Boston, Massachusetts

Wolters Kluwer | Lippincott Williams & Wilkins
Health

Philadelphia • Baltimore • New York • London
Buenos Aires • Hong Kong • Sydney • Tokyo

Acquisitions Editor: Charley Mitchell
Managing Editor: Stacey Sebring and Jessica Heise
Associate Production Manager: Kevin Johnson
Creative Director: Doug Smock
Compositor: Maryland Composition/ASI
Printer: RR Donnelley

The publisher is not responsible (as a matter of product liability, negligence, or otherwise) for any injury resulting from any material contained herein. This publication
contains information relating to general principles of medical care that should not be
construed as specific instructions for individual patients. Manufacturers' product
information and package inserts should be reviewed for current information, including contraindications, dosages, and precautions.

Printed in China
Library of Congress Cataloging-in-Publication Data
Blueprints neurology / Frank W. Drislane ... [et al.].
— 3rd ed.
        p. ; cm.
    Includes bibliographical references and index.
    ISBN 978-0-7817-9685-9
   1. Neurology—Examinations, questions, etc. 2. Physicians—Licenses—United
States—Examinations—Study guides. I. Drislane, Frank. II. Title: Neurology.
    [DNLM: 1. Nervous System Diseases. 2. Neurology. WL 140 B658 2009]
    RC336.B575 2009
    616.80076—dc22

                                                    2008025255

The publishers have made every effort to trace the copyright holders for borrowed material. If they have inadvertently overlooked any, they will be pleased to make the necessary
arrangements at the first opportunity.
To purchase additional copies of this book, call our customer service department at
(800) 638-3030 or fax orders to (301) 824-7390. International customers should call
(301) 714-2324.
Visit Lippincott Williams & Wilkins on the Internet: http://www.LWW.com. Lippincott
Williams & Wilkins customer service representatives are available from 8:30 am to
6:00 pm, EST.

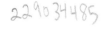

Contents

Reviewers

Catarina Castaneda, MD
Class of 2004
Drexel University College of Medicine
Philadelphia, Pennsylvania

Maureen Chase, MD
Resident, Emergency Medicine
Hospital of University of Pennsylvania
Jefferson Medical College
Thomas Jefferson University Hospital
Philadelphia, Pennsylvania

Suzanne Crandall
Class of 2005
Kansas City University of Medicine and Biosciences
Kansas City, Missouri

Alexis Dang, MD
Class of 2004
University of California—San Francisco
San Francisco, California

Lee S. Engel, MD, PhD
Fellow, Department of Infectious Diseases
Louisiana State University Health Sciences Center
New Orleans, Louisiana

Merritt Fajt, MD
Class of 2004
Temple University School of Medicine
Philadelphia, Pennsylvania
R1- Internal Medicine, Penn State University

Milton S. Hershey
Hershey Medical Center
Hershey, Pennsylvania

Baback Gabbay, MD
Class of 2005
David Geffen School of Medicine at UCLA
Los Angeles, California

Amir A. Ghaferi
Class of 2005
Johns Hopkins School of Medicine
Baltimore, Maryland

Hoda Ghanem, MD
Intern
UC Irvine—Internal Medicine
Irvine, California

Sarah Harper
Class of 2005
University of Pittsburgh School of Medicine
Pittsburgh, Pennsylvania

Gloria Hsu
Class of 2005
Stanford University School of Medicine
Stanford, California

Mark Lassoff, MD
Class of 2004
UMDNJ—New Jersey Medical School
Newark, New Jersey

Urology Resident
LAC+USC Medical Center
Los Angeles, California

Ryan Ley
Class of 2005
University of Nevada School of Medicine
Reno, Nevada

Meredith M. LeQuear, DO
Class of 2004
New York College of Osteopathic Medicine
Old Westbury, New York

Mark Naftanel
Class of 2005
Duke University School of Medicine
Durham, North Carolina

David J. Nusz, MD
Class of 2004
SUNY Downstate College of Medicine
Brooklyn, New York

Christi Otten
Class of 2005
University of Oklahoma Health Sciences Center—Physician Assistant program
Oklahoma City, Oklahoma

Pulak Ray
Class of 2005
University of Maryland School of Medicine
Baltimore, Maryland

Chris Reed
Class of 2005
Medical College of Wisconsin
Milwaukee, Wisconsin

Matheni Sathananthan
Class of 2006
SUNY at Buffalo School of Medicine
Buffalo, New York

Kamran Shamsa, MD
Class of 2004
University of California—San Diego
La Jolla, California

Victor Sung
Class of 2005
University of Texas Southwestern Medical Center
Dallas, Texas

Ahmet Tural, MD
Department of Infectious Diseases
Providence Physician Group
Everett, Washington

Alyssa Tzoucalis
Class of 2004
Hofstra University—Physician Assistant program
Hempstead, New York

Parham Yashar, MD
Neurological Surgery PGY-1
Albert Einstein College of Medicine
Bronx, New York

Ming Zhou, MD
Class of 2004
University of Nevada School of Medicine
Las Vegas, Nevada

Preface

In 1997, the first five books in the **Blueprints** series were published as board review for medical students, interns, and residents who wanted high-yield, accurate clinical content for USMLE Steps 2 and 3. Nearly a decade later, the **Blueprints** brand has expanded into a high-quality, trusted resource covering the broad range of clinical topics studied by medical students and residents during their primary, specialty, and subspecialty rotations.

The **Blueprints** were conceived as study aids created by students, for students. In keeping with this concept, the editors of the current editions of the **Blueprints** books have recruited resident contributors to ensure that the third edition of the series continues to offer the information and approach that made the original **Blueprints** a success.

Now in their third editions, each of the five specialty **Blueprints**—**Blueprints** Emergency Medicine, **Blueprints** Family Medicine, **Blueprints** Neurology, **Blueprints** Cardiology, and **Blueprints** Radiology—has been completely revised and updated to bring you the most current treatment and management strategies. The feedback we've received from our readers has been tremendously helpful in guiding the editorial direction of the second editions; for that, we are grateful to the hundreds of medical students and residents who have responded with in-depth comments and highly detailed feedback.

Each book has been thoroughly reviewed and revised accordingly, with new features being included across the series. An evidence-based resource section has been added to provide current and classic references for each chapter, and an increased number of current board-format questions with detailed explanations for correct and incorrect answer options are included in each book. All revisions to the **Blueprints** series have been made in order to offer you the most concise, comprehensive, and cost-effective information available.

Our readers report that **Blueprints** are useful for every step of their medical career, from their clerkship rotations and subinternships to a board review for USMLE Steps 2 and 3. Residents studying for USMLE Step 3 often use the books to review areas that were not their specialty. Students from a wide variety of health care specialties, including those in physician assistant, nurse practitioner, and osteopathic programs, use **Blueprints** either as a course companion or to review for their licensure examinations.

However you use **Blueprints**, we hope that you find the books in the series informative and useful. Your feedback and suggestions are essential to our continued success.

The Publisher
Lippincott Williams & Wilkins

Acknowledgments

We thank our patients for the opportunity of working with them and learning Neurology, our colleagues and teachers in the Beth Israel Deaconess Medical Center Neurology department for teaching us more fascinating concepts about the nervous system, and our families for tolerating the many hours spent writing and revising this book.

Abbreviations

A(β)	amyloid-beta		DM	dermatomyositis
ABP	abductor pollicis brevis		DMD	Duchenne muscular dystrophy
Abs	antibodies		DSD	detrusor-sphincter dyssynergia
AβPP	amyloid–beta protein precursor		DTRs	deep tendon reflexes
ACA	anterior cerebral artery		DWI	diffusion-weighted imaging
ACE	angiotensin converting enzyme		EA	episodic ataxia
AD	Alzheimer disease		ED	erectile dysfunction
ADEM	acute disseminated encephalomyelitis		EEG	electroencephalogram
ADHD	attention deficit–hyperactivity disorder		EMG	electromyography
ADM	abductor digiti minimi		ER	emergency room
AED	antiepileptic drug		ESR	erythrocyte sedimentation rate
AICA	anteroinferior cerebellar artery		ET	essential tremor
AIDP	acute inflammatory demyelinating polyradiculoneuropathy		EWN	Edinger-Westphal nuclei
			FDI	first dorsal interosseus
AIDS	acquired immunodeficiency syndrome		FEV$_1$	forced expiratory volume in 1 second
AION	anterior ischemic optic neuropathy		FLAIR	fluid-attenuated inversion recovery
ALS	amyotrophic lateral sclerosis		FTA	fluorescent treponemal antibody
ANA	antinuclear antibody		FTD	frontotemporal dementia
APP	amyloid precursor protein		FVC	forced vital capacity
APS	antiphospholipid syndrome		GAD	glutamic acid decarboxylase
AVM	arteriovenous malformation		GBS	Guillain-Barré syndrome
AZT	zidovudine		GCS	Glasgow Coma Scale
BMD	Becker muscular dystrophy		GTC	generalized tonic-clonic
BPPV	benign positional paroxysmal vertigo		HD	Huntington's disease
CBC	complete blood count		HIV	human immunodeficiency virus
cGMP	cyclic guanosine monophosphate		HNPP	hereditary neuropathy with liability to pressure palsies
CIDP	chronic inflammatory demyelinating polyradiculoneuropathy			
			HS	Horner's syndrome
CJD	Creutzfeldt-Jakob disease		HSAN	hereditary sensory and autonomic neuropathy
CK	creatine kinase			
CMAP	compound muscle action potential		HSV	herpes simplex virus
CMT	Charcot-Marie-Tooth disease		IBM	inclusion body myositis
CN	cranial nerve		ICA	internal cerebral artery
CNS	central nervous system		ICP	intracranial pressure
COMT	catechol O-methyl transferase		ICU	intensive care unit
CP	cerebral palsy		IIH	idiopathic intracranial hypertension
CPAP	continuous positive airway pressure		INO	internuclear ophthalmoplegia
CSF	cerebrospinal fluid		INR	international normalized ratio
CT	computed tomography		IVIg	intravenous immunoglobulin
DH	detrusor hyperreflexia		LEMS	Lambert-Eaton myasthenic syndrome
DI	detrusor instability		LGN	lateral geniculate nucleus
DLB	dementia with Lewy bodies		LMN	lower motor neuron

LND	light-near dissociation		PM	polymyositis
LP	lumbar puncture		PML	progressive multifocal leukoencephalopathy
MAG	myelin-associated glycoprotein			
MCA	middle cerebral artery		PN	peripheral neuropathy
MELAS	mitochondrial myopathy, encephalopathy, lactic acidosis, and stroke		PNS	peripheral nervous system
			POTS	postural orthostatic tachycardia syndrome
MERRF	myoclonic epilepsy with ragged red fibers		PP	periodic paralysis
			PPD	purified protein derivative
MFS	Miller Fisher syndrome		PPRF	paramedian pontine reticular formation
MG	myasthenia gravis		PS1	presenilin 1
MLF	medial longitudinal fasciculus		PS2	presenilin 2
MMN	multifocal motor neuropathy		PSP	progressive supranuclear palsy
MND	motor neuron disease		PT	prothrombin time
MRA	magnetic resonance angiography		PTT	partial thromboplastin time
MRC	Medical Research Council		PVR	post-void residual
MRI	magnetic resonance imaging		QSART	quantitative sudomotor axon reflex test
MRV	magnetic resonance venography		RAPD	relative afferent pupillary defect
MS	multiple sclerosis		REM	rapid eye movement
MSA	multiple system atrophy		RF	radiofrequency
MSLT	multiple sleep latency test		riMLF	rostral interstitial nucleus of the MLF
MuSK	muscle-specific kinase		RPR	rapid plasma reagin
nAChR	nicotinic acetylcholine receptor		rt-PA	recombinant tissue-type plasminogen activator
NCS	nerve conduction studies			
NCV	nerve conduction velocity		SAH	subarachnoid hemorrhage
NFTs	neurofibrillary tangles		SCA	spinocerebellar ataxia
NIF	negative inspiratory force		SCA	superior cerebellar artery
NMDA	*N*-methyl-D-aspartate		SE	status epilepticus
NMJ	neuromuscular junction		SLE	systemic lupus erythematosus
NMS	neuroleptic malignant syndrome		SMA	spinal muscular atrophy
NSAIDs	nonsteroidal anti-inflammatory drug		SNAP	sensory nerve action potential
OCD	obsessive-compulsive disorder		SPECT	single-photon emission computed tomography
ODS	optic disc swelling			
ON	optic neuritis		SSRI	selective serotonin reuptake inhibitor
PANDAS	pediatric autoimmune neurologic disorders associated with streptococcal infection		STT	spinothalamic tract
			TB	tuberculosis
			TCD	transcranial Doppler
PAS	periodic acid–Schiff		TE	time to echo
PCA	posterior cerebral arteries		TIA	transient ischemic attack
PCD	paraneoplastic cerebellar degeneration		TORCH	toxoplasmosis, other agents, rubella, cytomegalovirus, herpes simplex
PCNSL	primary central nervous system lymphoma			
			TR	time to repetition
PCR	polymerase chain reaction		TSC	tuberous sclerosis complex
PD	Parkinson's disease		UMN	upper motor neuron
PDC	paroxysmal (nonkinesogenic) dystonic choreoathetosis		VA	visual acuity
			VDRL	Venereal Disease Research Laboratory
PEO	progressive external ophthalmoplegia		VOR	vestibulo-ocular reflex
PET	positron emission tomography		VP	venous pulsation
PICA	posteroinferior cerebellar artery		VPL	ventroposterolateral
PKC	paroxysmal kinesogenic choreoathetosis		WD	Wilson's disease

Part 1

Basics of Neurology

The Neurologic Examination

To practicing neurologists, the neurologic exam reflects the uniqueness of the specialty. In a world of technology, it remains a purely clinical tool still unmatched in its ability to identify and localize abnormalities of the nervous system. To students, however, the exam can be both mystifying and bemusing, an endless series of maneuvers designed to elicit seemingly obscure and inexplicable findings.

When its principles and elements are presented simply, though, the exam is logical and elegant, reflecting the rational diagnostic process that characterizes not just Neurology but all of medicine.

PRINCIPLES

1. **The neurologic exam is not a standardized checklist.** Part of the intimidation of performing the exam is its sheer length; hours could be spent on examining the mental status alone. In reality, however, the exam is used in a focused and thoughtful way, depending on what hypotheses have been generated about the patient's disease from the history. A patient presenting with confusion may need quite a comprehensive mental status exam, whereas a patient presenting with a left foot drop may need detailed motor, sensory, and reflex testing of the left leg. In both cases general screening elements of the remaining parts of the exam may be sufficient.

2. **Observation is more important than confrontation.** Most abnormalities of the nervous system manifest themselves in ways visible to the observant examiner. A significant anomia becomes evident when a patient uses circumlocutions to relate the history, and proximal weakness is obvious when they have difficulty rising from a chair. It is often more useful to describe a patient's observed activities and capabilities than to describe the findings obtained upon formal testing. Confrontation testing is subjective and variable; the grading of muscle strength depends on the examiner's effort and expectations of what the patient's "normal" strength should be. The observation of a pronator drift, for example, is less subjective.

3. **The object is to localize.** The extent and complexity of the nervous system require that any attempt to formulate a concise differential diagnosis must begin with an accurate localization of the problem to a specific region of the nervous system. Left hand weakness may stem from carpal tunnel syndrome, a brachial plexus injury, cervical spondylosis, or a right middle cerebral artery stroke, all of which have different diagnostic workups, treatments, and prognoses. The alert physician thinks, "What signs would be present in a carpal tunnel problem that would not be present in a brachial plexus problem (and vice versa)?" Those signs are then sought and the exam further refined if necessary.

4. **Not all findings have equal importance.** A common difficulty is that completion of the exam results in a long list of many minor abnormalities of questionable importance, such as a 20% decrease in temperature sensation over a patch on the left thigh. Though certainly in some cases incidental findings may be the clue to a previously unsuspected diagnosis, in most cases the highest importance must be given to findings directly related to the patient's symptoms and to "hard" findings that require definitive explanation, such as a dropped reflex or a Babinski sign.

KEY POINTS

- The neurologic exam is not a standardized checklist.
- Observation is more important than confrontation.
- The object is to localize.
- Not all findings have equal importance.

ELEMENTS OF THE EXAM

As discussed earlier, the specific features to include in the neurologic exam should vary with each patient; however, commonly performed elements of the exam are described in this section and listed in Table 1-1.

■ **TABLE 1-1** Commonly Performed Elements of the Neurologic Examination	
Mental status	
Attention	Serial backward tasks (months of the year, digit span)
Language	Fluency of speech, repetition, comprehension of commands, naming objects, reading, writing
Memory	Three words in 5 minutes
Visuospatial function	Drawing clock, copying complex figure
Neglect	Line bisection, double simultaneous stimulation
Frontal lobe function	Generating word lists, learning a motor sequence
Cranial nerves	
II	Visual acuity, fields, pupils, funduscopic exam
III, IV, VI	Extraocular movements
V, VII	Facial sensation and movement
IX, X, XII	Palate and tongue movement
Motor	
Bulk	Palpation for atrophy
Tone	Evaluation for rigidity, spasticity
Power	Observational tests (pronator drift, rising from chair, walking on heels and toes), direct confrontation strength testing
Reflexes	
Muscle stretch reflexes	Biceps, brachioradialis, triceps, knee, ankle
Babinski sign	Stroking lateral sole of foot
Sensory	
Pinprick and temperature	Pin, cold tuning fork
Vibration and joint position sense	Tuning fork and moving digits
Coordination	
Accuracy of targeting	Finger-to-nose, heel-to-shin
Rhythm of movements	Rapid alternating movements, rhythmic finger or heel tapping
Gait	
Stance	Narrow or wide base
Romberg sign	Steadiness with feet together and eyes closed
Stride and arm swing	Assessment for shuffling, decreased arm swing
Ataxia	Ability to tandem walk

MENTAL STATUS

Neurologists use the mental status exam to identify cognitive deficits that help to localize a problem to a specific region of the brain. Thus the exam differs from that used by psychiatrists, whose objectives in performing the exam are different.

The first step in mental status testing is to assess the level of consciousness. This may vary from the alert wakefulness of a clinic outpatient to the coma of a patient in the intensive care unit. There is a tendency to use "medical" terminology—such as **stuporous**, **obtunded**, or **lethargic**—to describe the level of consciousness, but these have variable meanings; it is more useful to describe how well patients stayed awake or what stimulation was required to arouse them.

Next, assuming the level of consciousness allows for further testing of cognitive functions, attention is tested, typically with serial forward and backward tasks. These include digit span, reciting the months of the year, or spelling the word "**world**," all forward and backward. Attention is usually tested early, because significant inattention compromises the ability to perform subsequent cognitive tests and may render their interpretation difficult.

Next, language is assessed. As noted previously, listening to the patient tell their history may be all that is necessary to gauge language ability. Formal testing, however, includes assessing the fluency of spontaneous speech, the ability to repeat, the ability to comprehend commands, the ability to name both common and less common objects, and the ability to read and write.

For memory testing, most often the patient is given three words and asked to recall them several minutes later, with the aid of hints if necessary. More information can be gained by giving longer lists of words and charting the patient's learning (and forgetting) curve. Visual memory can be tested with three simple shapes for the patient to draw from memory in several minutes.

Visuospatial function can be tested in a variety of ways. Patients can be asked to draw a clock, a cube, or another simple figure; alternatively, they can be asked to copy a complex figure drawn by the examiner (Fig. 1-1).

Neglect is a mental status finding typically not sought by nonneurologists, yet its presence can be a very important sign. Patients with dense neglect may fail to describe items on one side of a picture or of their surroundings, or may fail to bisect a line properly. Subtle neglect may manifest as extinction to double simultaneous stimulation, in which a patient

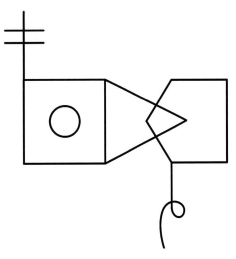

Figure 1-1 • Example of a complex figure to be copied by the patient as test of visuospatial function.

can sense a single stimulus on either side but when bilateral stimuli are presented simultaneously will sense only the one on the nonneglected side.

Tests of frontal lobe function include learning a simple motor sequence of hand postures, inhibiting inappropriate responses when following a "go/no-go" paradigm, or generating lists of words beginning with a particular letter or belonging to a particular category.

 KEY POINTS

- The mental status exam should begin with assessment of level of consciousness and attention, because these can affect the interpretation of subsequent tests.
- Language, memory, visuospatial function, neglect, and tests of frontal lobe function are other key elements of the mental status exam that can suggest focal brain lesions.

CRANIAL NERVES

It is usually easiest to test the cranial nerves (or at least to record the results) in approximate numerical order (Table 1-2).

Olfaction (cranial nerve I) is rarely tested, but when this is important, each nostril should be tested separately with a nonnoxious stimulus, such as coffee or vanilla.

Tests of optic nerve (II) function include visual acuity (using a near card), visual fields (tested by confrontation with wiggling fingers or with a small red

■ **TABLE 1-2** The Cranial Nerves

Nerve	English Name	Exit Through Skull	Function
I	Olfactory	Cribriform plate	Olfaction (test using nonnoxious substance)
II	Optic	Optic canal	Vision (acuity, fields, color), afferent limb of pupillary reflex
III	Oculomotor	Superior orbital fissure	Superior rectus, inferior rectus, medial rectus, inferior oblique, levator palpebrae, efferent limb of pupillary reflex
IV	Trochlear	Superior orbital fissure	Superior oblique (of contralateral eye)
V	Trigeminal	Superior orbital fissure (V_1), foramen rotundum (V_2), foramen ovale (V_3)	Muscles of mastication, tensor tympani, tensor veli palatini, facial sensation, afferent limb of corneal reflex
VI	Abducens	Superior orbital fissure	Lateral rectus
VII	Facial	Internal auditory meatus	Muscles of facial expression, stapedius, taste on anterior two-thirds of tongue, efferent limb of corneal reflex
VIII	Vestibulocochlear	Internal auditory meatus	Hearing, vestibular function
IX	Glossopharyngeal	Jugular foramen	Movement of palate, sensation over palate and pharynx, taste over posterior one-third of tongue, afferent limb of gag reflex
X	Vagus	Jugular foramen	Movement of palate, sensation over pharynx, larynx, and epiglottis, efferent limb of gag reflex, parasympathetic function of viscera
XI	Accessory	Jugular foramen	Sternocleidomastoid and trapezius movement
XII	Hypoglossal	Hypoglossal foramen	Tongue movement

object, which is more sensitive), and the pupillary light reflex, the afferent limb of which is mediated by this nerve. Funduscopic examination is the only means by which a part of the central nervous system (the retina) can be directly visualized.

Extraocular movements (III, IV, and VI) are tested in three ways: by having the patient pursue a moving target that is a drawing of the letter "H" in front of their face (pursuit), by directing their gaze rapidly to various stationary targets (saccades), and by fixating on an object while the head is being turned passively (vestibulo-ocular movements). The presence of nystagmus should be noted.

Muscles of mastication (V) are tested by assessing strength of jaw opening and palpating over the masseters bilaterally while the jaw is clenched. Facial sensation can be tested to all modalities over the forehead (V_1), cheek (V_2), and jaw (V_3). The afferent limb of the corneal reflex is mediated by this nerve.

Muscles of facial expression (VII) are tested by having patients raise their eyebrows, squeeze their eyes shut, or show their teeth. Though uncommonly tested, taste over the anterior two-thirds of the

tongue is mediated by this nerve and can be evaluated with sugar or another nonnoxious stimulus.

Hearing (VIII) may be evaluated in each ear simply by whispering or rubbing fingers; more detailed assessment of hearing loss may be accomplished with the Weber or Rinne tuning fork (512 Hz) test. Vestibular function can be tested in many ways, including evaluation of eye fixation while the patient's head is rapidly turned or by observation for drift in one direction while the patient is walking in place with the eyes closed.

Palatal elevation should be symmetric and the voice should not be hoarse or nasal (IX and X). Failure of the right palate to elevate implies pathology of the right glossopharyngeal nerve. The gag reflex is also mediated by these nerves.

Sternocleidomastoid strength is tested by having the patient turn the head against resistance; weakness on turning to the left implies a right accessory nerve (XI) problem. The trapezius muscle is tested by having the patient shrug their shoulders.

Tongue protrusion should be in the midline. If the tongue deviates toward the right, the problem lies with the right hypoglossal nerve (XII).

KEY POINTS

- Cranial nerve testing is most easily performed and recorded in approximate numerical order.
- Key elements of the cranial nerve exam include assessment of vision and eye movements, facial movement and sensation, and movements of the palate and tongue.

MOTOR EXAM

The motor exam includes more than just strength testing—in fact, strength should usually be the portion of the exam performed last.

First, bulk is assessed by observing and palpating the muscles and comparing each side to the other and the patient's overall muscle bulk to that expected for age. The presence of fasciculations or of adventitious movements such as tremor or myoclonus should also be noted.

Tone is one of the most important parts of the motor exam. In the upper extremities, tone is checked by moving the patient's arm at the elbow in both flexion-extension and circular movements, by moving the wrist in a circular fashion, and by rapidly pronating and supinating the forearm using a handshake grip. Abnormalities of tone such as spasticity and rigidity are discussed in subsequent chapters. Tone in the lower extremities can be tested well only with the patient supine. The examiner lifts the leg up suddenly under the knee; only in the presence of increased tone will the heel come off the bed.

Finally, strength or power is assessed, by both functional observation and direct confrontation (Fig. 1-2).

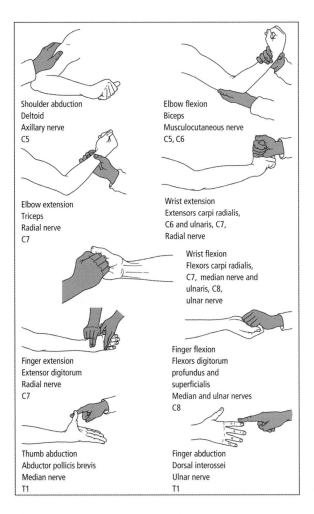

Shoulder abduction
Deltoid
Axillary nerve
C5

Elbow flexion
Biceps
Musculocutaneous nerve
C5, C6

Elbow extension
Triceps
Radial nerve
C7

Wrist extension
Extensors carpi radialis,
C6 and ulnaris, C7,
Radial nerve

Wrist flexion
Flexors carpi radialis,
C7, median nerve and
ulnaris, C8,
ulnar nerve

Finger extension
Extensor digitorum
Radial nerve
C7

Finger flexion
Flexors digitorum
profundus and
superficialis
Median and ulnar nerves
C8

Thumb abduction
Abductor pollicis brevis
Median nerve
T1

Finger abduction
Dorsal interossei
Ulnar nerve
T1

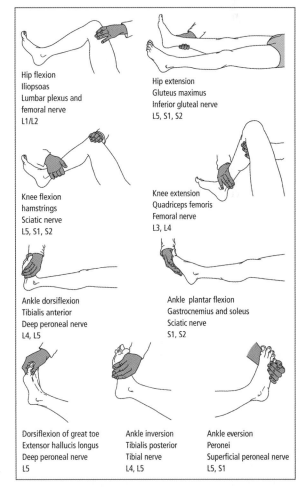

Hip flexion
Iliopsoas
Lumbar plexus and
femoral nerve
L1/L2

Hip extension
Gluteus maximus
Inferior gluteal nerve
L5, S1, S2

Knee flexion
hamstrings
Sciatic nerve
L5, S1, S2

Knee extension
Quadriceps femoris
Femoral nerve
L3, L4

Ankle dorsiflexion
Tibialis anterior
Deep peroneal nerve
L4, L5

Ankle plantar flexion
Gastrocnemius and soleus
Sciatic nerve
S1, S2

Dorsiflexion of great toe
Extensor hallucis longus
Deep peroneal nerve
L5

Ankle inversion
Tibialis posterior
Tibial nerve
L4, L5

Ankle eversion
Peronei
Superficial peroneal nerve
L5, S1

Figure 1-2 • Power testing of individual movements. For each movement, the predominant muscle, peripheral nerve, and nerve root are given.
(Reproduced with permission from Ginsberg L. *Lecture Notes: Neurology,* 8th ed. Oxford: Blackwell Publishing, 2005:40–41.)

■ TABLE 1-3 Medical Research Council Grading of Muscle Power	
0	No contraction of muscle visible
1	Flicker or trace of contraction visible
2	Active movement at joint, with gravity eliminated
3	Active movement against gravity
4	Active movement against gravity and some resistance
5	Normal power

A pronator drift may be observed in an arm held supinated and extended in front of the body. The patient may be asked to rise from a chair without using the arms or to walk on the heels or toes. The power of individual muscles assessed by direct confrontation testing is graded according to the Medical Research Council (MRC) scale (Table 1-3), although refinements of the scale (such as the use of 4−, 4, and 4+) or the use of a 10-point scale will increase precision.

KEY POINTS

- The motor exam begins with assessment of bulk and tone.
- Abnormalities of increased tone include both spasticity and rigidity.
- Strength testing involves both functional observation as well as confrontation testing of individual muscle's power.
- Strength is graded on the MRC scale from 0 to 5.

REFLEXES

Muscle stretch (or "deep tendon") reflexes can be useful aids in localizing or diagnosing both central and peripheral nervous system problems (Fig. 1-3).

In the upper extremities, the biceps, brachioradialis, and triceps reflexes are the ones commonly tested. Pectoral and finger flexor reflexes can also be tested. Hoffmann's sign is sought by flicking the distal phalanx of the middle finger while observing for flexion of the thumb.

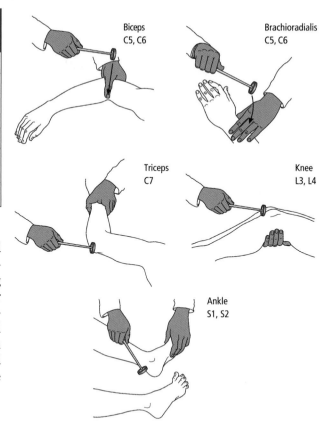

Figure 1-3 • Muscle stretch ("deep tendon") reflexes.
(Reproduced with permission from Ginsberg L. *Lecture Notes: Neurology*, 8th ed. Oxford: Blackwell Publishing, 2005:44.)

In the lower extremities, patellar (knee jerk) and ankle reflexes are the ones commonly tested. The adductor reflex can also be tested. The Babinski sign is sought by stroking the lateral sole of the foot while observing for extension of the great toe. Clonus, if present, can be elicited by forcibly dorsiflexing the ankle when it is relaxed.

SENSORY EXAM

The sensory exam can be frustrating to perform because of the tedium of potentially examining the entire body surface (see dermatome map in Chapter 6) as well as the inherent subjectivity and all-too-frequent inconsistencies in patients' responses.

In general, sensation should be tested in detail in areas relevant to a patient's complaints, especially if the complaints are sensory in nature. Otherwise, screening elements of the sensory exam that are targeted at the distal lower extremities, where most asymptomatic sensory abnormalities are likely to be found, may be sufficient.

Pinprick sensation is tested with a safety pin, the sharp edge of a broken-off cotton swab, or special pins designed for the neurologic exam.

Temperature sensation, mediated by the same pathway, is most easily tested with the side of a tuning fork, which, if freshly retrieved from an instrument bag, will be quite cold on the skin.

Vibration is tested by striking the 128-Hz tuning fork and placing its stem against the joint being tested, typically beginning at the toes.

Joint position sense, or proprioception, is tested beginning most distally by holding the patient's great toe by its sides and moving it slightly upward or downward.

Light touch is the least useful modality to test, because it is carried by a combination of pathways and is unlikely to provide clues to localization or diagnosis.

KEY POINTS

- The sensory exam is usually the most subjective portion of the neurologic exam.
- In a patient without sensory complaints, screening elements of the sensory exam that are targeted at the distal extremities may be sufficient.
- Pinprick and temperature are carried in one pathway; vibration and joint position sense in another.

COORDINATION

This portion of the exam, often incorrectly referred to as "cerebellar" testing, in fact serves to test coordinated movements whose successful completion requires the interaction of multiple components of the motor system, not just the cerebellum.

Finger-to-nose testing can identify the presence of dysmetria (inaccuracy of targeting) or intention tremor.

Heel-to-shin testing can elicit incoordination in the lower extremities.

Rapid alternating movements, rhythmic finger tapping, and heel tapping are particularly sensitive to coordination problems. Patients may have trouble with the timing or cadence of these movements. *Dysdiadochokinesis* is the term used to describe difficulty with rapid alternating movements.

GAIT

Aside from orthopedic surgeons, neurologists are among the only doctors to routinely test a patient's gait, yet the "normal" function of walking requires the proper functioning of so many different aspects of the nervous system that it is frequently a sensitive way to detect an abnormality. In addition, certain diseases, such as Parkinson disease, have quite distinctive gaits associated with them.

The patient with a normal stance maintains the feet at an appropriately narrow distance apart; a wide-based stance is abnormal.

The Romberg sign is present when the patient maintains a steady stance with feet together and eyes open but sways and falls with feet together and eyes closed. Its presence usually implies a deficit of joint position sense, not cerebellar function, as is commonly believed.

Stride length should be full. Short-stepped or shuffling gaits are characterized by a decrease in stride length and clearance off the ground.

Ataxia of gait results in an inability to walk in a straight line; patients may stagger from one side to the other or consistently list toward one side. Ataxia is typically associated with a wide-based stance. Ataxia can be brought out most obviously by having the patient attempt tandem gait, walking heel to toe.

The arms normally swing in the opposite direction from their respective legs during ambulation. Decreased arm swing is a feature of extrapyramidal disorders.

Finally, difficulty initiating ambulation or understanding the appropriate motor program for walking, leaving the feet "stuck to the floor" despite intact motor and sensory function, characterizes the gait of frontal lobe dysfunction, sometimes referred to as *gait apraxia*. Hydrocephalus is one etiology of such a gait disorder.

KEY POINTS

- Gait is one of the most important elements of the neurologic exam because it is sensitive for many deficits, and certain diseases have characteristic gait disorders.
- Stance, stride length, arm swing, ability to tandem walk, and initiation of walking should all be assessed in the gait exam.
- The Romberg sign suggests a deficit in joint position sense.

Neurologic Investigations

CEREBROSPINAL FLUID ANALYSIS

Cerebrospinal fluid (CSF) bathes the internal and external surface of the brain and spinal cord. It is produced by the choroid plexus of the ventricles and absorbed through the villi of the arachnoid granulations that project into the dural venous sinuses. CSF is produced continually at a rate of about 0.5 mL per minute; the total volume is approximately 150 mL. The entire CSF volume is thus replaced about every 5 hours. Lumbar puncture (LP) via the L3-4 interspace is the most commonly used means of obtaining CSF for analysis. LP is contraindicated by the presence of a space-occupying lesion that is causing mass effect, raised intracranial pressure, or local infection or inflammation at the planned puncture site.

TECHNIQUE

LP is best performed with the patient in the lateral recumbent position with the legs flexed up over the abdomen. Optimal positioning is the key to a successful and atraumatic LP. Ideally, a pillow should be placed between the legs, and the patient should lie on the edge of the bed where there is better support to keep the back straight. The anterosuperior iliac spine is at the level of the L3-4 vertebral interspace. The LP may be performed at this level, one interspace higher, or one to two interspaces lower. Remember that the spinal cord ends at the level of L1-2. The needle is inserted with the bevel facing upward, so that it will enter parallel to the ligaments and dura that it pierces rather than cutting them transversely. The needle is directed slightly rostrally to coincide with the downward angulation of the spinous processes. The needle

is advanced gently until CSF is obtained. To measure the opening pressure reliably, the patient's legs should be extended slightly and note should be made of fluctuation of the CSF meniscus within the manometer with respiration.

INTERPRETATION OF RESULTS

CSF is a clear, colorless fluid. The glucose content is about two-thirds that of blood, and it contains up to 40 to 50 mg/dL protein. Fewer than five cells are present, and these are lymphocytes. Measured by LP in the lateral recumbent position, the opening pressure is about 60 to 150 mm H_2O.

Xanthochromia refers to the yellow discoloration of the supernatant of a spun CSF sample. Its presence helps to distinguish an in vivo intrathecal hemorrhage from a traumatic tap [in which red blood cells (RBCs) have not lysed and the supernatant is still colorless].

The implications of various CSF findings are summarized in Table 2-1. The CSF findings in a variety of common conditions are summarized in Table 2-2. Special tests may be performed as indicated. Some examples include cytology for suspected malignancy, oligoclonal banding for suspected immune-mediated processes such as multiple sclerosis, 14,3,3-protein for Creutzfeldt-Jakob disease, and a variety of polymerase chain reactions and serologic tests for various infections.

SAFETY, TOLERABILITY, AND COMPLICATIONS

Cerebral or cerebellar herniation may occur when lumbar puncture is performed in the presence of

TABLE 2-1	Interpretation of CSF Findings	
Red blood cells	
No xanthochromia	Traumatic tap
Xanthochromia	Subarachnoid hemorrhage; hemorrhagic encephalitis
White blood cells	
Polymorphs	Bacterial or early viral infection
Lymphocytes	Infection (viral, fungal, mycobacterial); demyelination (MS, ADEM); CNS lymphoma
Elevated protein	Infection (fungal, mycobacterial); demyelination; tumor (e.g., meningioma, carcinomatous meningitis); sarcoidosis; age
Low glucose	Bacterial infection; mycobacterial infection
Oligoclonal bands	Demyelination (MS); CNS infections (e.g., Lyme disease); noninfectious inflammatory processes (e.g., SLE)
Positive EBV PCR	Highly suggestive of CNS lymphoma in patients with AIDS or other immunosuppressed states

ADEM, acute disseminated encephalomyelitis; AIDS, acquired immunodeficiency syndrome; CNS, central nervous system; EBV PCR, Epstein-Barr virus polymerase chain reaction; MS, multiple sclerosis; SLE, systemic lupus erythematosus.

either a supratentorial or infratentorial mass lesion. A computed tomography (CT) scan should be performed prior to an LP except in cases of suspected meningitis and when a CT scan cannot be performed. Radiologic contraindications to LP include closure of the fourth ventricle and quadrigeminal cistern. Low-pressure headache is the most common complication of lumbar puncture and is most effectively treated by having the patient lie flat and increase her intake of liquids and caffeine. Rarely, it may be necessary to administer an epidural blood patch (see Chapter 10).

TABLE 2-2	CSF Findings in Common Neurologic Diseases			
Disease	Cells (pleocytosis)	Protein	Glucose	Other
Bacterial meningitis	Polymorphs	High	Low	Culture and Gram stain may be positive
Viral meningitis/encephalitis	Lymphocytes	High	Normal	Viral PCR may be positive
Tuberculous meningitis	Lymphocytes	High	Very low	Positive for acid-fast bacilli
Guillain-Barré syndrome	None	High (degree depends on interval from symptom onset)	Normal	—
MS	Few lymphocytes	Slightly high	Normal	OCBs usually present
ADEM	Lymphocytes or polymorphs	Usually high	Normal	OCBs usually absent
Subarachnoid hemorrhage	Lymphocytes and many red blood cells	May be high	Normal	Xanthochromia

ADEM, acute disseminated encephalomyelitis; MS, multiple sclerosis; OCB, oligoclonal bands.

KEY POINTS

- A CT scan should be performed prior to lumbar puncture except when bacterial meningitis is suspected.
- Lumbar puncture is performed at or below the L2-3 interspace.
- Xanthochromia indicates recent intrathecal hemorrhage.

COMPUTED TOMOGRAPHY AND MAGNETIC RESONANCE IMAGING

TECHNICAL CONSIDERATIONS

CT measures the degree of x-ray attenuation by tissue. Attenuation is defined simply as the removal (by absorption or scatter) of x-ray photons and is quantified on an arbitrary scale (in Hounsfield units) that is represented in shades of gray. Differences in the shades directly reflect the differences in the x-ray attenuation of different tissues, a property that depends on their atomic number and physical density. Images are usually obtained in either an axial or a coronal plane. Three-dimensional reconstruction and angiography are possible with new-generation spiral CT scanners.

Magnetic resonance imaging (MRI) is similar to CT in that radiant energy is directed at the patient and detected as it emerges from the patient. MRI differs, however, in its use of radiofrequency (RF) pulses rather than x-rays. The images in MRI result from the varying intensity of radio-wave signals emanating from tissue in which hydrogen ions have been excited by an RF pulse. A detailed understanding of magnetic resonance physics is not necessary for the interpretation of routinely used MRI sequences. It is sufficient to understand that the patient is placed in a magnet and that an RF pulse is administered. Signal intensity is measured at a time interval, known as **time to echo** (TE), following RF administration. The RF pulse is administered many times in generating an image; the **time to repetition** (TR) is the time between these RF pulses.

Two basic MRI sequences in common usage are T1- (short TE and TR) and T2- (long TE and long TR) weighted images. Fat is bright on a T1-weighted image, which imparts a brighter signal to the myelin-containing white matter. Water (including CSF) is dark on T1 and bright on T2. T2 images are most

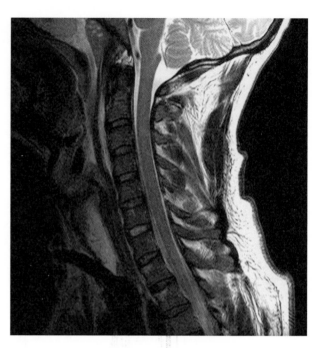

Figure 2-1 • T2-weighted MRI of the cervical spine.

useful in evaluating the spinal cord (Fig. 2-1). Gadolinium is the contrast agent used in MRI, and gadolinium-enhanced images are usually acquired with a T1-weighted sequence. Contrast-enhanced images are invaluable in determining the presence of brain tumors, abscesses, other areas of inflammation, and new multiple sclerosis lesions (see Fig. 19-2).

Other commonly used MRI sequences are fluid-attenuated inversion recovery (FLAIR) and susceptibility- and diffusion-weighted imaging (DWI). FLAIR is a strong T2-weighted image, but one in which the signal from CSF has been inverted and is thus of low rather than high intensity. FLAIR is the single best screening image sequence for most pathologic processes of the central nervous system (CNS). It is very useful in assessing the chronic lesion burden in multiple sclerosis (see Fig. 20-2). A susceptibility-weighted sequence is one that is sensitive to the disruptive effect of a substance on the local magnetic field. Examples of substances that exert such a susceptibility effect are calcium, bone, and the blood breakdown products ferritin and hemosiderin. Areas of increased susceptibility appear black on these images.

DWI demonstrates cellular toxicity with high sensitivity and is most commonly employed in the diagnosis of acute stroke, where it can be positive within half an hour of symptom onset. Areas of restricted

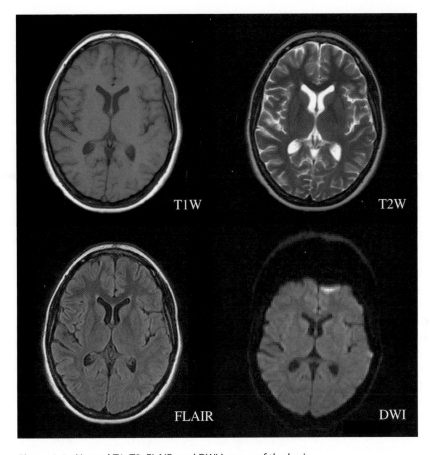

Figure 2-2 • Normal T1, T2, FLAIR, and DWI images of the brain.

diffusion appear bright on DWI. Figure 2-2 provides examples of T1, T2, FLAIR, and DWI images.

CLINICAL UTILITY

Head CT is often the initial investigation used in a variety of neurologic disorders, including headache, trauma, seizures, subarachnoid hemorrhage, and stroke. The sensitivity of a CT scan for detecting lesions depends on many factors, including the nature and duration of the underlying disease process. The sensitivity for detecting areas of inflammation, infection, or tumor may be increased by the administration of intravenous contrast. Contrast enhancement indicates local disruption of the blood-brain barrier. CT is the investigation of choice for demonstrating fresh blood.

Apart from providing better anatomic definition, MRI is particularly useful for imaging the contents of the posterior fossa and craniocervical junction, which are seen poorly on CT because of artifact from surrounding bone. DWI is the most sensitive technique

available for demonstrating early tissue ischemia and is therefore extremely useful in the evaluation of patients with suspected stroke.

SAFETY, TOLERABILITY, AND COMPLICATIONS

CT scanning employs x-rays and is thus relatively contraindicated during pregnancy. The use of RF waves in MRI makes this the imaging modality of choice in pregnant women. There is no cross-reactivity between the iodinated contrast agents used in CT and the gadolinium used as a contrast agent in MRI. When contrasted imaging is required, MRI may therefore be preferable when there is a history of allergy to intravenous contrast. Similarly, gadolinium does not have the nephrotoxicity of iodinated contrast. MRI may be used safely only in the absence of metal objects (foreign bodies, plates, and screws) and pacemaker and defibrillator devices. Some people with claustrophobia cannot tolerate MRI; under these circumstances, CT is preferred.

KEY POINTS

- CT is the imaging modality of choice for demonstrating acute intracranial bleeding.
- MRI is required for adequate imaging of the posterior fossa and craniocervical junction.
- DWI is the most sensitive MRI sequence for demonstrating early cerebral ischemia or infarction.

VASCULAR IMAGING STUDIES

Conventional angiography involves cannulation of the great vessels and injection of contrast dye to obtain an image of the vascular anatomy (Fig. 2-3). This is the most sensitive and specific imaging study of the intracranial and extracranial circulation. Risks of the procedure include contrast dye reaction, stroke due to plaque dislodged by the catheter, and bleeding from the cannulation site. Although the risks of the procedure, and developments in magnetic resonance angiography (MRA) (below), have decreased the number of conventional angiograms performed, it remains the "gold standard" in vascular imaging.

MRA uses blood flow as a contrast agent and MR technique to define vascular anatomy (Fig. 2-4).

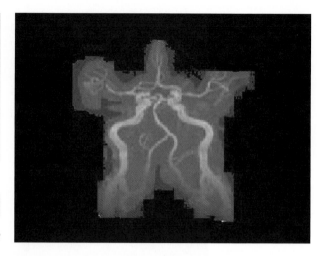

Figure 2-4 • MRA of the circle of Willis.

Compared with conventional angiograpy, MRA is less invasive and can be performed more quickly and less expensively, but it is not as sensitive or specific for cerebrovascular disease. MRA is performed commonly on the intracranial circulation of stroke patients to look for evidence of vascular narrowing or occlusion. "Fat-suppressed" MRA of the neck is useful for determining the presence of vertebral or carotid artery dissections. Magnetic resonance venography (MRV) can be used to demonstrate venous sinus thrombosis and other venous disease.

Extracranial Doppler sonography measures blood flow by determining the difference between emitted and received ultrasound frequencies. It is used commonly to detect stenosis or occlusion of the extracranial carotid circulation, especially in the planning stages for carotid endarterectomy. Transcranial Doppler (TCD) detects intracranial stenosis and emboli. Most of the intracranial circulation, however, is inaccessible to TCD. Although somewhat less accurate than MRA or conventional angiography, Doppler studies are noninvasive and virtually without contraindication.

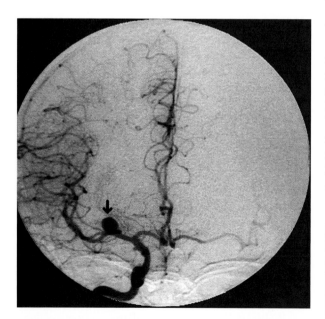

Figure 2-3 • Conventional cerebral angiogram demonstrating aneurysm of the right middle cerebral artery (*arrow*).
(Reproduced with permission from Patel PR. *Lecture Notes: Radiology,* 2nd ed. Oxford: Blackwell Publishing, 2005:278.)

KEY POINTS

- Conventional angiography is the gold standard for evaluating cerebrovascular anatomy.
- MRA is less invasive but also less accurate than conventional angiography.
- MRV is useful for assessing the presence of venous sinus thrombosis.

OTHER IMAGING STUDIES

Positron emission tomography (PET) scans measure regional brain metabolism. Hypermetabolism can be demonstrated during seizures (though it is rare to get the scan during a seizure), while hypometabolic regions may be evident interictally. Such a finding can be very useful in planning epilepsy surgery, especially in the temporal areas. Single-photon emission computed tomography (SPECT) uses a radioactive isotope to demonstrate increased blood flow during seizures. Both PET and SPECT scans have been studied in the evaluation of dementia. While regional patterns of abnormality help study disease processes, they are not specific enough for diagnosis in individual patients. Magnetic resonance spectroscopy is primarily a research tool used to demonstrate areas of neuronal damage or dysfunction and has been studied in the assessment of brain tumors, demyelinating disease, and infections of the CNS.

ELECTROENCEPHALOGRAPHY

The electroencephalogram (EEG) provides a record of the electrical activity of the cerebral cortex. Normal EEG patterns are characterized by the frequency and amplitude of the recorded electrical activity, and the patterns of activity correlate with the degree of wakefulness or sleep. The normally observed frequency patterns are divided into four groups: alpha (8 to 13 Hz), beta (14 to 30 Hz), theta (4 to 7 Hz), and delta (0.5 to 3.0 Hz) (Fig. 2-5). Under normal circumstances, alpha waves are observed over the posterior head regions in the relaxed awake state with the eyes closed. Lower-amplitude beta activity is more prominent over the frontal regions. Theta and delta activity is normal during drowsiness and sleep, and the different stages of sleep are defined by the relative proportions and amplitudes of theta and delta activity (see Chapter 13).

TECHNIQUE

The standard EEG is recorded from electrodes attached to the scalp in a symmetric array. The pattern in which these electrodes are connected to each other is referred to as the *montage*, of which there are essentially two types: bipolar and referential. In a bipolar montage, all electrodes are active and a recording is made of the difference in electrical activity between two adjacent electrodes. In a referential montage, the electrical activity is recorded beneath the active electrode relative to a distant electrode or common average signal. The signal recorded by an EEG is a sum of excitatory and inhibitory postsynaptic potentials of cortical neurons.

CLINICAL UTILITY

To appreciate the utility of the EEG, it is important to understand its limitations. First, the patterns of electrical activity recorded by the EEG are rarely (if ever) specific to their cause. For example, the presence of diffuse theta or delta activity during the awake state suggests an encephalopathy but does not indicate the etiology. Second, the EEG records the electrical activity of cortical neurons. Although subcortical structures influence cortical activity, the surface EEG may be insensitive to dysfunction of deep structures. For example, seizures originating in the medial frontal or temporal lobes may not be readily apparent on the surface EEG. Furthermore, the EEG provides a measure of the electrical activity of the cortex at the time of the recording and is therefore frequently normal in paroxysmal conditions such as seizures. The interictal EEG, for example, may be abnormal in only about 50% of adults with epilepsy. The frequency of interictal EEG abnormalities may be higher in certain forms of epilepsy.

Several common patterns of abnormal activity are recognized. Focal arrhythmic or polymorphic slow activity in the theta or delta range suggests local dysfunction in the underlying brain. Vascular disease is a common cause of such findings, but the slowing

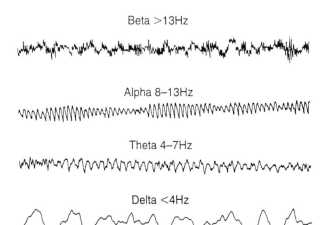

Beta >13Hz

Alpha 8–13Hz

Theta 4–7Hz

Delta <4Hz

Figure 2-5 • Electroencephalographic frequencies.

cannot specify the etiology. Generalized arrhythmic slow activity often indicates a diffuse encephalopathy. Interictal epileptiform findings include sharp- and spike-wave discharges, with or without an accompanying slow wave. Electrographic seizures may take various forms. The most common are rhythmic spike- or sharp- and slow-wave discharges or rhythmic slow waves. They may be focal or generalized. Activation procedures can be used to enhance the likelihood of finding abnormal EEG patterns: hyperventilation is useful for provoking EEG changes in patients with absence seizures, while photic stimulation can induce EEG changes in patients with myoclonic seizures.

KEY POINTS

- Alpha frequency (8 to 13 Hz) is the dominant posterior rhythm on the EEG in the awake restful state with the eyes closed.
- Epilepsy is a clinical diagnosis; interictal epileptiform EEG findings are demonstrable in about half of patients with epilepsy.

NERVE CONDUCTION STUDIES AND ELECTROMYOGRAPHY

Nerve conduction studies (NCS) and electromyography (EMG) are appropriately used as an extension of the clinical examination.

TECHNIQUE

In performing NCS, an electrical stimulus is applied over a nerve and recordings are made from surface skin electrodes. For motor studies, the recording electrodes are placed over the endplate of a muscle innervated by the nerve being stimulated. The nerve is stimulated in at least two locations (distal and proximal), and the distance between the two sites of stimulation is measured carefully. The distal latency, compound muscle action potential (CMAP), and conduction velocity are recorded. The CMAP is a recording of the contraction of the underlying muscle. The distal latency is the time interval between stimulation over the distal portion of the nerve and the initiation of the CMAP. Conduction velocity is calculated by measuring the difference in latency to CMAP initiation between proximal and distal sites of stimulation. For sensory studies, the nerve is stimulated at one site and the sensory nerve action potential (SNAP) is recorded either at a more proximal site (orthodromic study) or at a more distal site (antidromic study). Repetitive nerve-stimulation studies are used to demonstrate either decremental or incremental CMAP responses in disorders of the neuromuscular junction.

Electromyography involves the insertion of a needle into individual muscles. Recordings are made of the muscle electrical activity upon insertion (insertional activity), while the muscle is at rest (spontaneous activity), and during contraction (volitional motor unit potentials). To increase the strength of muscular contraction, motor units can fire more quickly (activation) or more motor units can be added (recruitment). Reduced activation is seen in CNS disease. Reduced recruitment suggests a lower motor neuron lesion, while early recruitment can be seen in myopathic disease. For routine EMG studies, activity is recorded from a group of muscle fibers simultaneously. Single-fiber EMG is the technique used in the investigation of disorders of the neuromuscular junction.

CLINICAL UTILITY

NCS and EMG are used primarily to assist in the localization of dysfunction within the peripheral

■ **TABLE 2-3** Electromyography in Neurogenic and Myopathic Disorders		
	Neurogenic	**Myopathic**
Insertional activity:	↑ (active denervation)	Usually normal ↑ (necrotizing myopathies)
Spontaneous activity:	↑ (active denervation)	Usually normal ↑ (necrotizing myopathies)
Volitional motor unit potentials: Recruitment:	Large amplitude; polyphasic Reduced	Small amplitude; polyphasic Usually normal early

■ **TABLE 2-4** Nerve Conduction Studies in Demyelinating and Axonal Neuropathies

	Demyelinating	Axonal
Distal latency:	Markedly prolonged	Normal, or mildly prolonged
Conduction velocity:	Markedly reduced	Normal; may be slightly slowed
CMAP amplitude:	Normal or mildly reduced	Reduced

CMAP, compound muscle action potential.

nervous system and to define pathophysiology more clearly. For example, NCS and EMG may help to differentiate a C8–T1 radiculopathy from a lower brachial plexopathy or an ulnar neuropathy in the patient who presents with numbness of the fourth and fifth fingers and weakness of the hand. Similarly, the combination of motor NCS, repetitive nerve stimulation, and EMG may help to localize motor dysfunction (i.e., weakness) to the peripheral nerve, the neuromuscular junction, or the muscle (Table 2-3). In a patient with a polyneuropathy, NCS may help to define the relative degree of motor and sensory involvement and to distinguish primary demyelinating from axonal disease (Table 2-4).

 KEY POINTS

- The goal of NCS and EMG is to localize the neurologic dysfunction within the peripheral nervous system.
- Repetitive nerve stimulation and single-fiber EMG are useful in the diagnosis of disorders of the neuromuscular junction.

Part 2

Common Neurologic Symptoms

The Approach to Coma and Altered Consciousness

The neurologic evaluation and management of a patient with coma or altered consciousness can be intimidating for the student, because such patients are usually critically ill and may require prompt intervention. The fundamental principles behind the evaluation of a neurologic problem, however, should not be discarded. On the contrary, an orderly and hypothesis-based approach may be even more important in a comatose patient than in others, given the need for timely diagnosis and the relative limitations on history and examination.

DEFINITION

Coma is defined as a state of unarousable unresponsiveness. Typically the patient lies with eyes closed and does not open them even to vigorous stimulation, such as sternal rub, nasal tickle, or nailbed pressure. Alterations in consciousness short of coma are often described using terms such as **drowsiness**, **lethargy**, **obtundation**, and **stupor**, but these terms tend to be used imprecisely and it is generally best to describe simply how the patient responded to various degrees of stimulation. The Glasgow Coma Scale assigns a numerical score to a patient's level of responsiveness and is commonly used by neurosurgeons in cases of head trauma (see Table 17-1). Its utility lies in its ease of use by nurses and paramedics, its interrater reproducibility, and its prognostic value following head injury.

KEY POINTS

- Coma is a state of unarousable unresponsiveness.
- It is important to describe a patient's responses to various degrees of stimulation.
- The Glasgow Coma Scale, which has prognostic value in patients with head trauma, is reproducible and easy to use.

CLINICAL APPROACH

An algorithm for approaching patients with coma or altered consciousness is presented in Figure 3-1. The initial steps of stabilization and evaluation culminate in the neurologic exam, which is performed with two goals in mind: to assess brainstem function and to look for focal signs. The differential diagnosis and further investigations stem from this clinical assessment.

1. **Remember the ABCs.** In any patient with altered consciousness, the airway, breathing, and circulation should be checked and maintained according to usual protocols, including intubation and mechanical ventilation if required.
2. **Look for obvious clues to etiology.** A brief history and general exam should be performed to search for obvious clues. A history of medical problems

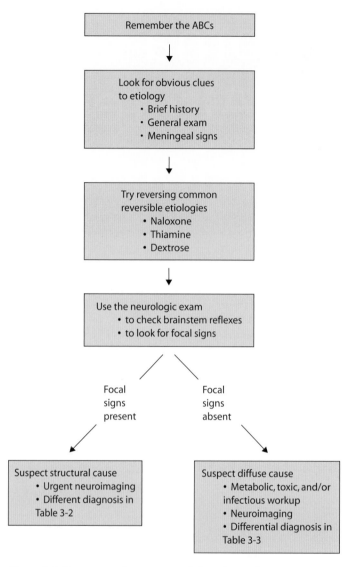

Figure 3-1 • The approach to coma and altered consciousness.

such as diabetes, hepatic failure, alcoholism, or a seizure disorder may be provided by the family, noted on a medical alert bracelet, or deduced from prescription labels. The circumstances in which the patient was found can offer clues to the onset or etiology of depressed consciousness. The general exam may yield telling signs, such as an odor on the breath, needle tracks on the skin, or a tongue laceration. It is important to check for meningeal signs in any unconscious patient because both bacterial meningitis and subarachnoid hemorrhage may lead to depressed consciousness.

3. **Try reversing common reversible etiologies.** Most emergency rooms (ERs) make it standard practice to administer naloxone, thiamine, and dextrose to any patient with depressed consciousness and no obvious etiology. Note that thiamine should always be given before glucose, because the latter can precipitate Wernicke encephalopathy if given alone.

4. **Check brainstem reflexes and look for focal signs.** These are the two primary goals of the neurologic exam in this setting, because the subsequent diagnostic and therapeutic steps will depend on these clinical findings.

KEY POINTS

- The clinical approach to the patient with altered consciousness begins with the ABCs: airway, breathing, and circulation.
- Look for obvious clues to etiology.
- Try reversing common reversible etiologies.
- Use the neurologic exam to check brainstem reflexes and look for focal signs.

EXAMINATION

It is important to proceed with the neurologic exam of a comatose patient in an orderly fashion—it is easy to be intimidated or distracted by the array of attached tubes and lines or by the intensity and anxiety of other clinicians. An appropriate way to begin is to progress systematically through the sequence of the usual neurologic exam, making adjustments as necessary for the patient's altered level of responsiveness.

Mental status testing in these patients begins with assessing the level of consciousness. An increasing gradient of stimulation should be applied and the patient's responses recorded. For example, does the patient lie with his or her eyes closed but open them slowly when spoken to in a loud voice? Does he or she groan but not open his or her eyes when sternal rub is applied? For many patients, further cognitive testing may not be possible. For those who can be aroused

even briefly, however, a short evaluation of attention, language, visuospatial function, and neglect is in order, because this may reveal a gross focal finding such as an aphasia or dense neglect of the left side.

Cranial nerves should be examined in detail, because this is the portion of the exam most relevant to the assessment of brainstem function. In an arousable patient, most cranial nerves can be tested in the usual manner. In a patient who is not arousable enough to follow commands, several important brainstem reflexes should be tested (Table 3-1), including the pupillary, corneal, oculocephalic, and gag reflexes. In addition, a funduscopic examination should always be performed. For many patients with altered consciousness, testing for a blink to visual threat may be the only way to judge visual fields. If the patient cannot move his or her face to command, the examiner may be restricted to looking for an asymmetry at rest, such as a flattened nasolabial fold on one side. The presence of an endotracheal tube may make such observation difficult.

Motor tone should be checked in all extremities. If the patient can cooperate with some testing, a gross hemiparesis can be ruled out by having the patient hold the arms extended or legs elevated and observing for downward drift. Otherwise, the examiner may be restricted to observing for asymmetry of spontaneous movements (or to asking caretakers whether all extremities have been seen to move equally). Failing that, noxious stimuli such as nailbed pressure or a pinch on a flexor surface can be applied

■ **TABLE 3-1** Brainstem Reflexes		
Reflex	**Cranial Nerves Involved**	**How to Test**
Pupillary	II (afferent); III (efferent)	Shine light in each pupil and observe for direct (same side) and consensual (contralateral side) constriction
Oculocephalic (doll's eyes)	VIII (afferent); III, IV, VI (efferent)	Forcibly turn head horizontally and vertically and observe for conjugate eye movement in opposite direction (contraindicated if cervical spine injury has not been ruled out)
Caloric testing (if necessary)*	Same	Inject 50 mL ice water into each ear and observe for conjugate eye deviation toward the ear injected
Corneal	V_1 (afferent); VII (efferent)	Touch lateral cornea with cotton tip and observe for direct and consensual blink
Gag	IX (afferent); X/XI (efferent)	Stimulate posterior pharynx with cotton tip and observe for gag

*Caloric testing should be performed if turning the head is contraindicated or does not result in eye movement. Never assume the eyes are immobile unless caloric testing has been done.

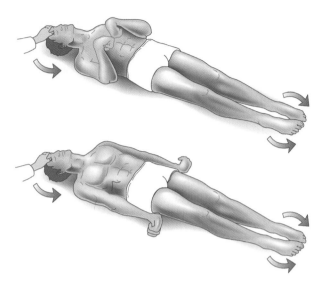

Figure 3-2 • Decorticate (*above*) and decerebrate (*below*) posturing in response to noxious stimuli. Both indicate brainstem dysfunction, although decorticate posturing suggests dysfunction slightly more superior than decerebrate posturing.
(Reproduced with permission from Kandel ER, Schwatz JH, Jessell TM. *Principles of Neural Science,* 4th ed. New York: McGraw-Hill, 2000:903.)

to each limb and the speed and strength of withdrawal noted, although abnormalities here may result from sensory loss as well as motor dysfunction. Decorticate and decerebrate posturing, signs of brainstem dysfunction, may be seen either spontaneously or in response to noxious stimuli (Fig. 3-2).

Muscle stretch reflexes can be tested in the usual manner, and a Babinski sign should be sought.

Sensory testing in most patients with altered consciousness is limited to testing of light touch or pain sensation. Noxious stimulation to each limb, as described previously, may be useful in looking for gross sensory abnormalities.

Coordination and gait may be tested in patients who are arousable enough.

KEY POINTS

* The mental status exam in patients with altered consciousness primarily assesses the level of responsiveness.
* The cranial nerve exam includes the testing of important brainstem reflexes, including the pupillary, corneal, and oculocephalic reflexes.
* The remainder of the examination should be dedicated to looking for focal abnormalities.

DIFFERENTIAL DIAGNOSIS

In theory, there are two main ways in which consciousness can be depressed: the brainstem can be dysfunctional or both cerebral hemispheres can be dysfunctional simultaneously. In fact, acute disease in the brainstem (e.g., pontine hemorrhage) can lead to coma, as can processes affecting both cerebral hemispheres at once (e.g., hypoglycemia). Unilateral cerebral hemispheric lesions, however, can also lead to coma if they are large or severe enough to cause swelling and compression of the opposite hemisphere or downward pressure on the brainstem.

Therefore most neurologists interpret the information obtained from the exam of the comatose patient using the following principle: the presence or absence of brainstem reflexes suggests how deep the coma is, while the presence or absence of focal signs narrows the differential diagnosis and guides the workup.

Thus, in milder cases of depressed consciousness, the pupillary, corneal, and gag reflexes may all be preserved. In more severe cases, some or all of these brainstem reflexes may be lost, no matter what the etiology. (Note that if a brainstem reflex is abnormal in an asymmetric fashion, such as a unilateral unreactive pupil, this would be interpreted as a focal sign and suggests compression of or primary disease in the brainstem.)

The presence of focal signs either on cranial nerve testing or in the remainder of the examination—including such findings as hemiparesis, aphasia, reflex asymmetry, facial droop, or a unilateral Babinski sign—suggests a structural cause of depressed consciousness (Box 3-1). Examples include a large unilat-

■ **BOX 3-1** Structural Causes of Depressed Consciousness
Acute ischemic stroke
Brainstem
Unilateral cerebral hemisphere (with edema)
Acute intracranial hemorrhage
Intraparenchymal
Subdural
Epidural
Brain tumor (with edema or hemorrhage)
Primary
Metastatic
Brain abscess

eral stroke or intracranial hemorrhage. The absence of focal signs suggests a diffuse cause of depressed consciousness, including metabolic, toxic, or hypoxic-ischemic etiologies (Box 3-2). Examples include coma from fulminant hepatic failure, barbiturate overdose, or anoxia following prolonged cardiac arrest.

 KEY POINTS

- In theory, consciousness can be depressed either by dysfunction of the brainstem or dysfunction of both cerebral hemispheres simultaneously; in reality, large unilateral hemispheric lesions (with pressure on the other side) qualify as well.
- The presence or absence of brainstem reflexes suggests how deep the coma is.
- The presence of focal signs suggests a structural cause of coma.
- The absence of focal signs suggests a diffuse cause of coma, such as metabolic, toxic, infectious or hypoxic-ischemic etiologies.

LABORATORY AND RADIOGRAPHIC STUDIES

The distinction between structural and diffuse causes of depressed consciousness, arrived at by interpreting the findings on exam, suggests different pathways of diagnostic workup.

The presence of focal findings on examination, suggesting a structural cause, demands urgent head imaging, almost always a noncontrast computed tomography (CT) scan. One should be looking for signs of a large acute stroke, an intracranial hemorrhage, or a mass lesion that may have enlarged rapidly or had hemorrhage within it. (Contrast-enhanced CT should be avoided if acute hemorrhage is possible.) Even in cases where focal brainstem signs are found, the initial choice of head imaging may have to be a CT scan rather than magnetic resonance imaging (MRI), despite the poor quality of the former in evaluating the brainstem, because of the possibility of a large cerebral hemispheric lesion compressing the brainstem as well as because of the more immediate availability of CT.

The absence of focal findings on examination, suggesting a diffuse cause, warrants an extensive workup for causes of metabolic, toxic, or infectious etiologies. Blood testing—including complete blood count (CBC), electrolytes, glucose, liver function tests, and

BOX 3-2 Diffuse Causes of Depressed Consciousness
Metabolic
Electrolyte abnormality
Hyponatremia, hypernatremia, hypocalcemia, hypercalcemia, hypomagnesemia, hypermagnesemia, hypophosphatemia
Glucose abnormality
Hypoglycemia, nonketotic hyperosmolar coma, diabetic ketoacidosis
Hepatic failure
Uremia
Thyroid dysfunction   Myxedema coma, thyrotoxicosis
Adrenal insufficiency
Toxic
Alcohol
Sedatives
Narcotics
Psychotropic drugs
Other exogenous toxins (carbon monoxide, heavy metals)
Infectious
Meningitis (bacterial, viral, fungal)
Diffuse encephalitis
Hypoxic-ischemic
Respiratory failure
Cardiac arrest
Other
Subarachnoid hemorrhage
Carcinomatous meningitis
Seizures or postictal state

toxicologic screen—may be necessary. If infection is suspected, a chest x-ray, urinalysis, and blood or urine cultures may be called for. There should be a low threshold for obtaining a lumbar puncture (LP). If a basic workup is unrevealing, one should search for more unusual causes (such as myxedema coma, by checking thyroid function tests). Head imaging is usually needed even in these cases of suspected diffuse cause because it may demonstrate signs of global hypoxic-ischemic injury, diffuse cerebral edema, or bilateral lesions mimicking a diffuse process, although the urgency is not as high as for patients with focal findings. Of course, a head CT should be performed before obtaining an LP almost without exception in the evaluation of a patient with depressed consciousness, given the risk of precipitating brain herniation if a large intracranial mass (particularly in the posterior fossa) is present. (If bacterial meningitis is suspected, empiric antibiotic treatment can be started if CT scanning is delayed.)

Frequently, an electroencephalogram (EEG) is ordered in patients with coma or altered consciousness. Although many of its findings may be nonspecific, the EEG can help to assess how deep a coma is based on the degree of background slowing. In addition, there are occasionally more specific patterns on EEG that suggest a particular diagnosis, such as hepatic encephalopathy or anoxic brain injury. Finally, the EEG can rule out nonconvulsive status epilepticus as a cause of coma in cases in which this is (or is not) clinically suspected.

KEY POINTS

- If a structural cause of coma is suspected, urgent head imaging, usually with a noncontrast head CT, should be performed.
- If a diffuse cause is suspected, an extensive workup for metabolic, toxic, or infectious causes should be undertaken.
- Head imaging in suspected diffuse cases may demonstrate cerebral edema, signs of global hypoxic-ischemic injury, or bilateral lesions mimicking a diffuse process.
- Almost without exception, head CT should be performed before LP.
- EEG can assess the depth of coma and can occasionally suggest a specific diagnosis.

TREATMENT AND PROGNOSIS

The treatment of coma and altered consciousness rests on the specific diagnosis. Metabolic, infectious, or toxic etiologies require mostly medical management, while some structural causes of coma may require neurosurgical intervention. Specific treatments for particular conditions are detailed in later chapters, in particular Chapter 14 for strokes and

hemorrhages, Chapter 17 for head trauma, Chapter 18 for systemic and metabolic disorders, Chapter 19 for brain tumors, and Chapter 21 for central nervous system (CNS) infections.

When increased intracranial pressure (ICP) is suspected clinically or radiographically, treatments aimed at lowering ICP should be applied. These include raising the head of the bed, hyperventilation, and the use of an osmotic diuretic such as mannitol. Corticosteroids tend to be useful only in cases of edema associated with brain tumors. The lowering of ICP may be a neurologic or neurosurgical emergency if the patient shows signs of brain herniation, which is discussed in more detail in Chapter 17.

The prognosis of depressed consciousness is mostly dependent on etiology—the patient with a barbiturate overdose may recover completely, whereas one with a severe anoxic injury likely will not. Age is an important prognostic factor as well. One of the most frequent reasons for admission to an intensive care unit (ICU) or neurologic consultation is to estimate the prognosis of a patient in coma following cardiopulmonary arrest. In these cases the circumstances and duration of the arrest are important, and published studies have correlated outcome with findings on neurologic examination performed at least 24 hours after the arrest.

KEY POINTS

- The treatment of coma or altered consciousness depends on etiology.
- The lowering of intracranial pressure may be a neurologic emergency if the patient shows signs of brain herniation.
- Prognostic factors for coma or altered consciousness include both etiology and patient age.

SPECIAL TOPICS

PERSISTENT VEGETATIVE STATE

Persistent vegetative state is a state in which patients have lost all awareness and cognitive function but may remain with their eyes open, exhibit sleep-wake cycles, and maintain respiration and other autonomic functions. Patients may progress into this state after being in coma for a prolonged period if their vital functions have been supported.

LOCKED-IN SYNDROME

Although a locked-in syndrome can be confused with coma at first glance, a patient with locked-in syndrome is awake and may be intact cognitively, with no abnormality of consciousness. Usually a consequence of large lesions in the base of the pons, the locked-in syndrome leaves patients unable to move the extremities and most of the face. If all other motor function is lost, they may be limited to communicating by vertical eye movements or blinks.

BRAIN DEATH

Death can be declared either when there has been irreversible cessation of cardiopulmonary function or there has been irreversible cessation of all functions of the entire brain, including the brainstem. A declaration of death based on the latter criterion is commonly referred to as **brain death**. Many institutions have specific guidelines for how brain death must be determined, but in general the patient must be comatose, have absent brainstem reflexes, and have no spontaneous respirations even when the P_{CO_2} has been allowed to rise (the apnea test). Confounding factors such as hypothermia or drug overdose must not be present. Confirmatory tests most commonly include an EEG, which can demonstrate electrocerebral silence ("flat line"), or cerebral angiography, which can demonstrate absence of blood flow to the brain. Local institutional guidelines for declaration of brain death should always be consulted.

KEY POINTS

- A persistent vegetative state may follow prolonged coma and is characterized by preserved sleep-wake cycles and maintenance of autonomic functions, with absence of awareness and cognition.
- Locked-in syndrome, in which awareness and cognitive function are preserved but almost complete paralysis occurs, is often caused by large lesions in the base of the pons.
- Brain death is a declaration of death based on irreversible cessation of all brain functions.

ACUTE CONFUSIONAL STATE

Definition

The terms **confusion**, **delirium**, and **encephalopathy** are often used nonspecifically to indicate a disturbance of mental status in which the patient is unable to carry out a coherent plan of thought or action. Most neurologists employ the terms **confusion** or **encephalopathy**, while **delirium** (commonly used by psychiatrists) often implies a state of encephalopathy characterized by a waxing and waning level of alertness.

At its core, an acute confusional state results from a problem of attention. Thus, a patient's failure to answer questions in a coherent manner or to carry out an intended series of actions in an expected way derives from an inability to maintain attention for long enough to proceed through the cognitive or motor steps required for the task. On formal mental status testing, therefore, patients with confusion typically do poorly on standard tests of attention, such as spelling the word "world" in reverse, reciting the months of the year backward, or completing serial subtractions. Such inattention may be significant enough to make impossible the performance of more detailed mental status testing. Depending on the underlying etiology of the acute confusional state, other associated features may be present on neurologic or general physical examination as well.

Differential Diagnosis

The differential diagnosis of acute confusion includes a number of different disorders, among them aphasia (particularly Wernicke), psychosis, and complex partial seizures. Patients with Wernicke aphasia may appear "confused" but in fact are attentive and able to carry out coherent series of actions; their deficit lies solely in their ability to communicate. Although patients with psychosis may also behave as if they were acutely confused, pure confusional states do not result in frank psychotic symptoms like hallucinations or delusions. Complex partial seizures can be characterized by behavior that appears "confused," but seizures are typically self-limited in duration and may be associated with clonic motor movements or automatisms such as lip-smacking.

Diagnostic Evaluation

An acute confusional state is most commonly caused by an underlying systemic or neurologic disorder, including infection, metabolic disturbance, inflammatory condition, or hypoxic-ischemic state, among many possibilities. Focal brain disorders, particularly acute right hemispheric lesions, can also lead to confusion. The appropriate diagnostic workup in a patient with confusion is therefore potentially quite extensive. Blood work and urinalysis to search for infectious or metabolic disturbances are often warranted. If there is clinical suspicion for a CNS infection, cerebrospinal fluid (CSF) analysis should be performed. Neuroimaging should be obtained if the neurologic history or examination suggests the possibility of an acute focal lesion. An EEG can help to determine whether there is a widespread dysfunction (encephalopathy) or focal abnormalities. It is unlikely to demonstrate the precise cause of an acute confusional state but can help to confirm a diagnosis, since characteristic findings of an encephalopathy may be present.

Treatment and Prognosis

The treatment and prognosis of acute confusional states depend largely on the underlying etiology. Most cases of confusion arise from a reversible underlying cause and will resolve if the underlying disorder is treated appropriately. Confusional states arising from structural neurologic lesions or more chronic underlying disturbances may be less likely to improve spontaneously.

KEY POINTS

- An acute confusional state, also sometimes called delirium, is characterized by an inability to carry out a coherent plan of thought or action.

- Acute confusion is primarily the result of a core problem with attention.

- Systemic infections and metabolic disturbances are common causes of an acute confusional state, although many possible etiologies exist.

4 Neuro-Ophthalmology

An understanding of visual impairment, pupillary disturbances, and oculomotor control is essential in the diagnosis of neurologic disorders. Maximal interpretation of our environment is accomplished through the integration of visual, somatosensory, motor, and auditory information.

A systematic approach to evaluating patients with "visual" problems includes the analysis of: vision, eye movements, and integration of visual information. This chapter covers the first two; the third constitutes part of higher cortical function, discussed elsewhere (see Chapter 11).

ANATOMY

Light enters the cornea and stimulates the rods and cones in the retina, where the visual stimuli are converted into electrical signals that are sent through the optic nerve to centers in the brain for further processing and visual perception. The visual pathway (with various field defects) is shown in Figure 4-1.

The more posterior parts of the cerebral hemispheres are involved in seeing and analyzing visual information, including written language, and the more anterior parts control looking at and exploring visual space.

Ninety percent of retinal axons terminate in a retinotopic fashion in the lateral geniculate nucleus, the principal subcortical structure that carries visual information to the cerebral cortex through the optic radiations. The primary visual cortex is visual area 1 (V1), corresponding to Brodmann's area 17, or striate cortex, which receives information from the contralateral visual hemifield. This information is then transferred to associative visual cortex, including areas 18 and 19, and to many higher-order centers in the posterior parietal and inferior temporal cortices, where the perception of motion, depth, color, location, and form takes place.

SYMPTOMS APPROACH TO NEURO-OPHTHALMOLOGIC DISTURBANCES

The most common neuro-ophthalmologic symptoms are loss of vision and diplopia. Other symptoms include eye pain, visual hallucinations, and oscillopsia. Two important signs discussed in this chapter are the abnormal optic disc and anisocoria (unequal pupils).

VISUAL LOSS

Visual disturbances can be described as positive or negative phenomena. Positive visual phenomena include brightness, shimmering, sparkling, hallucinations, shining, flickering, or colors, often suggesting migraine or seizures. Negative visual phenomena can be described as blackness, grayness, dimness, or shade-obscuring vision, as seen in patients with strokes or transient ischemic attacks.

When the complaint is loss of vision, ask the following questions:

1. Is this a monocular or binocular problem? Does the problem go away when one eye is closed?
2. Does it affect a portion or the entire visual field?
3. Is it transient or persistent?
4. Are there associated symptoms, such as headache, visual auras, motor or sensory disturbances, changes in mentation, seizures, or eye pain (e.g., with optic neuritis)?

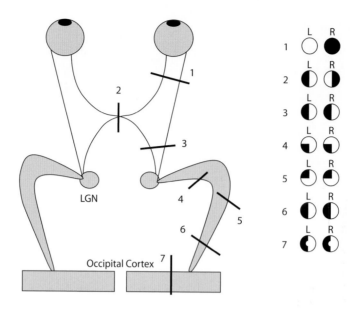

Localization	Visual field defect
1. Optic nerve	1. Right eye blindness
2. Chiasm	2. Bitemporal visual field defect
3. Optic tract	3. Left homonymous hemianopia
4. Optic radiations (parietal)	4. Left inferior homonymous quadrantonopia
5. Optic radiations (temporal or Meyer's loop)	5. Left superior homonymous quadrantonopia
6. Optic radiations (both)	6. Left homonymous hemianopia
7. Occipital cortex	7. Left homonymous hemianopia with macular sparing

Figure 4-1 • The visual pathway, with lesions and resultant visual field defects.

Diagnostic Evaluation

The evaluation of acquired visual loss (Box 4-1) begins with determining whether the problem is at the level of the eye, optic nerve, chiasm, optic tract, lateral geniculate nuclei (LGN), optic radiation, or occipital cortex. Once the site of dysfunction is determined, the workup is targeted to the specific cause.

The diagnostic evaluation includes assessment of visual acuity and color vision, test for afferent pupillary defects, testing of visual fields, and ophthalmoscopic evaluation. The ophthalmoscopic evaluation looks for damage to the retinal nerve fiber layer, optic atrophy, swollen disc, abnormal optic disc (hypoplastic, tilted, etc.), vascular lesions, and retinal emboli.

To test visual acuity (VA), use a distance chart with good illumination. At the bedside, the near chart (handheld Snellen chart) is often enough. If the VA is poor, try using a pinhole (one can be created by making small holes in a blank card). If the pinhole test improves the VA, the problem is in refraction. If

the patient is unable to read letters, try counting fingers, followed by perception of movement, and finally perception of a bright light. Impairment of VA is usually a problem in the refractive apparatus of the eye or the optic nerve, or both. Rarely, chiasmal or retrochiasmal lesions cause changes in VA.

Color vision is tested by using Ishihara plates. Another method is looking for red desaturation (decreased perception of red color), which can be seen early in optic nerve problems (particularly optic neuritis).

When testing pupils, report their size and reaction to light, both consensually and in accommodation. Use a bright light. Look for a relative afferent pupillary defect (RAPD), also known as a Marcus Gunn pupil. To perform this test, place the patient in a dimly illuminated room and ask for fixation in the distance. A bright light is flashed alternately for 2 to 3 seconds in each eye. If the light is directed toward one eye and the ipsilateral pupil appears to dilate, an RAPD is present (i.e., the dilating pupil is

■ BOX 4-1 Causes of Visual Loss

Retina	Chiasm
Detachment	Tumor: pituitary tumors such as adenoma, craniopharyngioma, and glioma
Infectious: CMV, toxoplasmosis	Sphenoid mucocele
Toxic: ethambutol	Internal carotid artery aneurysm
Degenerative: macular degeneration, retinitis pigmentosa	Trauma
Ischemic: embolic	Demyelination
Optic disc	Vascular
AION: vasculitic and nonvasculitic	Toxic
Optic neuritis	Retrochiasmal
Glaucoma	Tumor: glioma, meningioma, metastasis
Papilledema (late)	Stroke involving the visual pathway
Sarcoidosis	Demyelination
Tumor	Degenerative diseases
Optic nerve	
Demyelination	
Tumor, including meningioma, glioma, etc.	
Thyroid ophthalmopathy	
Trauma	

AION, anterior ischemic optic neuropathy; CMV, cytomegalovirus.

"deafferented": it does not constrict to direct light but constricts consensually to light shone in the other eye).

Visual field testing at the bedside is done by confrontation. Cover one eye at a time. Move your fingers or a small white or red object over the different quadrants and compare the patient's visual field to yours. Table 4-1 compares the clinical characteristics of visual loss according to localization.

KEY POINTS

- Organize your exam when examining vision. Remember to use a bright light.
- Examine one eye at a time.
- Monocular visual loss implies problems in the eye, optic nerve, or chiasm. Binocular visual loss implies a chiasmal or retrochiasmal lesion.
- The pattern of visual field loss helps in the localization of the site of the lesion (see Fig. 4-1).

DISORDERS OF THE PUPIL

Unequal pupil size (anisocoria) is common. The challenge is to distinguish a physiologic from a pathologic anisocoria.

ANATOMY

Light activates retinal ganglion cells, which send their axons through the optic nerve, chiasm, and optic tract to synapse in the pretectal midbrain nuclei, also known as **Edinger-Westphal nuclei** (EWN) in the rostral portion of the third nerve nucleus. Efferent parasympathetic fibers from the EWN travel with the third cranial nerve (CN). In the cavernous sinus, they run with the inferior division of the third nerve and ultimately synapse in the ciliary ganglion. The iris contains two muscles that regulate pupil size. The sphincter is a pupilloconstrictor innervated by parasympathetic fibers of the third nerve. The dilator (pupillodilator) is innervated by the cervical sympathetic system. The sympathetic system starts in the

■ TABLE 4-1 Comparison of Visual Loss According to Localization

Lesion Level	Causes	Symptoms/Signs	Visual Field Defect
Eye	Usually refractive error; central retinal artery occlusion; retinal detachment; central retinal vein occlusion	RAPD present; usually unilateral; vision improves with pinhole	Depends on the cause; only one eye affected
Optic nerve	Usually inflammatory lesions (MS and sarcoid); ischemic (vasculitis, atherosclerosis), such as AION; infiltrative (neoplasia)	Monocular visual loss; ipsilateral RAPD; discs swelling	Central, centrocecal, arcuate, or wedge field defect in the affected eye
Chiasm	Parasellar mass, including pituitary adenoma, craniopharyngioma, meningioma, aneurysm, etc.	Ipsilateral RAPD; binocular visual loss	Bitemporal hemianopia; central scotoma and centrocecal scotoma; important to evaluate contralateral superior temporal visual field
Lateral geniculate nucleus	Infarction, neoplasia, AVM	Binocular visual loss; no RAPD	Incongruous contralateral hemianopia
Optic radiation	Infarction, inflammatory, neoplasia, AVM	Binocular visual loss; ipsilateral smooth pursuit abnormalities; spasticity of conjugate gaze; no RAPD	
Temporal lobe			Superior contralateral quadrantanopia
Parietal lobe			Inferior contralateral quadrantanopia
Occipital lobe	Infarction (PCA strokes), inflammatory, neoplasia, AVM	Binocular visual loss; no RAPD	Congruous contralateral hemianopia with macular sparing

AION, anterior ischemic optic neuropathy; AVM, arteriovenous malformation; PCA, posterior cerebral artery; RAPD, relative afferent pupillary defect.

ipsilateral posterolateral hypothalamus (first-order neuron) and projects down the brainstem to the intermediolateral cell column at the C8–T1 spinal level. The second-order neurons synapse in the superior cervical ganglion and represent the preganglionic neurons. Third-order neurons (postganglionic) travel along the internal carotid artery into the cavernous sinus and from there into the orbit to the pupillodilator muscles.

DIAGNOSTIC EVALUATION

Document pupil reactivity and size in bright and dim illumination. Remember that up to 25% of normal people have asymmetric pupils without pathologic significance. In physiologic anisocoria, the amount of anisocoria does not change with different illumination. Pupils should respond normally to light and near stimulation. If the anisocoria is not physiologic, the next question to be answered is which pupil is abnormal, the dilated or the constricted one.

First, examine the pupils in the dark (turn the lights off and look at the pupils during the first 5 to 10 seconds). A dilation lag in the small pupil and anisocoria greater in darkness means a sympathetic defect in that pupil. Horner's syndrome (HS) is characterized by unilateral miosis, ptosis, and (sometimes) ipsilateral facial anhidrosis as a result of impaired sympathetic innervation. There are many different causes of HS, but in all of them cocaine eyedrops fail to dilate the abnormal pupil. If the cocaine test is negative, hydroxyamphetamine eyedrops will help to distinguish a preganglionic from a postganglionic HS (the pupil with a postganglionic HS fails to dilate with hydroxyamphetamine). The different causes of HS are summarized in Box 4-2.

Once you have established that the abnormal pupil is the larger one (mydriatic), localization of the prob-

■ **BOX 4-2** Etiology of Horner's Syndrome
First-order Horner's, or central Horner's:
Hypothalamic infarcts, tumor
Mesencephalic stroke
Brainstem: ischemia (Wallenberg syndrome), tumor, hemorrhage
Spinal cord: syringomyelia, trauma
Second-order Horner's, or preganglionic:
Cervicothoracic cord/spinal root trauma
Cervical spondylosis
Pulmonary apical tumor: Pancoast tumor
Third-order Horner's, or postganglionic:
Superior cervical ganglion (tumor, iatrogenic, etc.)
Internal carotid artery: dissection, trauma, thrombosis, tumor, etc.
Base of skull: tumor, trauma
Middle ear problems
Cavernous sinus: tumor, inflammation (Tolosa-Hunt syndrome), aneurysm, thrombosis, fistula

An Argyll Robertson pupil is classically associated with syphilis. Usually both pupils are small and irregular, with impaired light reaction and intact near response (light-near dissociation); pupils also dilate poorly to mydriatic agents.

KEY POINTS

- Horner's syndrome (HS) is characterized by ipsilateral miosis, ptosis, and facial anhidrosis.
- A complete third nerve palsy presents with mydriasis, ptosis, and ophthalmoplegia.
- An Adie's pupil is dilated, with segmental contraction and light-near dissociation.
- Argyll Robertson pupils are small and poorly reactive to light but have preserved near response; they are typically associated with syphilis.
- Light-near dissociation (LND): Normally the pupillary constriction to light is greater than to a near stimulus. The opposite is called LND. It implies a defect in light response, as in optic neuropathy, or the presence of aberrant regeneration, as in the Adie pupil. Other causes of LND include dorsal midbrain lesions and severe bilateral visual loss.

lem starts by following the course of the third nerve from the midbrain or third nerve nucleus to the iris muscle. If the problem is at the level of the midbrain, other neurologic signs are usually present (hemiparesis, nystagmus, loss of consciousness, tremor, etc.).

Third nerve palsy is characterized by ptosis, dilated pupil, and ophthalmoplegia. Because the parasympathetic fibers run in the outer part of the third nerve and the motor fibers are more internal, compression of the nerve initially produces a dilated pupil without compromising eye movements. On the other hand, vascular problems producing third nerve ischemia (e.g., diabetes) will produce a pupil-sparing third nerve lesion in which the pupil is normal and reactive but there is palsy of the ocular muscles innervated by the third nerve.

A tonic (Adie's) pupil results from interruption of the parasympathetic supply from the ciliary ganglion (cell bodies or postganglionic fibers). Symptoms include anisocoria, photophobia, and blurred near vision (because of some accommodation paresis). The exam shows a dilated pupil, poor light reaction (with the typical segmental contraction), and light-near dissociation. It can be confirmed by demonstrating supersensitivity of the affected pupil to 0.1% pilocarpine, which will produce more contraction in the affected pupil than in the normal pupil.

ABNORMAL OPTIC DISC

The term **papilledema** implies optic disc swelling resulting from increased ICP. Other forms of optic disc swelling due to local or systemic causes should just be called **optic disc swelling** (ODS).

The etiology of papilledema is a blockage of axoplasmic transport in the optic nerve. The clinical symptoms depend on the underlying cause (pain on eye movements with demyelinating optic neuritis, sudden visual loss in anterior ischemic optic neuropathy [AION], morning headache with space-occupying lesions, etc.). The most common symptom of ODS is transient visual obscurations, described as a dimming or "blacking out" of vision and usually lasting just a few seconds. They are usually precipitated by changes in posture (bending or straightening) and can occur many times per day.

The most common causes of unilateral optic disc edema are optic neuritis, AION, and orbital compressive lesions. As a rule, optic nerve function is abnormal in each. The appearance of the optic disc may be indistinguishable in these entities, but certain features of it may suggest a specific diagnosis. Disc hemorrhages, for example, are much more common in

AION than in optic neuritis or compressive lesions. The term **Foster-Kennedy syndrome** refers to ipsilateral optic disc atrophy due to compression by a space-occupying lesion in the frontal lobe and papilledema in the contralateral optic disc due to increased ICP.

Table 4-2 summarizes abnormalities of the optic disc and describes the most relevant clinical characteristics.

 KEY POINTS

- Always remember to carry your ophthalmoscope.
- An abnormal optic disc has many possible causes (see Table 4-2).
- LP measures intracranial pressure.

■ **TABLE 4-2** Assessment of Abnormal Optic Disc

Abnormality	Etiology	Clinical Manifestation and Fundoscopy	Diagnosis/Therapy
Increased intracranial pressure	Space-occupying lesion (tumor, AVM, aneurysm, edema, etc.) Idiopathic intracranial hypertension (IIH), also known as pseudotumor cerebri	Symptoms: morning headache, ataxia, and transient visual obscuration No RAPD, central acuity spared No color loss; enlarged blind spot Fundi show bilateral disc hyperemia	Clinical MRI/CT LP with opening pressure **Therapy:** specific to the cause **IIH:** acetazolamide, nerve decompression, shunt
Drusen (calcified hyaline bodies) or pseudopapilledema	Small hyaline concretions (familial, autosomal dominant)	Asymptomatic Enlarged blind spot with normal visual acuity (initially) Fundi: glistening hyaline bodies + VP No disc hyperemia or exudates	Clinical; CT and orbital ultrasound to see calcified hyaline bodies
Optic neuritis	Usually indicates demyelination (MS, SLE, adrenoleukodystrophy, sarcoidosis, tumor) Others: viral, meningitis, Behçet, Whipple, and Crohn diseases	Painful visual loss Uhthoff's phenomenon (worsening visual function during exercise, hot baths, etc.) RAPD Retro-orbital pain Loss of color discrimination Central scotoma is classic Fundi: variable: from normal optic disc to optic atrophy or papillitis.	Clinical; MRI looking for demyelination; LP Visual evoked potentials **Therapy:** IV methylprednisolone is indicated. If MRI of the head shows more than three demyelinating lesions, the probability of developing MS is up to 50% in 5 years
Ischemia (AION)	Vascular: carotid occlusion, embolic TIAs Inflammatory: temporal arteritis	Sudden painless visual loss Patients usually over age 50 Associated hypertension, diabetes Hypotensive episodes Variable visual field abnormalities and common RAPD Fundi: usually unilateral segmental disc edema	Medical workup for diabetes, hypertension, vasculitis MRA or ultrasound of the carotid artery TIA workup **Therapy:** specific to the cause

AION, anterior ischemic optic neuropathy; MS, multiple sclerosis; RAPD, relative afferent pupillary defect; VP, venous pulsation.

■ TABLE 4-3 Some Terms Used to Define Eye Misalignment	
Strabismus	Misalignment of the eyes
Comitant	Misalignment is constant in all directions of gaze, and each eye has full range of movement (usually an ophthalmologic problem)
Incomitant	The degree of misalignment varies with the direction of gaze (usually a neurologic problem)
Phoria	Misalignment of the eyes when binocular vision is absent
Tropia	Misalignment of the eyes when both eyes are opened and binocular vision is possible

DIPLOPIA

Double vision usually arises from a misalignment of the eyes, which may result from decompensation of a previous strabismus but in most cases is a symptom of neurologic disease. Abnormal eye movements can result from lesions in individual extraocular muscles, abnormalities of the neuromuscular junction, or dysfunction of the oculomotor nerves, their central nuclei, or central connections. Some useful concepts for understanding eye movements are summarized in Table 4-3.

ANATOMY OF EYE MOVEMENTS

The three CNs involved in eye movements are the oculomotor (III), the trochlear (IV), and the abducens (VI). CN III innervates the superior rectus, medial rectus, inferior rectus, levator palpebrae, pupil constrictor, and inferior oblique muscles. Its dysfunction produces ptosis, mydriasis, and ophthalmoparesis with the eye deviated down and out (when all parts of CN III are involved). In addition, depending on the site of the lesion, there may be one of the following patterns:

- **Nucleus of CN III:** Bilateral ptosis and weakness of contralateral superior rectus; failure of eye elevation
- **Subarachnoid space:** Meningismus, constitutional symptoms, and other CN defects
- **Tentorial edge compression:** Depressed level of consciousness, hemiparesis, and history of trauma or supratentorial mass lesion

CN IV innervates the superior oblique muscle that intorts and depresses the adducted eye. Fourth nerve lesions produce oblique diplopia, worse on downgaze when the affected eye is adducted. The patient usually complains of diplopia when reading or going down stairs. Patients compensate with a contralateral head tilt (in other words, the diplopia improves with head tilt away from the side of the lesion).

CN VI innervates the lateral rectus muscle. Lesions produce esotropia, especially on ipsilateral gaze. Sixth nerve palsy can be a nonlocalizing sign of increased ICP.

The most common causes of oculomotor nerve dysfunction in older adults include microvascular occlusion and ischemia, commonly associated with hypertension, diabetes mellitus, and atherosclerosis.

Destruction of the abducens nucleus in the brainstem leads to complete (binocular) ipsilateral conjugate gaze palsy because of simultaneous damage to the interneurons connected to the contralateral third nerve through the medial longitudinal fasciculus (MLF) (Fig. 4-2).

CLINICAL MANIFESTATIONS

Is it monocular or binocular? If binocular, is it horizontal or vertical? Is it worse at near or at far? And finally, is the problem localized to an extraocular muscle (paresis or fatigue), brainstem MLF (internuclear ophthalmoplegia), or the orbit itself?

The MLF connects the abducens nucleus with the contralateral third nerve nucleus. Lesions of the MLF produce an internuclear ophthalmoplegia (INO). The clinical characteristics of a right INO include inability to adduct the right eye in left lateral gaze plus nystagmus of the abducting left eye. Adduction during convergence is preserved because this action does not depend on the MLF. Bilateral INOs can be seen in Wernicke encephalopathy (along with gait ataxia or confusional state), botulism, myasthenia gravis, brainstem strokes, and demyelination.

"One-and-a-half syndrome" occurs as a consequence of a lesion involving the paramedian pontine

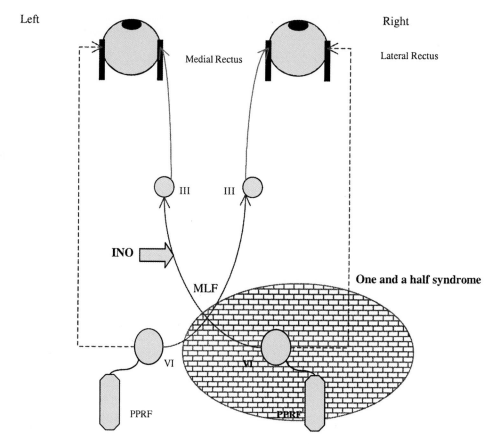

Left

Right

Medial Rectus

Lateral Rectus

III   III

INO

MLF

One and a half syndrome

VI   VI

PPRF   PPRF

Juan Acosta

Figure 4-2 • Damage to the PPRF, sixth nerve nucleus, and both MLF produces the "one-and-a-half syndrome syndrome" (patterned oval). The only eye movement present in the horizontal plane in this case is the abduction of the left eye. INO occurs after damage of the MLF. In this graphic, damage to the left MLF alone would produce a left INO, i.e., an inability to adduct the left eye and nystagmus in the right eye with right lateral gaze.

reticular formation (PPRF), or sixth nerve nucleus and the adjacent ipsilateral MLF. These produce an ipsilateral gaze palsy and INO on the contralateral side (the only eye movement present in the lateral plane is abduction of the contralateral eye) (Fig. 4-2).

Vertical eye movements are controlled by the rostral interstitial nucleus of the MLF (riMLF) located in the pretectal midbrain area, near the CN III nucleus. Fibers controlling upgaze from the riMLF cross to the contralateral side using the posterior commissure to communicate with the inferior oblique and superior rectus subnuclei of the CN III complex. The downgaze pathway is less well understood but does not travel in the posterior commissure. Abnormal vertical gaze movements can be found in dorsal midbrain syndromes. Parinaud syndrome is characterized by upgaze disturbance, convergence-retraction nys-

tagmus on attempted upgaze, and light-near dissociation of the pupils. It is generally produced by a pineal tumor compressing the dorsal midbrain.

Finally, skew deviation is a vertical tropia, generally caused by brainstem or cerebellar lesions. The hypotropic (lower) eye is often on the side of the lesion.

DIAGNOSTIC EVALUATION

The evaluation includes a careful history and a detailed neurologic exam. Some tests done to evaluate diplopia include the following:

• **Cover test:** Ask the patient to fixate on a small target. Cover one eye and watch the other eye. If the eye makes a refixation movement, this means that it was not aligned on the target. If the eye moves nasally, the patient has an exotropia; if it moves temporally, an esotropia. For example, a third nerve palsy produces exotropia and hypotropia of the paretic eye. Abducens palsy produces esotropia of the affected eye.

- **Alternate cover test:** Detects phoria (esophoria or exophoria). Phorias do not cause diplopia because the eyes are aligned when both are open simultaneously.
- **Park's three-step test:** Detects a fourth-nerve palsy:
  1. Hypertropia (relative upward deviation) of the paretic eye.
  2. Hypertropia increases when the patient looks to the opposite side.
  3. Hypertropia increases when the patient tilts the head to the same side.
- **Oculocephalic maneuver (doll's-eye test):** Useful in unconscious patients to evaluate the integrity of the vestibular and oculomotor apparatus. It is done by rapid horizontal and vertical movement of the head. The vestibulo-ocular reflex rotates the eyes in the direction opposite to head movement.
- **Saccades:** Rapid, conjugate movement of the eyes between objects (e.g., fingertips). In general, disorders of eye movement will produce slowness of saccades in the direction of the paretic muscle.
- **Pupillary size and reflexes**
- **Periocular signs or proptosis**

KEY POINTS

- The PPRF acts as the horizontal gaze center, activating the abducens nucleus in response to supranuclear gaze commands.
- The abducens nucleus contains motor neurons and internuclear neurons that travel with the MLF to the contralateral oculomotor nuclei in the midbrain.
- Lesions of the MLF produce an INO.
- Lesions of the PPRF and ipsilateral MLF produce the one-and-a-half syndrome (gaze palsy to the ipsilateral side and INO in contralateral gaze).
- The riMLF is the vertical gaze center, analogous to the PPRF for horizontal gaze.
- A gaze palsy may indicate a supranuclear or nuclear dysfunction. The doll's-eye maneuver or caloric testing will distinguish them. If doll's-eye movements are normal, the dysfunction is supranuclear.

SUPRANUCLEAR EYE MOVEMENTS

Saccades are rapid eye movements to redirect the eyes to a new fixation object. In general, voluntary saccades originate in the frontal eye field and superior colliculus contralateral to the direction of gaze. These areas have a direct connection with the contralateral PPRF and participate in saccadic movements. Other areas that contribute to saccadic control include the dorsolateral prefrontal cortex, supplementary eye field, and parietal lobe. Vertical saccades may also originate in frontal eye fields or superior colliculi and connect to the contralateral riMLF. Inability to produce saccades is called **oculomotor apraxia**.

Abnormal saccades include those that overshoot (hypermetric) or undershoot (hypometric) and unwanted saccades or saccadic intrusions (square wave jerks, ocular flutter, and opsoclonus).

Pursuit movements permit the eyes to conjugately track a moving visual target to keep it in focus. The control is hemispheric and ipsilateral. Visual cortex inputs reach the temporo-occipital region. The occipitoparietotemporal junction is responsible for integrating the movement data. The fibers course into the deep parietal lobe and continue to the ipsilateral dorsolateral pontine nucleus. Then they travel sequentially to the cerebellar vermis, nucleus prepositus hypoglossi, medial vestibular nuclei, and finally to the abducens nuclei for horizontal pursuit. Vertical pursuits are mediated by the interstitial nucleus of Cajal rather than the riMLF (as for vertical saccades).

Pursuit disorders may be difficult to identify. Neurologic diseases such as Parkinson disease, progressive supranuclear palsy, drugs, and aging can slow down pursuits. Deep parietal lobe lesions produce pursuit abnormalities as well. Because of the long pathway involved in this type of movement, its value in localizing a lesion is limited.

The vestibulo-ocular reflex (VOR) coordinates eye movements with head movement, preventing the visual image from slipping during movements of the head. Slow, passive head movements can elicit it. The pathway involves the semicircular canals (rotation) and otoliths (linear acceleration) and travels to the vestibular nuclei. From there, it proceeds to the abducens nuclei and then to CNs III and IV through the MLF. Abnormalities of the VOR result in nystagmus (see following section).

■ **TABLE 4-4** Types of Nystagmus

Type	Characteristics
Physiologic or nonpathologic	
Optokinetic nystagmus	Normal response to a continuously moving object.
Vestibulo-ocular	By rotations of the subject's head. Also irrigation of the ear (caloric test).
Endpoint nystagmus	Few beats of nystagmus in eccentric gaze.
Congenital nystagmus	Jerk or pendular, present after birth and remains throughout life.
Pathologic or acquired nystagmus	
Periodic alternating nystagmus	Horizontal jerk nystagmus that changes direction every 2 to 3 minutes. Acquired forms are associated with craniocervical junction abnormalities, multiple sclerosis, bilateral blindness, and toxicity from anticonvulsants.
Downbeat nystagmus	Present in primary position. Also seen in disorders of the craniocervical junction (Chiari malformation), spinocerebellar degeneration, multiple sclerosis, familial periodic ataxia, and drug intoxication.
Upbeating nystagmus	In primary position is associated with lesions of the anterior cerebellar vermis and lower brainstem. Also occurs with drug intoxication and Wernicke encephalopathy.
See-saw nystagmus	One eye elevates and intorts while the other depresses and extorts. Associated with third ventricle tumors and bitemporal hemianopsia, trauma, and brainstem vascular disease.
Gaze-evoked nystagmus	Similar to endpoint nystagmus but amplitude is greater and it occurs in a less eccentric position of the eyes. Most common cause is drug intoxication. Also seen in cerebellar disease and brainstem or hemisphere pathology.
Rebound nystagmus	Seen as a transient, rapid, horizontal jerk when eyes are moving to or from eccentric position. Usually associated with cerebellar or posterior fossa lesions.
Vestibular nystagmus	Usually horizontal with a rotatory component. Associated with peripheral inner ear disorders, Ménière disease, vascular disorder, and drug toxicity.

■ **TABLE 4-5** Tips for Differentiating Central from Peripheral Nystagmus

	Peripheral (vestibular)	Central (brainstem)
Direction	Unidirectional, fast phase away from the lesion	Bidirectional or unidirectional
Purely horizontal without rotatory component	Uncommon	Common
Vertical nystagmus	Never present	May be present
Visual fixation	Inhibits nystagmus and vertigo	No changes
Tinnitus or deafness	Often present	Rarely present
Romberg sign	Toward the slow phase	Variable
Vertigo	Severe	Mild
Duration	Short but recurrent	May be chronic
Causes	Vascular disorders, trauma, toxicity, Ménière disease, vestibular neuronitis	Vascular, demyelination, and neoplastic/paraneoplastic disorders

NYSTAGMUS

Nystagmus is a rhythmic to-and-fro movement of the eyes that can be congenital, physiologic, or a sign of CNS dysfunction, peripheral vestibular loss, or visual loss. It can be either pendular or jerking. In jerk nystagmus, the eye drifts away from fixation in a pursuit-like movement and returns with a fast, saccadic movement. The direction of the nystagmus is named by the direction of this fast component. Table 4-4 gives a brief description of physiologic and acquired nystagmus and possible causes.

Special attention needs to be paid to vestibular nystagmus. It is very common to be called to the ER to evaluate a patient with the acute onset of vertigo; the ER doctor immediately becomes concerned when the patient has nystagmus. Table 4-5 describes a few characteristics to help differentiate central from peripheral nystagmus.

KEY POINTS

- Peripheral nystagmus is often unidirectional, with the fast phase away from the lesion; it combines horizontal and torsional movements and is inhibited by fixation.

- Central nystagmus is normally bidirectional; often purely horizontal, vertical, or torsional; and not inhibited by fixation.

- Saccades are fast eye movements that redirect the fovea to a new target. Horizontal saccades are initiated in the contralateral frontal eye field or superior colliculus.

- Vertical saccades originate from bilateral frontal eye fields or the superior colliculus.

- Conjugate gaze deviation is observed in lesions of the frontal lobe with destruction of the frontal eye field; the eyes deviate toward the side of the lesion. During a seizure, the eyes often turn away from the frontal focus.

Weakness is one of the most common presenting neurologic complaints. Many patients may tolerate some degree of numbness, tingling, or even pain, but often it is when weakness sets in that medical attention is finally sought. Similarly, friends or family members will not notice a patient's sensory problems, but significant weakness will be obvious to all.

At the same time, weakness can be one of the most difficult neurologic problems to sort out, because the pathways that control motor function span the entire axis of the nervous system. Left leg weakness can arise from a peripheral nerve lesion, a lumbosacral plexus problem, or a stroke in the right cerebral hemisphere. Each of these has a different workup, prognosis, and treatment, and it is the job of the physician to use the history and examination to distinguish among them.

PRINCIPLES

Figure 5-1 presents a flowchart to aid in the diagnosis of weakness. The key steps in the clinical approach are outlined below.

1. **Make sure that true weakness is the complaint.** Sometimes patients will use the term *weak* to mean a general sense of fatigue; others will say a limb is "weak" when it is clumsy or numb. Having the patient confirm that decreased strength is the symptom may be useful. Likewise, a limb that is painful to move may seem "weak"; whether there is true underlying weakness may be difficult to discern.
2. **Identify which muscles are weak.** This seems like an obvious point but must be emphasized. It is not sufficient to know that a patient has left leg weakness. Testing must be done in enough detail to know which muscles in the left leg are weak or, if they are all diffusely weak, which are weaker than others.
3. **Determine the pattern of weakness.** This is frequently the crux of the entire diagnosis. It is the pattern of weakness that will reveal when left leg weakness is due to a peroneal nerve problem and not a right hemispheric stroke. Needless to say, one must be familiar with the different patterns of weakness and their implications.
4. **Look for associated signs and symptoms.** If a leg is weak, determine whether it is also numb, tingling, or painful. Check the reflexes carefully. Often the motor deficit overshadows other problems, whose presence may be helpful in supporting or excluding certain diagnoses.
5. **Use laboratory and electrophysiologic tests wisely.** Blood tests or neuroimaging studies can be useful in the appropriate settings, and electromyography/nerve conduction studies (EMG/NCS) can act as an extension of the clinical exam in localizing the problem to a particular segment of the peripheral nervous system. Tests are most useful in the setting of a complete clinical evaluation and formed diagnostic hypothesis, however.

KEY POINTS

- Weakness can be caused by lesions along the entire neuraxis, from brain to muscle.
- The diagnosis rests on determining what the pattern of weakness is, searching for associated signs and symptoms, and using laboratory tests and EMG/NCS to confirm clinical hypotheses.

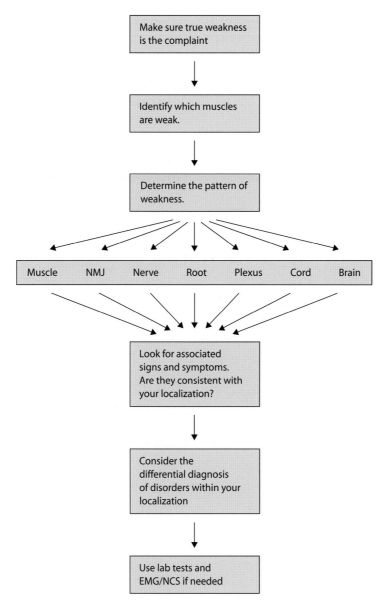

Figure 5-1 • The approach to weakness.

DIFFERENTIAL DIAGNOSIS

It is useful to consider the disorders that cause weakness in an anatomic order, from most distal in the nervous system (primary muscle disorders) to most proximal (disorders of the cerebral hemisphere). Below, each anatomic category is presented with the clues that might lead a clinician to suspect a disorder in that location. Individual diseases in each category are discussed in the later chapters covering specific neurologic disorders.

PRIMARY MUSCLE DISORDERS

Pattern of Weakness

Primary muscle problems tend to cause weakness predominantly in proximal muscles, in a symmetric fashion. Distal muscles are affected later or not as severely. In addition, neck flexors and extensors, which are not affected in most nerve or brain lesions, may be weak in a muscle disorder.

Associated Signs and Symptoms

Associated signs and symptoms may occasionally include muscle pain if the muscle disorder is inflammatory, such as polymyositis. By their nature, primary disorders of muscle should not cause sensory signs or other symptoms. Reflexes are characteristically preserved unless the process is so severe that the muscles are nearly paralyzed.

Laboratory Studies

Some disorders of muscle are characterized by an elevated serum creatine kinase (CK) level. The demonstration of characteristic "myopathic" changes on an EMG can help confirm a primary muscle disorder.

Differential Diagnosis

Primary muscle disorders, discussed in Chapter 24, include both acquired problems (myopathies), which can result from inflammatory or toxic etiologies among other causes, and congenital problems (muscular dystrophies).

KEY POINTS

- *Primary muscle disorders* typically cause symmetric proximal weakness and can affect neck muscles.
- Sensory signs and symptoms are not present in myopathies.
- Serum CK level is elevated in some muscle disorders, and EMG may show a characteristic "myopathic" pattern.

NEUROMUSCULAR JUNCTION DISORDERS

Pattern of Weakness

Neuromuscular junction (NMJ) problems can vary in the pattern of weakness they cause, though most affect proximal extremity muscles. Some NMJ disorders can lead to ptosis as well as weakness of extraocular, bulbar, and neck muscles. The characteristic feature of NMJ disorders is not the pattern of weakness, however, but the fluctuation. The degree of weakness may

change from hour to hour. Depending on the specific disease, strength may be worse after using the muscles or toward the end of the day; it may improve after resting or in the morning (fatigability). Alternatively, strength may paradoxically improve after exercise in other conditions.

Associated Signs and Symptoms

By their nature, NMJ problems, which affect only the junction between the motor axon terminal and the muscle, should not lead to sensory signs or symptoms. Some NMJ disorders may have associated autonomic features.

Laboratory Studies

EMG/NCS can demonstrate nearly pathognomonic findings for certain NMJ disorders on specialized testing. Some of the diseases in this category have specific serum markers, such as antiacetylcholine receptor antibodies in myasthenia gravis.

Differential Diagnosis

NMJ disorders are discussed in Chapter 24; they include myasthenia gravis and Lambert-Eaton myasthenic syndrome, among others.

KEY POINTS

- *NMJ disorders* can cause weakness of proximal muscles; some characteristically affect extraocular and bulbar muscles.
- The key to diagnosing NMJ disorders is fluctuation in the degree of weakness.
- Sensory signs and symptoms are not present in NMJ disorders.
- EMG/NCS can be nearly pathognomonic in some cases of NMJ disorders.

PERIPHERAL NERVE DISORDERS

Pattern of Weakness

Each muscle in the upper or lower extremity is innervated by an individual peripheral nerve (Table 5-1). A lesion involving a particular peripheral nerve will lead to weakness in the muscles innervated by that nerve while sparing other, often neighboring muscles.

Disorders affecting a single peripheral nerve are known as **mononeuropathies**. Certain systemic

■ TABLE 5-1 Commonly Tested Movements			
Movement	**Muscle**	**Nerve**	**Root**
Shoulder abduction	Deltoid	Axillary	C5
Elbow flexion	Biceps	Musculocutaneous	C5/C6
Elbow extension	Triceps	Radial	C7
Wrist extension	Wrist extensors	Radial	C7
Finger flexion	Finger flexors	Median, ulnar	C8/T1
Finger extension	Finger extensors	Radial	C7
Finger abduction	Interossei	Ulnar	C8/T1
Hip flexion	Iliopsoas	Nerve to iliopsoas	L1/L2/L3
Hip abduction	Gluteus medius, minimus	Superior gluteal	L5
Hip adduction	Hip adductors	Obturator	L3
Hip extension	Gluteus maximus	Sciatic	S1
Knee flexion	Hamstrings	Sciatic	L5/S1
Knee extension	Quadriceps	Femoral	L3/L4
Plantar flexion	Gastrocnemius, soleus	Tibial	S1
Dorsiflexion	Tibialis anterior	Peroneal	L5
Foot eversion	Peroneus muscles	Peroneal	S1
Foot inversion	Tibialis posterior	Tibial	L5
Great toe extension	Extensor hallucis longus	Peroneal	L5

conditions can lead to dysfunction of multiple peripheral nerves in succession, a disorder known as **mononeuropathy multiplex**. Finally, when peripheral nerves are all affected diffusely, in a **polyneuropathy**, dysfunction typically occurs in the longest nerves first. Thus, weakness from a polyneuropathy usually appears first in the distal muscles, symmetrically.

Associated Signs and Symptoms

Mononeuropathies may cause sensory symptoms—such as numbness, tingling, or pain—in the distribution of the relevant peripheral nerve. Mononeuropathy multiplex is characteristically associated with pain. Polyneuropathies, depending on etiology, usually have associated sensory loss and depressed or absent reflexes, particularly in the distal extremities.

Laboratory Studies

EMG/NCS can confirm the clinical suspicion of a problem localized to the peripheral nerves. NCS can identify whether the pathologic process affects primarily the axons or the myelin of the nerve, an essential step in formulating a differential diagnosis.

EMG may yield insight as to the relative acuity or chronicity of a nerve disorder.

Differential Diagnosis

Mononeuropathies most commonly occur as a result of entrapment (as in carpal tunnel syndrome). Mononeuropathy multiplex is associated with systemic vasculitis and other metabolic or rheumatologic diseases. Demyelinating polyneuropathies can be hereditary (such as Charcot-Marie-Tooth disease) or acquired (as in Guillain-Barré syndrome), while axonal polyneuropathies have many potential underlying causes. Peripheral nerve disorders are discussed in Chapter 23.

KEY POINTS

- *Mononeuropathies* lead to weakness in muscles innervated by a single peripheral nerve.
- Polyneuropathies first affect the muscles of the distal extremities symmetrically.
- EMG/NCS can confirm peripheral nerve involvement, identify axonal or demyelinating features, and evaluate the relative chronicity of a nerve disorder.

NERVE ROOT DISORDERS

Pattern of Weakness

Each nerve root relevant to the upper or lower extremity exits the spinal cord and eventually traverses a plexus (either brachial or lumbosacral) in which its fibers separate and become part of multiple different peripheral nerves, which then go on to innervate multiple different muscles. The result is that most muscles are innervated by fibers that originate from more than one nerve root, although some muscles are predominantly innervated by fibers from one nerve root (see Table 5-1). In any case, a lesion of a single nerve root will cause weakness in the muscles innervated predominantly by fibers from that root, while leaving other, often neighboring muscles unaffected.

A problem involving a single nerve root is termed a **radiculopathy**. Some processes lead to dysfunction of multiple nerve roots at once (**polyradiculopathy**), leaving a pattern of weakness that may be more diffuse and difficult to sort out because multiple muscles related to multiple nerve roots can be weak bilaterally.

Associated Signs and Symptoms

Radiculopathies often have associated tingling or pain, frequently radiating out from the neck or back. Objective sensory loss is rare in disorders affecting a single nerve root because there is overlap from neighboring roots. If the nerve root is one that subserves a particular muscle stretch reflex (Table 5-2), that reflex may be depressed or absent.

Laboratory Studies

EMG/NCS can confirm that nerve roots are the culprit in a weak patient and can be particularly useful for

■ **TABLE 5-2** Commonly Tested Muscle Stretch Reflexes

Reflex	Root
Biceps	C5
Brachioradialis	C6
Triceps	C7
Finger flexor	C8/T1
Patellar (knee jerk)	L4
Hip adductor	L3
Ankle jerk	S1

cases where clinical differentiation between a root problem and a peripheral nerve problem is murky. Single radiculopathies usually require MRI of the spine to rule out structural causes, whereas polyradiculopathies usually require lumbar puncture (LP) to look for infectious or inflammatory conditions.

Differential Diagnosis

Single radiculopathies can be caused by herniated discs or by reactivation of varicella-zoster virus (shingles), for example. Polyradiculopathies are often inflammatory or infectious. These disorders are discussed in Chapter 23.

KEY POINTS

- A *radiculopathy* causes weakness in the muscles innervated predominantly by fibers from one nerve root.
- Radiating pain and tingling are common symptoms.
- If the nerve root subserves a particular muscle stretch reflex, that reflex may be depressed or absent.
- A polyradiculopathy may lead to weakness of multiple muscles related to multiple nerve roots bilaterally.

PLEXUS DISORDERS

Pattern of Weakness

The intricacies of brachial and lumbosacral plexus anatomy (Fig. 5-2) are often quite intimidating for students, but it need not be, because—ironically—it is their complex anatomy that makes localizing lesions to a plexus more straightforward than expected. Put simply, if multiple muscles in a limb are weak and do not conform to the pattern of a particular nerve root or peripheral nerve, a plexus problem should be suspected.

In the leg, for example, weakness in both hip flexors and hip adductors would have to involve the L1, L2, and L3 roots or both the nerve to the iliopsoas and the obturator nerve (see Table 5-1); a much more likely explanation is a lesion in the upper part of the lumbosacral plexus.

Associated Signs and Symptoms

Because the plexus is where multiple nerve roots intermingle their fibers to form multiple peripheral

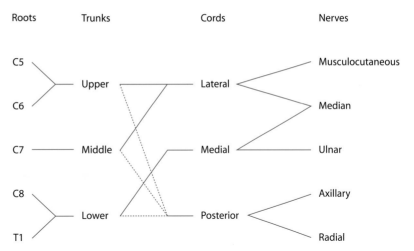

Figure 5-2 • Brachial plexus anatomy.

nerves, it is unsurprising that plexus disorders can have associated sensory findings (in the distribution of one or more roots or nerves) or dropped reflexes (subserved by one or more roots).

Laboratory Studies

EMG/NCS is frequently ordered in cases of clinically suspected plexopathies to help confirm the localization to the plexus, given the less than straightforward anatomy. MRI of the brachial plexus or pelvis (or lumbosacral plexus) may be necessary to rule out mass lesions.

Differential Diagnosis

Plexopathies can be caused by idiopathic inflammation, radiation, infiltration by metastases, hemorrhage, or trauma. They are discussed in Chapter 23. Diabetic patients are prone to develop a characteristic lumbosacral plexopathy known as **diabetic amyotrophy**.

KEY POINTS

- A *plexus* problem should be suspected when multiple muscles in a limb are weak and do not conform to a particular nerve root or peripheral nerve pattern.
- There may be associated sensory signs or reflex loss in plexus disorders.
- Plexopathies can be confirmed by EMG/NCS and have many potential causes.

SPINAL CORD DISORDERS

Pattern of Weakness

Spinal cord disorders cause weakness in two ways. First, the anterior horn cells located at the level of the lesion are affected, leading to weakness of the muscles innervated by the nerve root at that level. This mimics a radiculopathy, with weakness in a particular nerve root pattern. Second, there is weakness below the level of the lesion due to interruption of the descending corticospinal tracts. This weakness occurs in an upper motor neuron (UMN) pattern (Fig. 5-3).

Associated Signs and Symptoms

Depending on the extent of the lesion, there may be sensory findings due to interruption of the ascending tracts. There may be a sensory level (loss of sensation below a particular dermatomal level) on the torso. Typically, reflexes below the level of a spinal cord lesion are increased, and there may be Babinski signs. Bladder and bowel incontinence may occur.

Laboratory Studies

MRI of the spine can rule out structural etiologies or demonstrate intrinsic inflammation within the cord. LP may be needed to evaluate infectious, inflammatory, or neo-plastic possibilities.

Differential Diagnosis

Spinal cord disorders are discussed in Chapter 22; they may stem from inflammation (transverse myelitis),

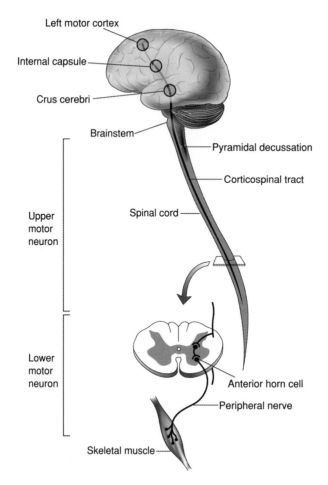

The descending motor pathway is divided into two parts.

The Upper Motor Neuron	The Lower Motor Neuron
Constitutes the neuron in the motor strip of the cerebral hemisphere and its descending axon all the way through the pyramidal decussation into the spinal cord.	Constitutes the anterior horn cell and its projecting axon all the way through the root and nerve to the neuromuscular junction of the innervated muscle.
Disorders of the UMN lead to a particular pattern of weakness: In the upper extremity, extensors and abductors become weaker than flexors and adductors. In the lower extremity, muscles that shorten the leg become weaker than muscles that extend the leg. In addition, UMN lesions lead to associated signs such as spasticity, hyperactive reflexes, and Babinski signs.	Disorders of the LMN lead to associated signs such as wasting and fasciculations.
In the face, lesions in the UMN (motor strip in cerebral hemisphere down to decussation in the pons) lead to weakness of the lower face but not the upper face, and weakness with volitional movements but not with emotional smile.	In the face, lesions in the LMN (peripheral facial nerve, as in Bell's palsy) lead to weakness of the upper and lower face, seen with all movements.

Figure 5-3 • Upper motor neuron (UMN) versus lower motor neuron (LMN).

infarction, compression, or other causes. Amyotrophic lateral sclerosis causes degeneration of both the corticospinal tracts and anterior horn cells.

KEY POINTS

- *Spinal cord disorders* lead to weakness in a UMN pattern below the lesion and weakness in a nerve root pattern at the level of the lesion.
- There may be sensory loss below the level of the lesion due to interruption of ascending tracts.
- Reflexes below the level of the lesion are typically increased, and Babinski signs may be present.
- Bladder and bowel incontinence may occur.

DISORDERS OF THE CEREBRAL HEMISPHERES AND BRAINSTEM

Pattern of Weakness

Lesions in the cerebral hemispheres lead to weakness of the contralateral body in a UMN pattern (see Fig. 5-3). Knowledge of the homunculus of the motor strip (Fig. 5-4) explains why lesions in the parasagittal part of the cerebral hemisphere cause weakness primarily in the leg, whereas lesions more laterally in the hemisphere cause weakness primarily in the face and arm. Deep hemispheric lesions, as in the internal capsule, may lead to weakness of all three parts of the contralateral body (face, arm, and leg), because motor fibers from all areas of the motor strip join together as they travel toward the brainstem.

Lesions in the base of the pons may lead to weakness of the ipsilateral face and contralateral arm and leg (crossed signs), because descending motor fibers to the face have crossed at that level but those to the body have not.

Associated Signs and Symptoms

Lesions of the cerebral hemispheres frequently have associated cognitive signs, such as those described in Chapter 11. Left hemispheric lesions may cause aphasia or apraxia, while right hemispheric lesions may cause neglect or visuospatial dysfunction. Lesions of the brainstem may cause cranial nerve problems, such as extraocular movement disorders.

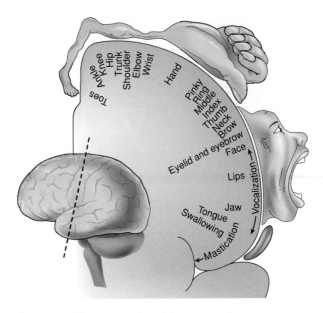

Figure 5-4 • The homunculus of the motor strip.

Laboratory Studies

Imaging of the brain is important to evaluate almost all of the potential etiologies in this category. The choice of MRI or CT depends on the suspected etiology and relative acuity.

Differential Diagnosis

The differential diagnosis includes such diverse etiologies as stroke (Chapter 14), demyelinating disease (Chapter 20), traumatic injury (Chapter 17), brain tumor (Chapter 19), and infection (Chapter 21).

KEY POINTS

- *Cerebral hemispheric lesions* lead to weakness of the contralateral side in a UMN pattern.
- Parasagittal lesions lead primarily to leg weakness, more lateral lesions lead primarily to face and arm weakness, and deep lesions may lead to weakness of all three parts.
- Cerebral hemispheric lesions may have accompanying cognitive signs, such as aphasia or neglect.
- *Brainstem lesions* may have accompanying CN findings.

The Sensory System

The sensory system includes somatosensory and special senses: smell, vision, taste, hearing, and vestibular sensation. The common characteristic in all is the presence of a receptor, an afferent nerve, and a dorsal root or cranial nerve ganglion that carries the information to the CNS.

Somatosensory abnormalities may be characterized by increase, alteration, impairment, or loss of feeling. The diagnosis of these problems includes analysis of the nature, location, characteristics, and distribution of symptoms.

ANATOMY OF THE SENSORY PATHWAYS

Each sensory modality has a receptor. Information from the receptor is then carried to the CNS by individual fibers in the nerve (peripheral or cranial) known as first-order neurons. Pain and temperature are carried by thinly myelinated and unmyelinated slowly conducting fibers (A-delta and C fibers, respectively) that synapse at the level of the dorsal horn of the spinal cord. From here, the axons from the second-order neurons cross and travel contralaterally in the spinothalamic tract (STT), also called the anterolateral system (Fig. 6-1). Proprioception, vibration, and light touch run ipsilaterally in heavily myelinated fibers (A-alpha and A-beta fibers) in the dorsal column system, reaching the second-order neuron at the level of the medulla in the nuclei gracilis and cuneatus. Axons from these nuclei cross at the lower medulla to form the medial lemniscus (Fig. 6-2).

There is a somatotopic arrangement of fibers in these tracts.

- **Spinothalamic tract:** At the level of the spinal cord, sacral segments are located laterally, lumbar fibers more medially, and cervical segments in the most medial locations.
- **The dorsal columns:** The medial fibers are from the legs and lateral fibers from the arms. At the level of the medial lemniscus, the upper body fibers become medial and those of the lower body lateral.

Facial sensation is carried to the brainstem by the trigeminal nerve. The STT and the trigeminal tract terminate in the thalamus (ventroposterolateral and ventroposteromedial, respectively), with further cortical projections through the third-order neurons to the postcentral cortex in a somatotopic arrangement similar to that in the motor cortex, with the face in the lowest area and the leg in the parasagittal area. Fine sensory discrimination and localization of pain, temperature, touch, and pressure require normal functioning of the sensory cortex.

EXAMINATION OF THE SENSORY SYSTEM

This is a difficult part of the neurologic exam and requires the patient's cooperation. The evaluation of different primary sensory modalities (temperature, pain [pinprick], light touch, vibration, and proprioception) is necessary to characterize sensory loss and its extent. In some instances, it is difficult to demonstrate sensory abnormalities in a patient with sensory symptoms; in others, the exam shows sensory findings in an asymptomatic patient. Whatever the situation, the sensory examination must be organized and methodical.

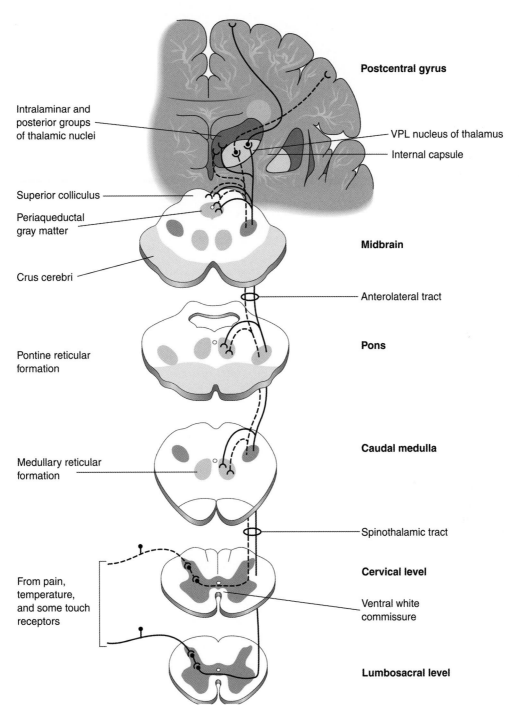

Figure 6-1 • Anterolateral system.

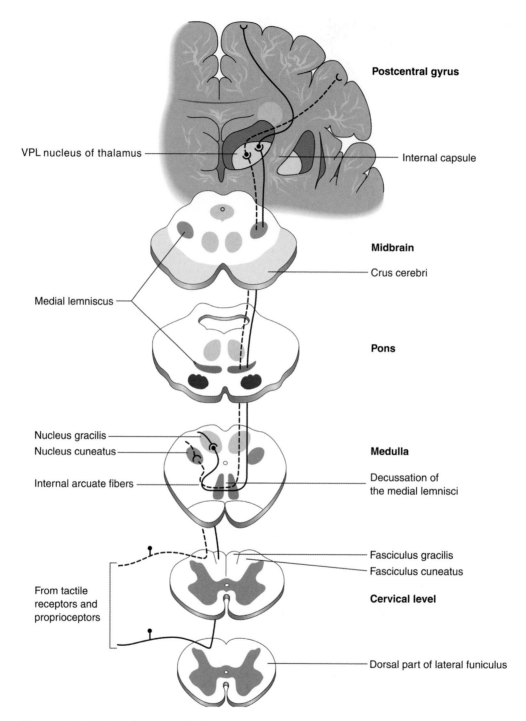

Postcentral gyrus

VPL nucleus of thalamus

Internal capsule

Midbrain

Crus cerebri

Medial lemniscus

Pons

Nucleus gracilis
Nucleus cuneatus

Medulla

Internal arcuate fibers

Decussation of
the medial lemnisci

Fasciculus gracilis
Fasciculus cuneatus

From tactile
receptors and
proprioceptors

Cervical level

Dorsal part of lateral funiculus

Figure 6-2 • Posterior column—medial lemniscal system.

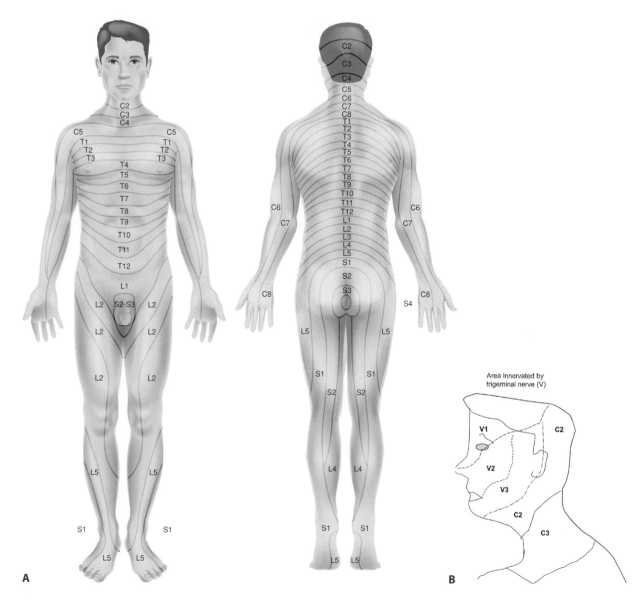

Figure 6-3 • Dermatome map.

Touch sensation is tested with a wisp of cotton, using a very soft stimulus. Pain sensation is tested with a pin. Thermal modalities are tested using objects with a temperature range between 10° and 50°C, because beyond those limits the stimulus becomes painful. Moving the great toe up and down and asking the patient to indicate the direction of movement test joint position sense. Proprioception can also be tested by moving an object up or down on the skin and asking the patient the direction of the movement. The testing of vibration sense requires a tuning fork (128 Hz) to be applied to toes and other bony prominences.

The next step is to record the sensory abnormalities using accepted definitions. It is important to register the patient's own words rather than using the terms below. Not only the presence or absence of sensation but also slight differences and gradations should be recorded. The following list defines some of the terminology used to describe sensory abnormalities:

- **Paresthesias** are abnormal sensations described by the patient as tingling, prickling, pins, and needles, etc.
- **Dysesthesias** are unpleasant sensations triggered by painless stimuli.

TABLE 6-1 Patterns of Sensory Loss According to Localization

Site of the Lesion	Sensory Findings	Other Neurologic Abnormalities	Examples
Peripheral nerve	Loss of LT, T, PP, and proprioception in the influenced area; associated weakness in muscles innervated by that nerve	Distal muscle weakness, atrophy, areflexia	Peroneal neuropathy; median and ulnar neuropathies
Root	Loss of all sensory modalities in a dermatomal distribution	Weakness in a myotomal distribution, atrophy, segmental hyporeflexia	L5 radiculopathy; cervical radiculopathy
Plexus	Sensory loss in the distribution of two or more peripheral nerves	Muscle weakness that cannot be localized to a single nerve or root	Brachial plexopathy due to trauma, inflammation, infiltration, etc.
Spinal cord	Sensory level: bilateral loss of all sensory modalities. Sensory dissociation. Contralateral hypesthesia and ipsilateral loss of proprioception (Brown-Séquard syndrome). Proprioceptive loss and corticospinal tract involvement. Saddle anesthesia	Paraplegia, tetraplegia; initially areflexia, then hyperreflexia below the lesion; Babinski sign	Myelopathy; central cord syndromes; Brown-Séquard syndrome; subacute combined degeneration
Brainstem	Ipsilateral facial numbness and contralateral body numbness	Alternating hemiplegia; cranial nerve findings; INO, ataxia	Posterior circulation strokes; tumor
Thalamus	Hemibody anesthesia	May have motor findings	Lacunar stroke; hemorrhage
Posterior limb of internal capsule	Hemibody anesthesia	Hemiplegia	Lacunar stroke; hemorrhage; tumor
Cortex	All modalities affected on the contralateral side	Sensory neglect; agraphesthesia	Parietal stroke; hemorrhage; AVM
Psychogenic	Hyperesthesia for one modality in one area with anesthesia for another modality in the same area; changing sensory findings. Nonphysiologic sensory level changes (abrupt midline changes, vibration asymmetry over the forehead, etc.)	Any	Psychogenic (this is a rule-out diagnosis; therefore, all other explanations need to be excluded before reaching this conclusion.)

AVM, arteriovenous malformation; INO, internuclear ophthalmoplegia; LT, light touch; PP, pinprick; T, temperature.

- **Hyperesthesia** is increased sensitivity to sensory stimuli. The opposite is **hypesthesia**.
- **Allodynia** is pain provoked by normally innocuous stimuli.
- **Dissociated sensory loss** refers to the loss of one of the sensory systems with preservation of another. For example, in a syrinx, the STT is compromised early, with loss of pain and temperature in the dermatomes involved but preservation of posterior column function and therefore a normal response to light touch and normal proprioception. This occurs frequently with central cord syndromes (see Chapter 22).

APPROACH TO THE PATIENT WITH SENSORY LOSS

Sensory dysfunction becomes manifest through two types of symptoms: **negative**, such as numbness, loss of cold or warm sensation, blindness, and deafness; or

positive, such as pain, paresthesias (tingling, pins and needles), visual sparkles, and tinnitus. The former usually means disruption of nerve excitation; the latter in general means excitation or disinhibition.

In a patient complaining of sensory disturbances, the first goal is to establish the presence or absence of a neurologic lesion and then, if present, to establish its location. Sometimes the sensory problems accompany other symptoms—such as weakness, neglect, visual field cuts, behavioral problems, or seizures—that may help to determine the lesion's location.

The goal is to recognize sensory abnormalities by modality and to judge the level at which they are produced. Although in theory it is easy to distinguish peripheral nerve from segmental nerve or root, spinal cord, or other CNS locations, this is in fact often not possible or at best imprecise. In general, compression of a peripheral nerve has a distribution of sensory loss in the territory of that specific nerve. Root problems give a dermatomal pattern of loss (Fig. 6-3). Spinal cord disease leads to a characteristic loss of sensation below a certain level. In brainstem lesions, the sensory abnormalities may occur on the ipsilateral side of the face and contralateral side of the body. Central sensory loss involving the thalamus or sensory cortex will generally affect the contralateral face, arm, and leg.

Once the location of sensory loss has been characterized, it is important to determine what sensory modality is involved, because different pathologic processes can affect different sensory systems.

The last step in evaluating these sensory abnormalities is to establish the cause. There are many primary neurologic diseases as well as systemic diseases that can present with sensory symptoms. They are explored in more detail in Chapter 23 on peripheral neuropathies.

The different patterns of sensory loss and the location of the respective neurologic problem are represented in Table 6-1. This table provides a guide to the process of diagnosis based on clinical symptoms and the physical exam, without the need for further technologic resources.

KEY POINTS

- It is important to obtain a good history of the sensory abnormalities and direct the exam according to it.
- Nerve damage produces sensory problems in the distribution of the damaged nerve; root damage produces sensory problems in a dermatome; and plexus damage produces sensory problems in a group of nerves in the same limb.
- Spinal cord lesions produce a sensory level; brainstem lesions cause a crossed sensory loss; and thalamus and cortex lesions produce sensory loss in the contralateral face, arm, and leg.

Dizziness, Vertigo, and Syncope

Because "dizziness" means different things to different people, it is not a useful term in describing one's symptoms. Broadly speaking, the possibilities include vertigo, light-headedness, dysequilibrium, and a fourth category of ill-defined dizziness. Vertigo is an illusion or hallucination of movement that is usually rotatory but may be linear. Light-headedness may also be described as feeling faint and may refer to a presyncopal state. This chapter focuses on these two categories.

Dysequilibrium is a sensation of imbalance or unsteadiness that is usually referable to the legs rather than to a feeling inside the head. The neurologic abnormalities responsible for this symptom are outlined in detail in Chapter 8. Finally, there are people who simply cannot define their symptoms accurately, as well as those with anxiety.

VERTIGO

Most vertigo is caused by an acute asymmetry or imbalance of neural activity between the left and right vestibular systems. Vertigo does not result from symmetric bilateral loss of vestibular function (as with ototoxic drugs) or from a slow unilateral loss of vestibular function (e.g., with an acoustic neuroma); the brain appears to habituate to slow changes. A useful approach (Box 7-1) to sorting out the etiology is to determine the periodicity and duration of the symptoms and whether they are positional or spontaneous. A determination should also be made as to whether the vertigo is of peripheral or central origin; the most helpful features in this regard are the presence and nature of the associated symptoms and signs. Tinnitus or hearing loss suggests a peripheral

cause, whereas diplopia, dysarthria, dysphagia, or other symptoms of brainstem dysfunction indicate a central process. Accompanying nausea and vomiting is often more prominent with peripheral causes of vertigo, and the ability to walk or maintain posture may be more impaired with central disease. Neither of these latter features, however, is very reliable. Finally, the nature of the nystagmus may suggest the source of the vertigo. Vertical and direction-changing gaze-evoked nystagmus indicates a central process. Unidirectional nystagmus may arise from either central or peripheral dysfunction.

Vestibular neuronitis presents as an acute unilateral (complete or incomplete) peripheral vestibulopathy. The designation **neuronitis** is inaccurate because there is no evidence of inflammation, but the term is retained here because of its common usage. Patients develop a sudden and spontaneous onset of vertigo, nausea, and vomiting. The onset is usually over minutes to hours; symptoms peak within 24 hours and then improve gradually over several days or weeks. Complete recovery may not occur for months. Nystagmus is strictly unilateral and may be suppressed by visual fixation. Recovery represents central compensation for the loss of peripheral vestibular function.

Labyrinthine concussion may result from head injury irrespective of whether there is an associated skull fracture. Vertigo is sometimes accompanied by hearing loss and tinnitus.

Infarction of the labyrinth, brainstem, or cerebellum. The blood supply to the central and peripheral vestibular apparatus and the cerebellum is via the vertebrobasilar system (posterior and anterior inferior cerebellar arteries and the superior cerebellar artery). Blood supply to the inner ear is via the internal

■ BOX 7-1 Approach to the Patient With Vertigo

Spontaneous vertigo
Single prolonged episode
Vestibular neuronitis
Labyrinthine concussion
Lateral medullary or cerebellar infarction
Recurrent episodes
Ménière disease
Perilymph fistula
Migraine
Posterior circulation ischemia
Positional vertigo
Peripheral
Benign positional paroxysmal vertigo (BPPV)
Central

auditory artery, a branch of the anteroinferior cerebellar artery. Infarction of the inner ear presents with a sudden onset of deafness, vertigo, or both.

Brainstem or cerebellar stroke is the most important differential diagnosis in patients with suspected acute vestibular neuronitis. The type of nystagmus and the presence of associated neurologic signs are the main distinguishing factors. A central-type nystagmus results from cerebellar or brainstem infarction, and almost invariably there are associated cranial nerve signs, weakness, ataxia, or sensory changes that clearly indicate a central process.

Ménière disease is characterized by episodic vertigo with nausea and vomiting; fluctuating, but progressive hearing loss; tinnitus; and a sensation of fullness or pressure in the ear. It is caused by an intermittent increase in endolymphatic volume.

A **perilymph fistula** results from disruption of the lining of the endolymphatic system. Typically, the patient reports hearing a "pop" at the time of a sudden increase in middle ear pressure, with sneezing, nose-blowing, coughing, or straining. This is followed by the abrupt onset of vertigo.

Patients with **benign positional paroxysmal vertigo** (BPPV) have episodes of vertigo that are precipitated by changes in position, such as turning over in bed or looking upward. The attacks are brief, usually lasting seconds to minutes, and symptoms typically begin after a few seconds' latency following the

change in position. Attacks occur most frequently when the individual is reclining in bed at night or upon awakening in the morning. There may be associated severe nausea and vomiting. Attacks may occur in clusters, with patients remaining asymptomatic for months or years in between.

BPPV results from freely moving crystals of calcium carbonate within one of the semicircular canals. When the head is stationary, these crystals settle in the most dependent part of the canal (usually posterior). With head movements, the crystals move more slowly than the endolymph within which they lie; once the head comes to rest, their inertia causes ongoing stimulation of the hair cells, resulting in the illusion of movement (vertigo). Diagnosis is established by demonstrating the characteristic downbeating and torsional nystagmus with the Dix-Hallpike test (Fig. 7-1, upper). The offending ear is the one that is toward the ground when vertigo occurs during the test. A positioning (Epley) maneuver (Fig. 7-1, lower) can be used to remove the crystals from the posterior semicircular canal. The head is turned in the direction of the offending ear. The illustration demonstrates treatment for BPPV originating from the left ear.

KEY POINTS

- Vertigo is a hallucination of movement that results from acute unilateral vestibular dysfunction.
- Tinnitus and hearing loss often accompany peripheral vertigo; diplopia, dysarthria, or other symptoms of brainstem dysfunction indicate a central cause.
- Isolated vertigo is almost never caused by brainstem ischemia.
- Recurrent episodes of vertigo lasting seconds to minutes triggered by a change in head position are typical of benign positional paroxysmal vertigo.

SYNCOPE

Syncope is a transient loss of consciousness and postural tone that results from brain hypoperfusion. Prior to losing consciousness, patients often report light-headedness and a variety of visual symptoms (blurred or tunnel vision, graying or blacking out). The term **presyncope** is used when patients experience this prodrome of symptoms but do not subsequently lose consciousness. Observers may note that

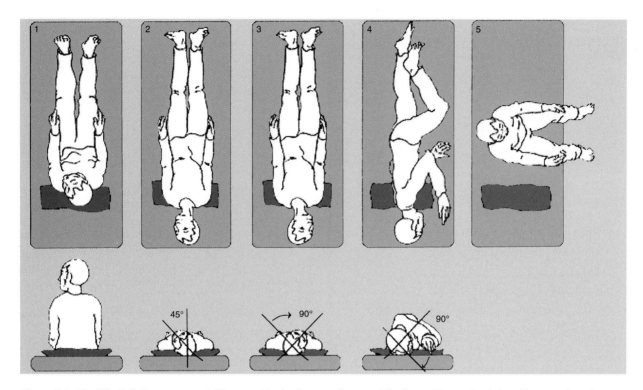

Figure 7-1 • The Dix-Hallpike maneuver is illustrated in the first two frames of the figure. The patient's head is rotated 45 degrees to one side and then extended 30 degrees over the edge of the bed. The examiner looks for a rotatory and down-beating nystagmus. The Epley positioning maneuver begins with the positioning used for the Dix-Hallpike maneuver and continues with a series of other positions, as illustrated.
(Reproduced with permission of the Department of Neurology, Charité, Humbolt University, Berlin.)

the patient appears pale or is sweating. Syncope is most commonly a manifestation of hypotension due to cardiac causes, low intravascular volume, or excessive vasodilation. Cardiac causes include asystole, third-degree heart block, tachyarrhythmias, outflow obstruction, valvular disease, or myocardial infarction. Low intravascular volume can result from dehydration, blood loss, or Addison disease and can result in either syncope or orthostatic hypotension. Excessive vasodilation usually has a neurologic cause. There are essentially two neurologic varieties of syncope, both involving some dysfunction of the autonomic nervous system that results in excessive vasodilation. The more common is neurogenic syncope, in which acute hypotension results from a sudden reflex change in autonomic cardiovascular control. Less commonly, orthostatic hypotension and syncope may result from autonomic failure.

Neurogenic syncope is an acute hemodynamic reaction produced by a sudden change in the activity of the autonomic nervous system. Its pathophysiology involves a reflex triggered by excessive afferent discharges from arterial (including cardiac or great vessel) or visceral mechanoreceptors. Afferent impulses via the vagus nerve lead to cardioinhibition and vasodepression, resulting in hypotension and bradycardia. Different terms are used to describe this reflex, depending on the trigger (Table 7-1).

Autonomic failure is characterized by an inability to activate efferent sympathetic fibers appropriately, particularly on assumption of the upright posture.

■ TABLE 7-1 Reflex Syncope	
Type of Syncope	**Pathophysiologic Trigger**
Micturition syncope	Rapid emptying of a distended bladder
Carotid sinus hypersensitivity	Compression of the carotid sinus
Neurocardiogenic syncope	Vigorous contraction of an underfilled ventricle
Vasovagal syncope	Strong emotions or acute pain

This usually leads to orthostatic hypotension, but syncope can also result. The underlying pathologic process can be either central (e.g., spinal cord injury or degenerative neurologic conditions that affect the autonomic nervous system, such as multiple system atrophy and Parkinson disease) or peripheral (e.g., diabetes resulting in autonomic neuropathy), but the hallmark of both is the failure to release norepinephrine on standing. Patients usually complain of light-headedness and presyncopal symptoms in response to a sudden change in posture or prolonged standing. There may be associated weakness, fatigue, cognitive slowing, headache, neck pain, or buckling of the legs.

In evaluating patients with syncope or orthostatic hypotension, a thorough history and medical and neurologic examinations are warranted. The history is critical in detailing the precipitating circumstances of the event and excluding other conditions, such as seizures, that can be confused with syncope. If a cardiac cause is suspected, an electocardiogram or more prolonged cardiac monitoring with a Holter monitor may be indicated in order to exclude an underlying arrhythmia. An echocardiogram is indicated if a structural cardiac lesion (e.g., valvular) is suspected. In addition, clinical findings, orthostatic signs, and blood work (hemoglobin, hematocrit, blood urea nitrogen, and creatinine) can indicate intravascular volume depletion and its causes, such as blood loss or dehydration. If a neurologic cause for syncope is suspected, the exam can demonstrate a degenerative neurologic condition or a peripheral neuropathy. If no clear cause for syncope can be identified, tilt-table testing may be helpful in documenting autonomic dysfunction and diagnosing neurogenic syncope, particularly when the clinical history is unclear.

In managing patients with symptomatic orthostatic hypotension or syncope, it is important to recognize the potential contribution of drugs such as diuretics, antihypertensives, vasodilators, and antidepressants. Raising the head of the bed will reduce nocturnal diuresis, and patients should be advised to move gradually from the supine to standing position. A variety of drugs are available to ameliorate the symptoms of orthostatic hypotension, with midodrine and fludrocortisone being most commonly used. Beta blockers can be used to treat neurogenic syncope by suppressing overactive cardiac mechanoreceptors.

KEY POINTS

- Presyncopal symptoms include light-headedness, headache, neck pain, blurring of vision, cognitive slowing, and buckling of the knees.
- Syncope results from cerebral hypoperfusion.
- The two main neurologic causes of syncope are neurogenic syncope and autonomic failure (central or peripheral).
- Neurogenic syncope results from inappropriate activation of a cardioinhibitory and vasodepressor reflex, which may be triggered by micturition, deglutition, carotid sinus compression, sudden underfilling of the ventricle, or heightened vagal tone.
- The hallmark of autonomic failure is the failure to release norepinephrine on standing.
- Orthostatic hypotension may result from intravascular volume depletion, autonomic failure, or medications.

Chapter

8 Ataxia and Gait Disorders

Ataxia is a term derived from Greek meaning "irregularity" or "disorderliness"; it is a general term often used to describe the manifestations of diseases of the cerebellum or its connections. It is important, however, to recognize that not all ataxia is cerebellar in origin. For example, the deafferentation due to the loss of position sense also results in an ataxia. Hence it is appropriate to distinguish cerebellar ataxia from sensory ataxia.

The cerebellum controls the force, direction, range, rate, and rhythm of movements; a disturbance of these elements results in the signs and symptoms characteristic of cerebellar disease (Box 8-1). Ataxia is not the only process that may underlie a gait disorder; these other causes are described separately below.

ATAXIA

DIAGNOSTIC APPROACH

The spectrum of disorders characterized by prominent ataxia is diverse. A limited differential diagnosis can often be generated by considering the acuity with which symptoms begin and whether the disorder is temporary, episodic, or progressive. It is also helpful to consider the age of onset, family history, and mode of inheritance. A classification based on this approach is outlined in Box 8-2. The details of a few of these disorders are specified below. Associated symptoms and signs may also provide useful diagnostic information; some of these are summarized in Table 8-1. Finally, at a clinical level, a distinction can often be made between lesions of the vermis and those of the cerebellar hemispheres. Vermal lesions typically produce prominent truncal and gait ataxia. Hemispheric

lesions, however, typically manifest with ipsilateral limb ataxia.

CEREBELLAR HEMORRHAGE OR INFARCTION

Cerebellar hemorrhage or infarction typically presents with the abrupt onset of vertigo, vomiting, and inability to walk. Level of arousal may be depressed if there is compression of the fourth ventricle with hydrocephalus or if there is pressure on the brainstem. Cerebellar stroke should be considered a medical emergency because neurosurgical intervention may be required for decompression if there is brainstem compression or risk of herniation.

ALCOHOLIC CEREBELLAR DEGENERATION

Alcoholic cerebellar degeneration is a consequence of long-standing alcohol abuse and is usually accompanied by an alcoholic polyneuropathy. Alcohol is the most common cause of acquired cerebellar degeneration. The vermis bears the brunt of the damage; the presentation, therefore, is usually with progressive gait and truncal ataxia that evolves over a period of weeks or months. Cessation of drinking and supplementation of nutrition offer the best (although limited) chance of improvement.

POSTINFECTIOUS CEREBELLITIS

Postinfectious cerebellitis typically affects children between the ages of 2 and 7 and usually follows a

■ BOX 8-1 Signs and Symptoms of Cerebellar Disease

Dysmetria: Abnormality of the range and force of a movement; manifests as erratic, jerky movements with over- and undershooting the target (hence limb or ocular dysmetria)

Intention tremor: Rhythmic side-to-side oscillations of the limb as it approaches the target

Dysdiadochokinesia: Abnormality of the rate and rhythm of a movement demonstrated by asking the patient to perform a rapid alternating movement

Gait ataxia: Broad-based and unsteady, with an inability to walk in a straight line and a tendency to lurch from side to side

Truncal ataxia: Impaired control of truncal posture; when severe, unable to even sit unsupported

Dysarthria: Slow scanning and monotonous speech

Nystagmus

■ BOX 8-2 Classification of the Ataxias

Acute or subacute onset with resolution or episodic course

Postinfectious and infectious cerebellitis

Cerebellar hemorrhage or infarction

Drugs (e.g., phenytoin, barbiturates, antineoplastic agents)

Multiple sclerosis

Hydrocephalus*

Posterior fossa mass*

Foramen magnum compression*

Dominantly inherited episodic ataxias

Childhood metabolic disorders (e.g., aminoacidurias, disorders of pyruvate and lactate metabolism)

Acute or subacute onset with progressive course

Paraneoplastic cerebellar degeneration

Alcoholic or nutritional cerebellar degeneration

Chronic onset and progressive course

Autosomal dominant spinocerebellar degenerations

Autosomal recessive cerebellar degenerative disorders

Infectious (e.g., Creutzfeldt-Jakob disease)

Vitamin E deficiency

Hypothyroidism

Childhood metabolic disorders (e.g., mitochondrial encephalomyelopathies, Wilson disease, ataxia-telangiectasia)

*May also cause insidious onset and chronically progressive ataxia.

varicella or other viral infection. Children present with acute onset of limb and gait ataxia as well as dysarthria. Severity ranges from mild unsteadiness to complete inability to walk. The diagnosis is one of exclusion; this usually requires a careful search for underlying drug intoxication and for a mass lesion in the posterior fossa. The illness lasts a few weeks and recovery is usually complete.

PARANEOPLASTIC CEREBELLAR DEGENERATION

Paraneoplastic cerebellar degeneration (PCD) typically presents with the acute or subacute onset of a pancerebellar syndrome with truncal, gait, and limb ataxia; dysarthria; and disturbances of ocular motility (ocular dysmetria, nystagmus). The disease usually evolves to its maximal extent over a period of weeks and then stabilizes, leaving the patient with profound disability. PCD is typically associated with an underlying gynecologic or small cell lung cancer and may become manifest prior to diagnosis of the tumor. MRI is usually normal. The CSF may have an elevated protein or a lymphocytic pleocytosis but is frequently normal. A variety of autoantibodies (e.g., anti-Yo, anti-Hu) have been described in this condition.

FRIEDREICH ATAXIA

Friedreich ataxia is an autosomal recessive disorder characterized by a progressive ataxia that usually affects the arms more than the legs as well as by severe dysarthria. Onset is usually in childhood. Classic associated findings are loss of reflexes, spasticity and extensor plantar responses, and impaired vibration and position sense.

INHERITED EPISODIC ATAXIA

The episodic ataxia (EA) syndromes are characterized by brief episodes of ataxia, vertigo, nausea, and vomiting. EA-1 is caused by mutations in a voltage-gated

■ **TABLE 8-1** Associated Symptoms and Signs in Cerebellar Ataxia	
Associated Symptom or Sign	**Diagnostic Possibilities**
Vomiting	Cerebellar stroke, posterior fossa mass
Fever	Viral cerebellitis, infection, or abscess
Malnutrition	Alcoholic cerebellar degeneration or vitamin E deficiency
Depressed consciousness	Cerebellar stroke, childhood metabolic disorders
Dementia	Creutzfeldt-Jakob disease, inherited spinocerebellar ataxia
Optic neuritis or atrophy	Multiple sclerosis
Ophthalmoplegia	Wernicke encephalopathy, Miller Fisher syndrome, multiple sclerosis, cerebellar stroke, posterior fossa mass
Extrapyramidal signs	Wilson disease, Creutzfeldt-Jakob disease, olivopontocerebellar atrophy
Hyporeflexia or areflexia	Miller Fisher syndrome, Friedreich ataxia, alcoholic cerebellar degeneration, hypothyroidism
Downbeat nystagmus	Foramen magnum lesion, posterior fossa mass

potassium channel. Episodes are brief, and an interattack skeletal muscle myokymia is associated. EA-2 is caused by mutations in the pore-forming α_1 subunit of the P/Q-type voltage-gated calcium channel. Attacks are longer, lasting several minutes; there is interictal nystagmus; and a progressive irreversible ataxia may develop late in the disease.

AUTOSOMAL DOMINANT SPINOCEREBELLAR DEGENERATIONS

The clinical diagnosis is based on the occurrence of cerebellar ataxia, with or without additional neurologic signs, and a family history consistent with autosomal dominant inheritance. The typical presentation is the insidious onset of progressive impairment of gait and dysarthria in early adult life. Associated neurologic abnormalities (e.g., oculomotor, pyramidal, or extrapyramidal signs) may suggest the underlying genotype. Mild to moderate cognitive decline is a late feature in most of the spinocerebellar ataxias (SCAs). Many SCAs for which the genetic defect has been identified have been shown to be caused by trinucleotide (CAG) expansions. SCA6 is allelic to EA-2, with the mutated gene being the pore-forming α_1 subunit of the P/Q-type voltage-gated calcium channel. The normal function of the other SCA genes is presently unknown.

MILLER FISHER SYNDROME

The Miller Fisher syndrome (MFS) is a disorder characterized by the triad of ataxia, areflexia, and

ophthalmoplegia. The ataxia is due to proprioceptive loss rather than to cerebellar dysfunction. MFS is thought to be a variant of the Guillain-Barré syndrome; as such, it is most likely mediated by a postinfectious immune process. IgG anti-GQ_{1b} antibodies are detectable in the serum of over 90% of patients with this syndrome. It is usually a self-limiting disorder with a relatively good prognosis for full recovery.

KEY POINTS

- Sudden onset of cerebellar ataxia with associated vomiting and depressed level of consciousness suggests a cerebellar stroke.
- Alcoholic cerebellar degeneration typically affects the vermis and manifests itself with gait and truncal ataxia.
- Postinfectious cerebellitis is a relatively common cause of ataxia in children.
- Paraneoplastic cerebellar degeneration is a pancerebellar syndrome and is most often associated with small cell lung cancer or a gynecologic malignancy.
- The inherited episodic ataxias are caused by mutations in calcium and potassium channel genes.
- The autosomal dominant SCAs are a group of degenerative disorders caused by trinucleotide expansions.

■ **TABLE 8-2** Etiology of Various Abnormal Gaits		
Gait Disorder	**Anatomic Location**	**Pathology**
Hemiplegic	Brainstem, cerebral hemisphere	Stroke, tumor, trauma
Paraplegic	Spinal cord	Demyelination (e.g., multiple sclerosis), transverse myelitis, compressive myelopathy
	Bihemispheral	Diffuse anoxic injury
Akinetic-rigid	Basal ganglia	Parkinson disease; other parkinsonian syndromes
Frontal	Frontal lobes	Hydrocephalus, tumor, stroke, neurodegenerative disorder
	Subcortical	Binswanger disease
Waddling	Hip-girdle weakness	Muscular dystrophy, spinal muscular atrophy, acquired proximal myopathy
Slapping	Large-fiber neuropathy	Vitamin B_{12} deficiency
	Dorsal columns	Tabes dorsalis

OTHER GAIT DISORDERS

Abnormalities of gait are common and frequently multifactorial. This is especially true in the elderly, in whom falls often result. Not all gait disorders are the result of disease of the nervous system. For example, local mechanical factors such as pain and arthritis may impair ambulation. These factors are not discussed further here.

Clues to the etiology of the gait disorder may be derived from the presence of other neurologic abnormalities, such as weakness, spasticity, rigidity, bradykinesia, ataxia, or frontal lobe dysfunction. Sometimes, however, an abnormal gait is sufficiently characteristic to permit identification of the underlying disorder based solely on the features of the gait. The following sections are devoted to descriptions of the different types of gait disorders. The differential diagnosis of each type of gait is presented in Table 8-2.

HEMIPARETIC GAIT

The affected leg is stiff and does not flex at the hip, knee, or ankle. The leg is circumducted, with a tendency to scrape the floor with the toes. The arm is held in flexion and adduction and does not swing freely. A spastic (paraparetic) gait is essentially that of a bilateral hemiparesis. The adductor tone is increased, and the legs tend to cross during walking (scissoring gait).

AKINETIC-RIGID GAIT

Posture is stooped, with flexion of the shoulders, neck, and trunk. Gait is narrow-based, slow, and shuffling with small steps and reduced arm swing. Instead, the arms are carried flexed and slightly ahead of the body. There is often difficulty with gait initiation. Postural reflexes are impaired, and the patient may take a series of rapid small steps (festination) forward (propulsion) or backward (retropulsion) in an effort to preserve equilibrium. The foregoing description is typical of patients with idiopathic Parkinson disease, but these features may also be seen in other extrapyramidal disorders. One difference in progressive supranuclear palsy is that posture tends toward extension rather than flexion.

FRONTAL GAIT

Posture is flexed, and the feet may be slightly apart. Gait initiation is impaired; the word "magnetic" is used to describe the patient's difficulty in lifting the feet off the ground. The patient advances with small, shuffling, and hesitant steps. With increasing severity, the patient may make abortive stepping movements in one place without being able to move forward.

WADDLING GAIT

A waddling gait is characteristic of hip-girdle weakness. During normal walking, the hip abductors contract to fix the weight-bearing leg and thus allow the opposite leg to rise and the trunk to tilt toward the fixed leg. Weakness of the abductors and consequent failure to stabilize the weight-bearing hip cause the pelvis and trunk to tilt toward the opposite side during walking.

SENSORY ATAXIA

Loss of proprioceptive input from the feet impairs the patient's ability to determine his position in space. Gait, therefore, becomes cautious. It is wide-based, and steps are slow. Contact with the ground is made by the heel, and the forefoot then strikes the floor with a slapping sound (hence **slapping gait**). Walking on uneven surfaces or in the dark is particularly difficult for such a patient.

PSYCHOGENIC GAIT

There is no single typical characteristic to this gait. Instead, a range of abnormalities may be seen. With psychogenic leg weakness, for example, the patient tends to drag her leg behind or push it ahead of her. The circumduction characteristic of the genuine hemigait (described earlier) is absent. Another feature is that the patient may adopt extreme postures and lurch wildly in all directions but without falling, thus demonstrating good strength and more than adequate postural reflexes. The term **astasia-abasia** is used to describe this sort of acrobatic psychogenic gait.

KEY POINTS

- Hemiparetic gait suggests hemispheric dysfunction, most often stroke.
- Paraparetic gait typically suggests spinal cord disease.
- Akinetic-rigid gait is a feature of parkinsonian syndromes.
- Frontal gait suggests hydrocephalus (including normal-pressure hydrocephalus), neurodegenerative process, or bifrontal or diffuse subcortical disease.
- Waddling gait suggests proximal muscle (hip girdle) weakness.
- Slapping gait indicates large-fiber sensory or dorsal column dysfunction.

Urinary and Sexual Dysfunction

Urinary bladder dysfunction is associated with a wide variety of neurologic diseases including stroke, dementia, Parkinson disease, multiple sclerosis, and diabetes. An understanding of how these diseases cause incontinence is important in both diagnosis and management.

BLADDER INCONTINENCE

ANATOMY AND PHYSIOLOGY

Neural circuits in the brain and spinal cord coordinate the activity of visceral smooth muscle (bladder and urethra) and striated muscle (external urethral sphincter) to control micturition (voiding). These circuits act as on-off switches to shift the lower urinary tract between storage (sympathetic) and elimination (parasympathetic) modes (Fig. 9-1).

Bradley has defined the different neuroanatomic connections important for bladder control as "circuits." The first circuit connects the dorsomedial frontal lobe to the medial (M) region in the pons, providing the volitional control of micturition. The second, or spinobulbospinal circuit, is a reflex arc that starts in the urinary bladder and projects to the M region of the pons, with outflow connections to the parasympathetic sacral spinal motor nuclei. The third circuit is a spinal segmental reflex arc with afferent fibers from the detrusor muscle to the pudendal nucleus in the sacral spinal cord and efferent fibers to the striated sphincter muscles (see Fig. 9-1).

M-region stimulation produces a decrease in urethral pressure, followed by a rise in detrusor muscle pressure and voiding. The M region projects to the intermediolateral columns of the sacral cord. The lateral (L) region is at the same level of the pons; its stimulation produces a powerful contraction of the urethral sphincter (storage). Damage at the level of the pontine micturition center will produce a loss of inhibitory control over spinal reflexes. As the bladder becomes distended, the micturition reflex is automatically activated without the patient's awareness or control, and detrusor hyperreflexia and incontinence occur.

DIAGNOSTIC EVALUATION

The first objective in the evaluation of bladder incontinence is to determine if the problem is neurogenic or not. A detailed history is essential. It is important to obtain information about initiation; voiding problems such as frequency, stream characteristics, urine volume, fullness, and urgency; effects of posture, cough, Valsalva maneuver, and medications; and associated bowel and sexual dysfunction.

Thorough physical and neurologic examinations are necessary. The examiner seeks signs of frontal lobe dysfunction, parkinsonian features, sensory level, myelopathy, and so forth. Laboratory evaluation includes basic urinalysis to rule out infection. Measurement of the postvoid residual (PVR) by bladder ultrasound or catheterization is important in the characterization of bladder dysfunction. The PVR represents the residual volume in the bladder after voiding. A normal PVR is less than 50 mL. Urodynamic studies can clarify the characteristics of the incontinence, determine the underlying neurologic abnormality, categorize the vesicourethral dysfunction, and provide a basis for appropriate therapy.

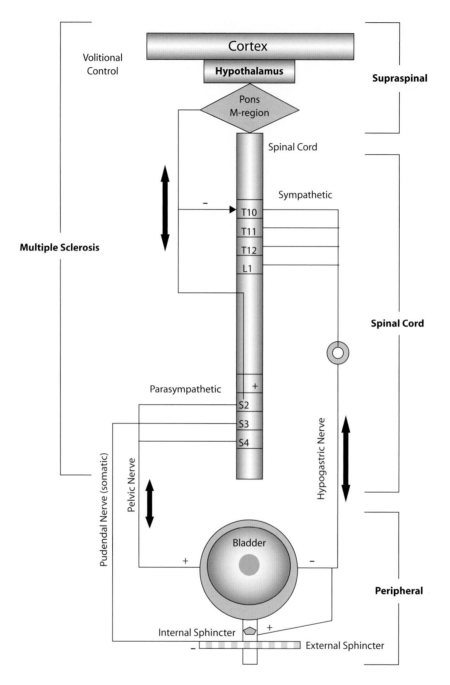

Figure 9-1 • The control of bladder function.
(Figure by Dr. Juan Acosta.)

■ TABLE 9-1 Urodynamic Findings in Neurogenic Bladder

Type	Capacity	Compliance	Others
Spastic bladder	Decreased	Reduced	Uninhibited detrusor contractions
Atonic bladder	Increased	Increased	Low voiding pressure and flow rate

Some urodynamic studies include the following:

- **Cystometry:** Provides information about bladder compliance, capacity, and volume at first sensation and at urge to void; voiding pressure; and the presence of uninhibited detrusor contractions.
- **Cystourethroscopy:** Assesses the integrity of the lower urinary system and identifies important urethral and bladder lesions.
- **Retrograde urethrography**
- **Neurophysiologic studies:** These include EMG of the sphincter and pelvic floor.

Urodynamic findings in various types of neurogenic bladder dysfunctions are listed in Table 9-1.

KEY POINTS

- The M region in the pons is the site of activation of micturition.
- History and a complete neurologic exam are important in the evaluation of bladder incontinence.
- PVR should be less than 50 mL. Increased PVR implies poor bladder emptying. Sphincter dyssynergia and atonic bladder are common neurogenic causes of elevated PVR.

CLASSIFICATION

This classification is based on symptoms.

Urge incontinence is an involuntary loss of urine associated with a strong desire to void (urgency), usually associated with detrusor instability (DI). When the DI is the result of a neurologic problem, the term **detrusor hyperreflexia** (DH) is used; its clinical expression is a spastic bladder. DH is common in patients with strokes, suprasacral spinal cord lesions, and multiple sclerosis. It is usually accompanied by detrusor-sphincter dyssynergia (DSD), which is inappropriate contraction of the external sphincter with detrusor contraction. This can result in urinary retention, vesicoureteral reflux, and subsequent renal damage.

Stress incontinence is an involuntary loss of urine during coughing, sneezing, laughing, or other physical activities that increase intra-abdominal pressure (in the absence of detrusor contraction or an overdistended bladder). This is common in multiparous women who have cystoceles or weakened muscles of the pelvic floor. Other causes include urethral hypermobility; significant displacement of the urethra and bladder neck; and intrinsic urethral sphincter deficiency due to congenital weakness in patients with myelomeningocele or epispadias or who have had prostatectomy, trauma, or radiation.

Mixed incontinence is a combination of urge and stress incontinence.

Overflow incontinence is an involuntary loss of urine associated with overdistention of the bladder, reflecting a lower motor neuron problem. Patients report constant dribbling or urge or stress incontinence symptoms. The resultant atonic bladder can be produced by an underactive or acontractile detrusor (due to drugs, diabetic neuropathy, lower spinal cord injury, or radical pelvic surgery that interrupts innervation to the detrusor muscle). Bladder outlet and urethral obstruction can also cause overdistention and overflow.

KEY POINTS

- Spastic bladder implies an upper motor neuron problem due to lesions involving the frontal lobes, pons, or suprasacral spinal cord. Symptoms include incontinence with urgency. Urodynamics show decreased capacity and reduced compliance.
- Atonic bladder implies a lower motor neuron lesion at the level of the conus medullaris, cauda equina, or sacral plexus; or it may reflect peripheral nerve dysfunction. It is characterized by overflow incontinence and increased capacity and compliance.
- Sphincter dyssynergia produces an increased PVR with fluctuating voiding pressures and varying flow rate.
- A small PVR is good; a large PVR with spastic or atonic bladder is not. It can cause increased intrabladder pressure with deleterious effect on the ureters and kidneys.

INCONTINENCE IN THE NEUROLOGIC PATIENT

The evaluation of urinary incontinence in the neurologic patient requires a detailed physical and neurologic exam in an attempt to define the level of the lesion: supraspinal, spinal, peripheral, or mixed.

Supraspinal Diseases

Supraspinal diseases usually result in a hyperreflexic bladder, causing urge incontinence, reduced bladder capacity, and small PVR, with no deleterious effects on the upper urinary tract because voiding is unobstructed.

Cerebrovascular Disease

Large strokes (particularly frontal or pontine) produce an upper motor neuron bladder (hyperreflexic and small with urgency and frequency). Urinary incontinence after stroke is common and is associated with overall poor functional outcome.

Parkinson Disease

Voiding dysfunction occurs in 40% to 70% of patients with Parkinson disease. DH is the most common finding. Pseudodyssynergia occurs as a consequence of sphincter bradykinesia. Urologic causes, such as benign prostatic hypertrophy, are frequently associated.

Spinal Cord Diseases

Spinal cord diseases are the most common cause of neurogenic bladder dysfunction. In a clinical study, 74% of patients with neurogenic bladder dysfunction had some form of spinal cord disease.

Following disconnection from the pons, the sphincter tends to contract when the detrusor is contracting (dyssynergia). New reflexes emerge to drive bladder emptying and cause DH. During spinal shock, the bladder is acontractile, but gradually, over weeks, reflex detrusor contractions develop in response to low filling volumes.

Spinal Cord Injury

Spinal cord injury produces DH, loss of compliance, and detrusor-sphincter dyssynergia.

Multiple Sclerosis

About 75% of patients with multiple sclerosis (MS) have bladder dysfunction. About 65% complain of irritative symptoms, 25% of obstructive symptoms, and 10% of mixed symptoms. DH occurs in 50% to 90% of patients, among whom 50% also have detrusor-sphincter dyssynergia.

Peripheral Nerve Diseases

Because of the bladder's extensive autonomic innervation, its dysfunction is most often seen in those generalized polyneuropathies involving small (autonomic) nerve fibers. Urodynamic studies show impaired detrusor contractility, decreased bladder sensation, decreased flow rate, and increased PVR. A classic example is diabetic cystopathy, in which a progressive loss of bladder sensation and impairment of bladder emptying eventually results in chronic low-pressure urinary retention. The situation is similar in other types of neuropathies such as amyloidosis, immune-mediated polyneuropathies (25% of Guillain-Barré patients have bladder symptoms), and inherited neuropathies. Injury to pelvic nerves (e.g., by local radiation or surgery) can produce similar symptoms.

KEY POINTS

- Stroke and spinal cord disease usually produce an upper motor neuron bladder or spastic bladder with or without sphincter dyssynergia.
- Small-fiber neuropathies can produce a neurogenic atonic bladder with high PVR.

TREATMENT

Therapy for a neurogenic bladder includes pharmacologic and nonpharmacologic approaches. Some of the behavioral techniques that may help with the treatment of this condition include toileting assistance, bladder retraining, and pelvic muscle rehabilitation.

Pharmacologic agents are available to treat bladder dysfunction. The choice of therapy is based on an understanding of the underlying mechanism of the dysfunction and therefore the site of the neural injury. Table 9-2 summarizes treatments for urinary incontinence.

■ TABLE 9-2 Treatment of Urinary Incontinence

Type	Therapy	Notes

Urge incontinence (spastic bladder)	1. Anticholinergic agents
	  a. Tolterodine (Detrol), 2 mg tid
	  b. Oxybutynin (Ditropan), 2.5 to
	    5.0 mg po tid/qid
	  c. Propantheline, 7.5 to 30.0 mg tid/qid
		Tolterodine is tolerated better than oxybutynin. Most frequent side effect: dry mouth. Others include headache, dyspepsia, dizziness, and urinary tract infections

	2. Tricyclic antidepressants a. Imipramine, 25 mg po tid/qid	
	3. Desmopressin (DDAVP) spray or tablets	Desmopressin is used to treat diabetes insipidus; however, it produces a significant reduction in voiding frequency in the 6 hours following treatment. Use only *once* a day.
	4. Intravesical capsaicin	Intravesical capsaicin is used for intractable detrusor hyperreflexia. It has a neurotoxic effect on the afferent C fibers that drive volume-determined reflex detrusor contractions. Lessening of urgency and frequency may last up to 6 months.

Stress incontinence	1. Alpha-adrenergic agonist drugs
	  a. Phenylpropanolamine, 25 to
	    100 mg bid
	  b. Pseudoephedrine, 15 to
	    30 mg tid
		Alpha-adrenergic agonist drugs stimulate smooth muscle alpha-adrenergic receptors. Estrogen therapy is adjunctive for postmenopausal women with stress or mixed incontinence.

	2. Estrogen therapy, oral or vaginal	
Atonic bladder with overflow incontinence	1. Credé's maneuver or Valsalva maneuver to empty the bladder	
	2. Intermittent self-catheterization is perhaps the mainstay of long-term treatment.	
	3. Pharmacotherapy is usually not an effective treatment modality. The cholinergic agent bethanechol (25 to 100 mg qid) is used.	Bethanechol stimulates cholinergic receptors, increasing detrusor muscle tone. Side effects include bronchospasm, diarrhea, abdominal pain, and flushing.
Detrusor dyssynergia	1. Intermittent catheterization	
	2. Suprapubic catheterization	
	3. Sacral nerve stimulation	

bid, twice a day; po, by mouth; qid, four times a day; tid, three times a day.

KEY POINTS

- Therapy of urinary incontinence is individualized and often requires adjustments.
- The main management goals are preservation of upper urinary tract function and improvement of the patient's urinary symptoms that impair quality of life.
- ED affects an estimated 10 to 20 million men in the United States.

ERECTILE DYSFUNCTION

The sexual response cycle of excitement, plateau, orgasm, and resolution requires the integrated and coordinated activity of the somatic and autonomic nervous systems innervating the reproductive system. Erectile dysfunction (ED) is defined as the persistent inability to attain or maintain penile erection sufficient for sexual intercourse.

An estimated 10 to 20 million American men have some degree of ED. Biologic or organic causes are demonstrated in up to 80% of cases, though psychiatric or psychogenic factors are important.

ANATOMY AND PHYSIOLOGY

The pudendal nerves carry both motor and sensory fibers that innervate the penis and clitoris. The parasympathetic nerves are located in the sacral cord (S2 through S4) and participate in erection. The sympathetic nerves arise from cells in the T11 to T12 levels of the spinal cord through the hypogastric plexus and are important in ejaculation.

Local tissue mediators such as nitric oxide and cGMP are primarily released by parasympathetic activity, contributing to sustained erection.

CAUSES OF SEXUAL DYSFUNCTION

The etiology of sexual dysfunction can be multifactorial. Neurogenic causes include neuropathy, myelopathy, cauda equina lesions, and CNS dysfunction. Other causes include vascular disease, pelvic trauma, and endocrine disorders such as hypothyroidism, hypogonadism, and hyperprolactinemia. Chronic illness, psychogenic illness, and drugs (i.e., antihypertensives, anticholinergics, antidepressants, sedatives, and narcotics) are frequent causes. Metabolic and toxic disorders such as alcohol abuse, liver disease, and renal failure are also common causes.

DIAGNOSTIC EVALUATION

The evaluation of a patient with ED includes a complete history and physical exam. Neurologic examination may provide evidence of cerebral, spinal cord, or peripheral nerve dysfunction. Laboratory evaluation includes an endocrine panel with levels of prolactin, testosterone, and gonadotropins. Sleep studies can be helpful (erection usually occurs with each episode of rapid-eye-movement [REM] sleep). EMG and somatosensory evoked potentials can help in cases of myelopathy or peripheral nerve disease. Vascular studies evaluate the response of the penis to the injection of vasoactive agents such as papaverine.

TREATMENT

The management of ED requires recognition of the etiology and treatment of the underlying disease. Endocrine, metabolic, vascular, and psychogenic causes must be treated when present. If drugs are responsible, changes in medication may be beneficial. Discussion of most available medical and surgical treatments is beyond the scope of this chapter.

Pharmacologic therapy of ED includes selective inhibitors of cGMP-specific phosphodiesterases like sildenafil (Viagra) and vardenafil (Levitra), intraurethral suppositories, and intracavernosal injections of alprostadil (Caverject).

KEY POINTS

- ED is often multifactorial. Many neurogenic diseases can produce ED, including strokes, multiple sclerosis, and diabetes.
- Medical and surgical therapies are available.

Headache and Facial Pain

Headache is the most common reason for referral to a neurologist. People are often concerned that a headache is symptomatic of an underlying brain tumor or some other mass lesion, but these are in fact rare causes of headache. In general, we make a distinction between what are referred to as *primary* and *secondary* headache disorders. The latter are conditions in which the headache is due to some other intracranial process such as a mass lesion, raised intracranial pressure or some inflammatory or infectious process. In considering possible secondary causes of headache it is helpful to recall that the brain parenchyma itself is insensitive to pain. Pain-sensitive structures include the meninges (pia mater), the cranial nerves, the arteries that make up the circle of Willis and its proximal branches, meningeal vessels, the external carotid artery, the scalp, pericranial muscles, the mucosa of the paranasal sinuses, the teeth, and cervical nerve roots. Diseases that involve or affect these structures have the propensity to cause a secondary headache. Primary headache disorders are those in which the headache is the primary problem rather than due to some other disease process. Migraine and tension-type headache are the most common primary headache disorders; other examples include cluster headache and paroxysmal hemicrania.

EVALUATION OF THE HEADACHE PATIENT

THE HEADACHE HISTORY

The clinical evaluation of the patient with a headache begins with a careful and detailed history.

For most causes of headache, and certainly for the primary headache disorders, the examination will be normal and a judgment about the nature and cause of a headache will be based on the patients' subjective description of the headache and associated symptoms. It is necessary to ask about the tempo with which the headache evolves. Did it begin suddenly and reach maximal intensity shortly after it began? Or did it evolve gradually over a period of many minutes or several hours? The clinician should also ask about the location and quality of the headache. Is it unilateral or bilateral? Is the pain mostly located behind the eye or does it seem to radiate up from the neck? What does the pain feel like? Patients often respond to this question with a description of the *severity* of the pain, but it is necessary to emphasize that what is needed is a description of the *quality* of the pain. Is the headache throbbing, pressing, or stabbing? As with any complaint of pain, the physician should ask about factors that alleviate and aggravate the pain. Related to these questions is the matter of the patient's behavioral response to the headache. Is there a tendency to go and sit or lie quietly in a room somewhere or does the patient feel like getting out for some exercise when the headache is present? What about the duration of the headache and its periodicity? Does it last only a few minutes, several hours, several days, or even perhaps persist without relief? How frequently does the headache recur? Finally, it is important to ask about other symptoms that may be associated with the headache. Is it accompanied by nausea, vomiting, or sensitivity to light or sound? What about visual symptoms such as flashing lights or other associated symptoms such as paresthesias, weakness, or difficulty with concentration or speech? Space does not permit a detailed exploration of all of the questions that one might ask of someone complaining of a headache, but this short introduction should provide a sense of the approach that should be adopted. The physician must develop a clear picture in the mind's eye of all aspects of the headache.

The student of neurology should appreciate that some headaches are sufficiently characteristic that their nature and cause can be identified with confidence based on the history alone. Examples include migraine, cluster headache, and some of the paroxysmal hemicranias. Other headaches, particularly those due to some other underlying disease process, may be less distinctive and require both physical examination and the judicious use of ancillary diagnostic tests.

THE EXAMINATION

The neurologic examination is typically normal in patients with primary headache disorders. Exceptions include people with complicated forms of migraine in whom visual field defects or motor weakness are occasionally present during, or persist following, the headache. The examination, therefore, is focused on identifying focal neurologic deficits that might suggest a secondary cause for the headache. Examples include the presence of papilledema that suggests raised intracranial pressure, temporal artery tenderness suggestive of giant cell arteritis, or nuchal rigidity (neck stiffness) that points toward a meningeal inflammatory process as the cause of the headache.

KEY POINTS

- The headache history should focus on the location, quality, tempo, duration, and periodicity of the headache; the presence or absence of associated symptoms; and the factors that alleviate and aggravate the headache.
- The neurologic examination is typically normal in patients with primary headache disorders.
- Important clinical signs to look for in patients with headache are neck stiffness, papilledema, limitation of eye movements, visual field defects, and other focal neurologic deficits.

PRIMARY HEADACHE DISORDERS

MIGRAINE HEADACHE

Migraine is one of the most common causes of headache, second in frequency only to tension-type headache. Migraine headaches are recognized as such based on their characteristics. These are typically unilateral headaches that are throbbing or pulsating in quality; often associated with nausea and vomiting; typically exacerbated by movement, light (photophobia), or sounds (phonophobia); and typically last from several to 72 hours. Two forms of migraine are recognized—migraine with aura (also known as classic migraine) and migraine without aura (also known as common migraine). The aura of migraine is most commonly visual. Patients usually complain of some positive visual phenomenon (e.g., flashing or zig-zag lines) that bounds or borders on a negative visual phenomenon (i.e., a scotoma), hence the use of the term *scintillating scotoma* to describe the visual aura of migraine. Another typical feature of the migraine aura is a characteristic tempo—marching or progressing across the visual field over 15 to 20 minutes. The aura may precede, accompany, or even follow the headache.

The pathophysiology of migraine has been under intense investigation in recent years. One widely accepted hypothesis is that migraine begins with a process known as cortical spreading depression (CSD). CSD is a wave of hyperpolarization (followed by a wave of depolarization) that spreads across a region of the cortex at a rate of 2 to 3 mm/min. CSD itself is thought to underlie the visual aura of migraine, and it is proposed that CSD also leads to the release of chemical substances (potassium, arachidonic acid, hydrogen ions, and nitric oxide) that activate trigeminal nerve afferents, and that this orthodromic transmission in the trigeminovascular system leads to activation of the trigeminal nucleus caudalis and brainstem parasympathetic efferent projections. Although the precise mechanism of pain in migraine is unclear, it is thought to result somehow from this increased activity within the trigeminal nucleus caudalis and parasympathetic efferents.

The diagnosis of migraine is a clinical one. When a characteristic history is elicited and the neurologic examination is normal, the diagnosis can be made without any investigations. There are two approaches to the pharmacologic management of migraine. The first entails abortive therapy, i.e., therapy to alleviate the headache during an attack. The second approach is prophylactic, i.e., treatment to reduce the frequency of future attacks. Pharmacologic therapy should be undertaken in conjunction with an effort to identify and avoid potential environmental triggers. Triptans (drugs that are agonists of the 5-hydroxytryptamine 1B, 1D, and 1F receptors) are the mainstay of therapy, and these are available in several formulations (oral, sublingual, nasal, and subcutaneous). They are most effective when administered early in the course of an attack and should be used with caution in subjects with a history of, or at risk for, coronary artery disease. There are, however, several other classes of drugs that may be effective for abortive therapy. These include ergotamine derivatives, caffeine containing compounds, and intravenous antiemetics such as metoclopramide and prochlorperazine. Drugs of many different classes have been used for prophylactic therapy, including β-blockers, tricyclic antidepressants, and anticonvulsants. Prophylactic therapy is generally indicated when headaches occur more frequently than once per month.

KEY POINTS

- Migraine headaches are characteristically unilateral and throbbing, accompanied by nausea, photophobia and/or phonophobia, and a behavioral response that involves retreat to a quiet dark place.
- Cortical spreading depression is the mechanism thought to underlie migraine pathophysiology.
- Triptans are the mainstay of abortive therapy for acute migraine attacks.

TENSION-TYPE HEADACHE

Tension-type headache is the most common form of headache. This is a specific form of primary headache that is characterized by recurrent attacks of bilateral or holocranial headaches of a pressing, squeezing, or tightening sensation. The quality of the pain has been likened to that of having a band or vice around the head. The duration of headaches may be from 30 minutes to several days. In contrast to migraine, tension-type headaches are not accompanied by nausea or neurologic symptoms and are not exacerbated by physical activity. In the past, tension-type headaches have been described as muscle contraction headaches, but the role of muscle contraction in headache pathogenesis remains unclear. Cervical or

paracervical muscle spasm and tenderness may be present on examination, but it is important to recognize that tension-type headaches have a particular character, and the term should not be used as a "grab-bag" for all ill-defined headaches. The diagnosis of tension-type headache is again a clinical one, with little need for neuroimaging unless the history is atypical or focal neurologic deficits are identified on examination. Treatment may be challenging and includes both nonpharmacologic measures and simple forms of analgesia. Over-use of caffeine and barbiturate-containing compounds should be avoided, given their propensity to cause medication-withdrawal or rebound headaches.

CLUSTER HEADACHE

Cluster headache is the best known, albeit rare, member of a group of primary headaches known as the trigeminal autonomic cephalgias (TAC). The TACs are a group of disorders characterized by unilateral trigeminal nerve distribution pain, accompanied by prominent ipsilateral autonomic symptoms. Cluster headache derives its name from its temporal pattern—affected individuals experience periods that may last several days, weeks, or months in which headaches occur with a high frequency, followed by headache-free periods that may last many months or even years. Also, the headaches are strictly unilateral (although may occasionally alternate sides between headaches within a cluster) and are most commonly located over the orbital or temporal region. Headaches are almost invariably accompanied by cranial autonomic symptoms such as lacrimation, conjunctival injection, facial or forehead swelling, eyelid edema, nasal congestion, rhinorrhea, and signs of a Horner syndrome (miosis, ptosis). With the exception of the Horner syndrome, these symptoms and signs occur only in conjunction with a headache. The pain is typically excruciating, and affected individuals are often restless and feel the need to be up and moving around (in contrast to patients with migraine who prefer to lie still in a quiet, dark place). There are several (often overlapping) approaches to management. Triptans are the most effective abortive agents. Steroids (e.g., prednisone) may shorten the duration of a cluster and the frequency of headaches during a cluster. Patients should be advised to avoid alcohol. For those with frequent clusters, agents such as verapamil and lithium may offer effective long-term prophylaxis.

PAROXYSMAL HEMICRANIA

Paroxysmal hemicrania is another unusual, but very characteristic primary headache disorder. Also classified among the TACs, paroxysmal hemicrania is also strictly unilateral with accompanying autonomic symptoms. Paroxysmal hemicrania, however, differs from cluster headache in two important respects. Firstly, the episodes of headache are typically of much shorter duration (typically 10 to 30 minutes) and occur with greater frequency (anywhere from several to 40 attacks per day). The other striking feature of these headaches is their responsiveness to the nonsteroidal anti-inflammatory agent indomethacin.

SECONDARY HEADACHE DISORDERS

SUBARACHNOID HEMORRHAGE

Almost everyone is familiar with the phrase "the worst headache of my life" that is often used to characterize the headache that accompanies a subarachnoid hemorrhage (SAH). This phrase is misleading, however, primarily because all people who have ever had headaches (and that's a lot of people) have, at some stage, had the worst headache of their lives. Very few of these people have had an SAH. A better characterization of the headache that accompanies an SAH is a headache that begins suddenly and peaks in intensity within seconds of its onset, also known as a thunderclap headache. Not every thunderclap headache is due to an SAH, but this possibility should always be considered. A head CT followed by a lumbar puncture to demonstrate the presence of blood or blood break-down products (that produce yellow or xanthochromic CSF) are the primary investigations required for the diagnosis of an SAH. The scope of this chapter does not permit a discussion of the importance of angiography in identifying the cause of an SAH or the complex issues surrounding the selection of open surgery or an endovascular approach to the treatment of a ruptured intracranial aneurysm.

LOW PRESSURE HEADACHES

Low pressure within the subarachnoid space or cerebrospinal fluid (CSF) is an important cause of secondary headache. The characteristic feature of a low pressure headache is that the symptoms are worse in the upright position and alleviated by recumbency (i.e., the headache is orthostatic). The headache may or may not be throbbing and is typically bilateral. Low pressure headaches are usually iatrogenic, occurring as a complication of a lumbar puncture. Low pressure is the consequence of low CSF volume, which results from a persistent leak of CSF from the subarachnoid space following insertion of a spinal needle. Low pressure headaches, however, may also arise spontaneously, typically caused by spontaneous rupture of a CSF pouch or cyst that surrounds a nerve root. The consequence is again low CSF volume, as production of CSF fails to keep pace with loss from the leak. The postural headache following a lumbar puncture is sufficiently characteristic that no further tests are needed for diagnosis. The mechanism of the headache in syndromes of low CSF volume is complex, but likely relates at least in part to the descent of the brain that occurs as a consequence of low CSF volume, which in turn leads to traction or distortion of pain-sensitive structures. The treatment of both forms of CSF hypovolemia and low CSF pressure is recumbency, aggressive fluid replacement, caffeine, and occasionally an epidural blood patch.

IDIOPATHIC INTRACRANIAL HYPERTENSION

Elevated pressure within the subarachnoid space may also cause headaches that are often characterized by increasing severity when recumbent, with some relief in the upright position. Headaches are often worse in the mornings and may be accompanied by pulsatile tinnitus and transient visual obscurations (fleeting visual symptoms such as blurring or loss of vision lasting just seconds) that are often precipitated by activities such as the valsalva maneuver that transiently increase intracranial pressure further. Examination may disclose papilledema, as well as unilateral or bilateral sixth nerve palsies. Idiopathic intracranial hypertension (IIH), previously referred to as pseudotumor cerebri, is a disorder that primarily affects young overweight women, who frequently report menstrual irregularities. The etiology and pathophysiology of this disorder are hotly debated, with some suggesting impaired resorption of CSF through damaged arachnoid granulations in the dural venous sinuses, and others invoking clot formation within dural venous sinuses, secondarily impairing CSF drainage. The important diagnostic feature of IIH is the finding of elevated

CSF pressure in the absence of identifiable intracranial pathology. Venous sinus thrombosis is an important mimic of this syndrome and should always be excluded with venous sinus imaging. Treatment comprises measures to reduce CSF volume including repeated lumbar puncture and diuretics, as well as optic nerve fenestration, and occasionally lumboperitoneal shunting. The most important complication of this disorder is visual loss due to a compressive optic neuropathy from persistently elevated CSF pressures, and the goal of long-term treatment is avoidance of this complication.

TEMPORAL ARTERITIS

Temporal arteritis, also known as giant cell arteritis (GCA), is a systemic granulomatous arteritis that affects medium and large caliber arteries, typically in individuals over the age of 50. The inflammatory process primarily targets the extra-cranial carotid vasculature. The headache that accompanies GCA does not have any identifiable characteristics but may be associated with tenderness of the scalp as well as thickening, nodulation, and tenderness of the temporal arteries to palpation. Associated symptoms may include claudication of the jaw with chewing and systemic symptoms such as fever, weight loss, and fatigue. The most feared complication is visual loss from an anterior ischemic optic neuropathy. The diagnosis should be considered in all subjects over the age of 50 who present with a new headache. The erythrocyte sedimentation rate and C-reactive protein levels are typically elevated, and temporal artery biopsy should show characteristic pathologic findings of a vasculitis with mononuclear cell infiltration and granulomatous changes. Since the pathology is segmental, the diagnosis is possible even in the face of a normal temporal artery biopsy. Treatment consists of high dose steroids.

 ## KEY POINTS

- The headache of SAH is characterized by maximal intensity very shortly after the onset of headache.
- Both elevated and low CSF volume and pressure are important causes of secondary headache.
- New headache in someone over the age of 50 should raise concern for the possibility of giant cell arteritis.

CHRONIC DAILY HEADACHE

Unlike the other headache disorders discussed so far, chronic daily headache (CDH) is not a single entity, but rather should be conceptualized as a clinical syndrome with many different causes. The defining feature of CDH, as its name implies, is that headache is present every day or almost every day. Operationally, it is defined on the basis of the occurrence of a headache on at least 15 days per month. The causes of CDH include chronic forms of the primary headache disorders discussed above—chronic (or transformed) migraine, chronic cluster headache, chronic tension-type headache, chronic paraoxysmal hemicrania—as well as secondary causes of headache such as chronic meningitis, head injury, giant cell arteritis (temporal arteritis), medication overuse, and medication withdrawal headache. Of these, transformed migraine, chronic tension-type headache, and medication overuse or withdrawal are certainly the most common. The management is both simple and complicated. The essence of management is to exclude secondary causes, taper and withdraw medications if overuse is suspected, and recognize the nature of the underlying primary headache disorder. The details of how this can be accomplished are, however, beyond the scope of this chapter.

FACIAL PAIN

Facial pain has many causes, including neurologic, vascular, and dental conditions. It is important to remember that dental causes (including temporomandibular joint disease) are common whereas neurologic and vascular causes of facial pain are rare. The neurologic causes of facial pain include (but are not limited to) trigeminal neuralgia, glossopharyngeal neuralgia, and postherpetic neuralgia. Giant cell arteritis and cluster headache may occasionally manifest with more facial pain than headache.

TRIGEMINAL NEURALGIA

Trigeminal neuralgia is a syndrome characterized by paroxysms of severe neuropathic pain in the distribution of one or more branches of the fifth (trigeminal) cranial nerve. Affected individuals typically complain of short paroxysms of an electrical-like painful sensation in the face that may be triggered by some tactile stimulus such as combing hair, brushing teeth, shaving, eating, drinking, or even a gentle breeze against the face. The disorder is thought to result from compression of the trigeminal nerve root at the cerebellopontine angle, most often by an aberrant vascular loop. MRI is typically required to exclude other compressive lesions, but is usually normal. Carbamazepine is the treatment of choice, but if this does not provide adequate relief then other anticonvulsant drugs may be tried. Surgical measures such as percutaneous radiofrequency ablation and microvascular decompression are usually reserved for refractory cases.

POSTHERPETIC NEURALGIA

Postherpetic neuralgia (PHN) describes the neuropathic pain that may accompany and follow an acute attack of varicella zoster (shingles). Shingles typically results from re-activation of a dormant infection of the virus that causes chickenpox within the dorsal root ganglion and is characterized by a herpetic rash (crops of vesicles on an erythematous base) within the distribution of one or several nerve root segments. The pain is typically described as burning, itching, and hypersensitivity to light touch. There is good evidence that early treatment of shingles with antiviral therapy (acyclovir) reduces the risk of PHN. Once present, management is symptomatic, with tricyclic antidepressants and gabapentin being most efficacious.

KEY POINTS

- Dental and temperomandibular joint diseases are far more common as causes of facial pain than neurologic disease.
- An important clue to a neurologic cause of facial pain is a history of pain that has a neuropathic quality. Neurologic examination is typically normal in both neurologic and nonneurologic causes of facial pain.

Part 3

Neurologic Disorders

Aphasia and Other Disorders of Higher Cortical Function

Disorders of higher cortical function are among the most interesting in Neurology to both physicians and laypersons. Stories of patients who have lost particular aspects of language or who mistake a wife for a hat, for example, continue to intrigue medical students and residents.

It is not hard to understand why this might be. Although primary vision, sensation, and motor control are clearly brain functions that are essential for day-to-day survival, it is the more developed cognitive functions that allow us to carry out the activities that seem **human**. The fact that these functions reside in some fairly discrete areas of the brain and can be quite selectively damaged by lesions in these areas contributes to our fascination with them.

APHASIA

Aphasia refers to any acquired abnormality of language, usually from a focal brain lesion. The problem must be a primary disorder of language; not everyone who cannot communicate properly is aphasic. For example, diffuse problems with consciousness, attention, or initiative may prevent a patient from communicating by oral or written means, but this would not necessarily qualify as aphasia. Likewise, problems with speech, such as dysarthria (slurring) or stuttering, or problems with motor control of the mouth may prevent oral communication, but articulation deficits should not be confused with aphasia.

DIAGNOSTIC EVALUATION

There are several recognized forms of aphasia (Table 11-1) that are typically caused by lesions in particular brain locations (Fig. 11-1) and can be distinguished from each other by testing certain aspects of language, such as fluency, comprehension, and repetition (Table 11-2).

A sensitive test for detecting an aphasia of any kind is to test naming, since **anomia** (impaired naming) is a feature of essentially all aphasias. Severely aphasic patients may not be able to name common or high-frequency objects (e.g., watch, necktie), while less severely afflicted patients may have trouble only with low-frequency objects or parts (e.g., dial of the watch, lapel). In addition, no aphasic patient writes normally. Screening for aphasia by asking patients to write a paragraph is quite effective.

KEY POINTS

- **Aphasia** is an acquired abnormality of language, usually from a focal brain lesion.

- Other causes of impaired communication—including problems with attention, initiative, or articulation— are not truly aphasias.

- Problems with naming or writing are features of almost all types of aphasias.

■ TABLE 11-1 Aphasias

Type	Fluency	Repetition	Comprehension	Commonly Associated Signs	Lesion Location
Broca	Impaired	Impaired	Relatively preserved	Right hemiparesis (especially face)	Broca's area
Wernicke	Preserved	Impaired	Impaired	Right upper visual field cut	Wernicke's area
Conduction	Preserved	Impaired	Preserved	—	Arcuate fasciculus
Transcortical motor	Impaired	Preserved	Preserved	Right hemiparesis	Near Broca's area
Transcortical sensory	Preserved	Preserved	Impaired	—	Near Wernicke's area
Global	Impaired	Impaired	Impaired	Severe right hemiparesis	Large left hemisphere lesion
Subcortical	Variable	Preserved	Variable	Hypophonia	Left basal ganglia, thalamus

BROCA'S APHASIA

Broca's aphasia is primarily a problem of language production. Speech is nonfluent, meaning that the patient cannot produce a reasonably long string of words. Attempted speech output is punctuated by hesitations and ill-fated attempts at beginnings of words ("tip-of-the-tongue" phenomenon). A Broca's aphasia patient's speech may be telegraphic, in that conjunctions, prepositions, and the like may be omitted and only key nouns and verbs are strung together (e.g., "want go store"). Patients' speech may include paraphasias (word substitution errors), often of the phonemic type (substitution based on sound, like "spool" for "spoon"). An important feature of Broca's aphasia is that patients are quite aware of and almost invariably frustrated by their language problem. Oddly, overused phrases (e.g., "how do you do?"), expletives, and lyrics sung to music may be relatively preserved. Broca's aphasia patients cannot repeat phrases said to them. Although the most prominent deficit is with language output, Broca's aphasia patients have subtle deficits of comprehension, particularly for complex grammatical constructions involving prepositions or the passive voice. For example, Broca's aphasia patients may not be able to follow a command such as "under the paper put the pen" or understand which animal is dead if "the lion was killed by the tiger."

Classically, Broca's aphasia arises from lesions that include the posterior part of the inferior frontal gyrus in the dominant (usually left) hemisphere, a region known as Broca's area. Most often these are relatively large strokes in the territory of the superior division of the middle cerebral artery (MCA), although tumors, hemorrhages, and other lesions in this area can cause an identical syndrome. Strokes here typically are associated with some weakness of the contralateral side, particularly involving the face and arm.

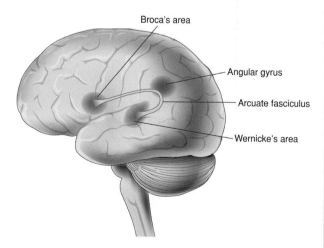

Broca's area

Angular gyrus

Arcuate fasciculus

Wernicke's area

Figure 11-1 • Higher cortical centers in the left hemisphere.

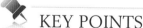

KEY POINTS

- **Broca's aphasia** is a problem of language production.
- Patients are frustrated and have nonfluent, hesitant, telegraphic speech output, with an inability to repeat but relatively preserved comprehension.
- Broca's aphasia is typically caused by lesions in the posteroinferior frontal lobe (Broca's area).

TABLE 11-2 Examination of Language Function	
Function	**Testing**
Fluency	Listen to patient's spontaneous speech to see if words are strung together into phrases.
	Overused phrases (e.g., "how do you do?") do not count.
Repetition	Least challenging: Ask patient to repeat single words.
	Most challenging: Ask patient to repeat complex sentence, such as "no ifs, ands, or buts about it."
Comprehension	Least challenging: Ask patient to follow simple midline commands, such as "close your eyes" or "open your mouth."
	Most challenging: Ask patient to follow multistep appendicular commands that cross the midline, such as "point to the ceiling, then touch your left ear with your right hand."
Naming	Least challenging: Ask patient to name high-frequency objects, like watch or tie.
	Most challenging: Ask patient to name low-frequency objects or parts of objects, like dial of watch or lapel.
Reading	Ask patient to read written material aloud, and to follow written instructions.
Writing	Ask patient to write a spontaneous sentence, or a sentence dictated by the examiner. Simply having the patient write his name does not count, as that is an overlearned task.

WERNICKE'S APHASIA

Although Wernicke's aphasia is often characterized as a problem with language comprehension, it features difficulty with both the output and input of language. Patients cannot understand what is said to them and thus may not be able to follow even the simplest commands. Their spontaneous speech is fluent but nonsensical, so that they can string words together, but the sequence or content may not make sense ("word salad"). Wernicke's aphasia patients produce many paraphasias, particularly of the semantic type (substitution based on meaning, like "fork" for "spoon") as well as neologisms (nonexistent words). The cadence and fluency of speech are preserved, but the content is often incomprehensible. One might not be able to recognize that a speaker of a foreign language had a Wernicke's aphasia, because all but the content of language would be intact. Wernicke's aphasia patients cannot repeat. Unlike patients with Broca's aphasia, those with Wernicke's aphasia seem unaware of their deficit initially and can become quite angry or paranoid when it becomes obvious that others have difficulty understanding them.

Classically, Wernicke's aphasia arises from lesions in the posterior part of the superior temporal gyrus in the dominant hemisphere, known as Wernicke's area. Most commonly, these are strokes involving the inferior division of the MCA, and a high percentage of them are due to emboli from proximal locations such as the heart or the internal carotid artery. However, other nonvascular lesions in this area can cause an identical syndrome. Lesions causing Wernicke's aphasia may not be accompanied by weakness or sensory loss, but there may be a contralateral homonymous superior quadrantanopia.

KEY POINTS

- **Wernicke's aphasia** is a problem with language comprehension that results in difficulties with both output and input of language.
- Patients have fluent but very abnormal speech output ("word salad"), frequent paraphasias and neologisms, and an inability to comprehend or repeat.
- Wernicke's aphasia is typically caused by lesions involving the posterior part of the superior temporal gyrus (Wernicke's area).

OTHER APHASIAS

A distinct form of aphasia called **conduction aphasia** is characterized by an inability to repeat what is said, with preserved fluency and comprehension. Classic teaching states that the lesion responsible lies in the arcuate fasciculus, the white matter connections between Broca's and Wernicke's areas. However, there is little anatomic evidence to support this idea, and in fact lesions involving the temporal or parietal lobes (but sparing Wernicke's area) can lead to this syndrome. Patients with conduction aphasia also make many paraphasic errors, which we all normally correct "on the fly" as we monitor our own speech—a function they cannot perform.

Lesions in the frontal lobe slightly superior to Broca's area can cause a nonfluent aphasia very similar to Broca's aphasia except that repetition is preserved, because the path between and including Broca's and Wernicke's areas is unaffected. Such a **transcortical motor aphasia** can also be caused by lesions in the supplementary motor area and in the anterior portions of the basal ganglia.

Similarly, a **transcortical sensory aphasia** is caused by lesions in the inferior portion of the left temporal lobe and is characterized by fluent speech with impaired comprehension but preserved repetition. Infarcts in the territory of the left posterior cerebral artery (PCA) as well as small temporal lobe hemorrhages and contusions are the most common causes.

A distinction, therefore, is made between perisylvian (around the sylvian fissure) aphasias (Broca, Wernicke, and conduction), in which repetition is impaired, and transcortical aphasias (motor and sensory), in which repetition is preserved.

 KEY POINTS

- **Conduction aphasia**, primarily characterized by an inability to repeat, is caused by lesions involving the temporal and parietal lobes but sparing Wernicke's area.
- **Transcortical motor and sensory aphasias** resemble Broca and Wernicke aphasias, respectively, except that repetition is preserved.

Global aphasia, typically caused by large dominant hemispheric lesions affecting the frontal and temporal lobes including Broca's and Wernicke's areas, results in problems with language production, comprehension, and repetition.

Subcortical aphasias are acquired language deficits associated with lesions in deep dominant hemispheric structures, such as the basal ganglia and thalamus. These typically do not fall easily into the aphasia classification given above, although more anterior subcortical lesions have a tendency to produce aphasias that resemble Broca's aphasia and more posterior lesions lead to aphasias that resemble Wernicke's aphasia. Often, subcortical aphasias are accompanied by hypophonia of the voice.

DISORDERS OF WRITTEN COMMUNICATION

Reading and writing are commonly affected in all of the aphasias. Typically, reading parallels comprehension of spoken language, while writing parallels production of spoken language, although the respective difficulties with written language are typically much worse than those with spoken language. Thus Broca's aphasia patients may be able to understand simple commands by reading them, though they cannot read them aloud or write them.

A unique syndrome called **alexia without agraphia**, or **pure alexia**, is characterized by an inability to read despite a preserved ability to write. This leads to the surprising finding that patients may not be able to read back the words they have just written well. The responsible lesion is situated in the dominant occipital lobe but also involves the splenium of the corpus callosum. In this way the fibers connecting visual cortex (on either side) to Wernicke's area in the dominant hemisphere are interrupted, thus preventing input of language through visual means. A contralateral homonymous hemianopia is typically an associated finding.

APRAXIA

Apraxia is defined as an inability to carry out a learned motor task despite preservation of the primary functions needed to carry out the task, such as comprehension, motor ability, sensation, and coordination.

A patient with an apraxia, for example, might not be able to demonstrate how to hammer a nail, despite sufficient language comprehension to understand the command and sufficient motor strength, sensation in the hands, and coordination to carry out the command. It is as if the patient could not imagine or execute the motor program for the task.

Terminology regarding different types of apraxias—including names such as **ideational**, **ideomotor**, and **limb-kinetic**—is confusing. It is more enlightening simply to describe what the patient can and cannot do. In one type of apraxia, patients can recognize when others are carrying out the task correctly rather than incorrectly, but they cannot perform the motor task themselves. Sometimes these patients can carry out the task with the actual objects given to them (e.g., using a real hammer and nail), but they cannot mimic the task without the actual objects. In another type of apraxia, patients cannot even recognize when others are carrying out the task correctly.

DIAGNOSTIC EVALUATION

There are three basic ways to test for apraxia: asking patients to pretend they are performing an action, to mimic the examiner performing an action, or to use actual objects in performing an action. Examples of bedside tests include asking the patient to wave goodbye, salute, brush his or her teeth, or comb his or her hair. Two-handed tasks, such as hammering in a nail or slicing a loaf of bread, are more demanding. Some patients who have a specific form of apraxia involving oral movements may be unable to demonstrate whistling or blowing out a match. Many patients with apraxia will have a tendency to use their limbs as objects (e.g., running their fingers through their hair when asked to demonstrate how to use a comb).

ETIOLOGY

Apraxias are typically associated with either frontal or parietal lesions in the dominant hemisphere. Frontal lesions typically cause apraxias in which patients are able to recognize the task done correctly by others but cannot perform it themselves, whereas parietal lesions typically result in apraxias in which patients cannot recognize the task done correctly.

KEY POINTS

- **Apraxia** is the inability to perform a learned motor task despite preservation of the necessary basic motor, sensory, and cognitive capacities.
- Examples of bedside tests for apraxia include asking a patient to mimic the motions necessary to brush the teeth, comb the hair, hammer in a nail, or slice a loaf of bread.
- Apraxia is typically caused by lesions in the frontal or parietal lobes of the dominant hemisphere.

AGNOSIA

Agnosia refers to an inability to recognize objects through one or more sensory modalities despite the preserved functioning of those primary sensory modalities.

DIAGNOSTIC EVALUATION

Patients with visual agnosia, for example, might not be able to recognize objects placed in his or her vision, though all other aspects of their vision, such as acuity and fields, are intact. The same patients would be able to recognize those objects when allowed to touch them. With his or her vision, he or she might be able to describe specific features of the object, but he or she would not be able to recognize the object as a whole.

ETIOLOGY

Agnosias are typically caused by lesions in the sensory association areas of the brain, processing areas that lie next to the primary sensory areas and are responsible for integrating primary sensory information into higher-order complex forms. For example, the visual association area lies in the occipitotemporal region anterior and inferior to the primary visual cortex and is responsible for the recognition of objects using primary visual information. Lesions here can cause a visual agnosia. A specific form called **prosopagnosia**, an inability to recognize faces, can occur with right hemispheric or bilateral lesions in the visual association area.

KEY POINTS

- **Agnosia** is the inability to recognize objects despite preservation of the basic sensory modalities being used.
- Agnosia is typically caused by lesions in the sensory association areas.

GERSTMANN'S SYNDROME

Lesions in the inferior parietal lobule of the dominant hemisphere, and specifically in the angular gyrus (see Fig. 11-1), can cause **Gerstmann's syndrome**, a constellation of problems in higher cortical function. These are agraphia, the inability to write; acalculia, the inability to calculate; right-left confusion; and finger agnosia, the inability to recognize one's own or the examiner's individual fingers. One explanation is that this area of the parietal lobe is responsible for the symbolic representation of body parts as well as orthographic and numerical symbols.

KEY POINTS

- **Gerstmann's syndrome** is characterized by four elements: agraphia, acalculia, right-left confusion, and finger agnosia.
- Gerstmann's syndrome is typically caused by lesions in the angular gyrus of the dominant hemisphere.

NEGLECT

There are times when it seems that all interesting higher cortical functions reside in the dominant hemisphere. Neglect, however, one of the most fascinating cortical disorders, is usually the result of damage to the nondominant (usually right) hemisphere.

Neglect is directed inattention, or a relative lack of attention, paid to one hemispace. Patients with neglect will tend to be less aware (or completely unaware) of objects or actions in one side of the world (usually the left). It is not that a patient has a hemianopia and cannot see that side or a primary motor or sensory deficit for that side; rather, there is decreased attention toward the left side.

DIAGNOSTIC EVALUATION

Those with the most severe forms of neglect ignore the left side completely and deny that such a side even exists. They may leave their left side ungroomed, unshaven, and undressed; they may leave food on the left side of their plates untouched. They may deny having a left hand, and when confronted with it, may claim that it is actually the examiner's. When asked to describe their surroundings or draw a picture, they may omit items on the left side (Fig. 11-2).

Patients with milder neglect may not have such gross abnormalities but may perform actions involving the left side only with encouragement or after repeated prodding. When asked to bisect a line, they may err toward the right. When asked to cross out letters scattered across a page, they may leave some on the left side unmarked.

The most sensitive sign of neglect, which may be the only finding seen in patients with the mildest form, is extinction to double simultaneous stimulation. This phenomenon occurs when sensory stimuli applied singly to either side are felt properly; but when both sides are stimulated simultaneously, only the stimulus on the nonneglected side is felt. Extinction may exist with tactile, visual, or auditory stimulation.

ETIOLOGY

Neglect is typically caused by lesions in the right hemisphere, particularly the right frontal or parietal lobes. It is most commonly seen as an acute finding after a stroke, though other lesions in these areas can cause a similar clinical syndrome. Lesions in the right frontal lobe may cause more of a motor neglect, in which the patient has a tendency to not use the left side for motor actions, whereas lesions in the right parietal lobe may cause more of a sensory neglect, in which stimuli from the left side tend to be ignored.

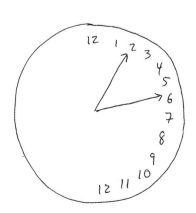
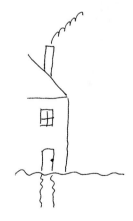

Figure 11-2 • Drawing demonstrating neglect of the left side.

KEY POINTS

- **Neglect** is directed inattention or a relative lack of attention paid to one hemispace, usually the left.

- Patients with severe neglect may fail to describe objects on the left, may fail to dress or shave the left side, or may even deny that their left arms are theirs.

- Those with milder forms may not bisect lines or cancel out letters properly, or they may exhibit extinction to double simultaneous stimulation.

- Neglect is usually caused by lesions in the right frontal or parietal lobe.

OTHER NONDOMINANT HEMISPHERIC SYNDROMES

The semantic elements of language (those associated purely with meaning) reside in the language-dominant (usually left) hemisphere, as described in the discussion on aphasias above. However, some of the other elements of successful oral communication, such as changing the inflection of one's voice when asking a question or when making an angry statement, reside in the nondominant (usually right) hemisphere. These elements are collectively referred to as *prosody*, and patients with right hemispheric lesions may have difficulty with this part of communication. Some may have difficulty applying the proper inflection to their own speech output, for example, and sound fairly monotone. Others may have difficulty understanding the speech inflections of those speaking to them and cannot distinguish between a statement said to them in anger or in jest.

Some patients with right hemisphere lesions have a tendency to be unaware of their deficits, a condition termed **anosognosia**. A patient with a complete left hemiplegia, for example, may insist on immediate discharge from the hospital because he or she feels that nothing is wrong. A patient with a dense left hemianopia may wonder why he or she keeps bumping into others when he or she notices nothing wrong with his or her vision. As expected, these patients tend to have more difficult and unsuccessful rehabilitations.

Dementia

Dementia is a common cause of morbidity and mortality in the elderly and has many different etiologies. It implies an intellectual and cognitive deterioration of sufficient severity to interfere with normal functioning. Memory, orientation, visuospatial perception, language, and higher executive functions (planning, organizing, and sequencing) may be impaired in dementia.

The terms **delirium** and **acute confusional state** imply a global disturbance of mental functions, in general reversible, accompanied by altered level of consciousness. These conditions are often acute and reversible; they are discussed further in Chapter 3.

EPIDEMIOLOGY

Dementia is most common in the elderly but can occur at a younger age (particularly in those with a hereditary component). Approximately 5% of people between ages 65 and 70 have dementia; this increases to more than 45% above age 85. Alzheimer disease accounts for 50% to 70% of cases of dementia. Cerebrovascular disease accounts for about 15% to 20%, and the other causes presented in Box 12-1 account for most of the rest. Dementia has a considerable social cost (over $50 billion in the United States every year).

CLINICAL MANIFESTATIONS

There is a known cognitive decline with old age, and sometimes the differentiation between a dementing illness and age-related cognitive decline is difficult. In general, most patients with dementia start having problems with short-term memory, followed by an indolent deterioration of cognitive functions that may involve language, praxis, and so forth. Many dementing illnesses manifest characteristic symptoms and clinical findings that are helpful in establishing an etiologic diagnosis.

DIAGNOSTIC EVALUATION

The initial recognition of dementia is difficult. Normal aging can mimic some of its features. Rarely, the patient is aware of cognitive deterioration; in most cases, the family brings the patient to the doctor months or years after problems have started. The most important information in the diagnosis of dementia is the clinical history (including reports by relatives) and the physical exam (with a very detailed mental status examination). Then, the diagnosis of the cause of dementia consists of matching the major clinical features of the individual patient with characteristics of known dementing illnesses.

It is important to rule out an underlying depression, because depression can mimic dementia ("pseudodementia"), and the associated cognitive abnormalities of depression can constitute a true dementia. Not rarely, when a patient complains of features suggesting dementia, depression is the problem. Correspondingly, it is often a family member who brings a patient with dementia to the physician.

The use of laboratory tests depends on the clinical history and exam, the tentative diagnosis, and the possibility of finding reversible causes. Box 12-2 summarizes some tests to consider. Most are used to rule out reversible causes of dementia.

■ BOX 12-1 Causes of Dementia

Degenerative
Alzheimer disease
Huntington disease
Parkinson disease
Lewy body dementia
Pick disease
Progressive supranuclear palsy
Spinocerebellar degeneration
Amyotrophic lateral sclerosis with dementia
Olivopontocerebellar atrophy
Frontotemporal dementia associated with chromosome 17 (FTD-17)
Metabolic
Wilson disease
Hypothyroidism
Vitamin B$_{12}$ deficiency
Hypercalcemia
Addison disease
Lipid storage diseases and leukodystrophies
Toxic
Drug intoxication
Alcohol
Arsenic, mercury, and lead intoxication
Infectious
Creutzfeldt-Jakob disease
AIDS
Syphilis
Subacute sclerosis panencephalitis (postmeasles)
Neoplastic and paraneoplastic
Vascular
Vascular dementia
Vasculitis
Hydrocephalus
Traumatic
Severe head injury
Boxer encephalopathy (punch drunk)
Chronic subdural hematoma
Undetermined
Mixed (Alzheimer plus vascular)

■ BOX 12-2 Tests to Consider in a Patient With Dementia

Hematologic screening, including ESR
Vitamin B$_{12}$ and folate
Blood calcium
Liver function tests, including ammonia
Electrolytes
Serum urea nitrogen and creatinine levels
Infection workup, including syphilis, HIV, TB, etc.
Thyroid function tests
EEG: Should not be ordered routinely in a dementia assessment. Its use is justified when the patient has evidence of fluctuations in cognitive status that could represent seizures. The EEG may be useful at the initial presentation in patients with suspected CJD.
CT or MRI of the brain (rule out structural abnormalities such as tumor, subdural hematoma, and hydrocephalus and evaluate cortical atrophy).
Neuropsychological assessment: Useful in early stages to establish the diagnosis of dementia and to use as a comparison tool in the progression of the disease.
Brain biopsy: Only indicated in specific cases such as CJD, HIV, CNS vasculitis, and so on, to confirm the diagnosis and find or exclude possible treatable causes.

KEY POINTS

- Symptoms and signs of dementia include memory loss, abnormalities of speech, difficulties with problem solving and abstract thinking, impaired judgment, personality changes, and emotional lability.
- The diagnosis of the cause of dementia requires a detailed history and neurologic and physical examination.

CAUSES OF DEMENTIA

ALZHEIMER DISEASE

In 1907, Alois Alzheimer, a German clinician and neuropathologist, published the landmark case of a 51-year-old woman with deterioration of her mental state. Her autopsy disclosed the classic pathology of Alzheimer disease (AD): neurofibrillary tangles and senile plaques in the cerebral neocortex and hippocampus.

Epidemiology

Nearly 4% of people older than 65 years have severe AD and are incapacitated. Recent estimates suggest that more than 2 million people have AD in the United States alone. Because of increased life expectancy, the population at risk for AD is the fastest-growing segment of society. Annually, approximately 100,000 people die of Alzheimer disease and more than $25 billion is spent on the institutional care of patients with AD.

Etiology and Risk Factors

Many factors are associated with an increased frequency of AD, including age, female sex, history of severe head trauma, and Down syndrome.

There are also many putative genetic risk factors. The gene for ApoE4 (on chromosome 19) has been shown to be associated with both early- and late-onset AD of both sporadic and familial varieties. Early-onset AD has been associated with mutations in the amyloid precursor protein (APP) on chromosome 21, and presenilin 1 (PS1) and presenilin 2 (PS2) on chromosomes 14 and 1, respectively. More than 65 mutations in these genes are described. Another mutation in a gene on chromosome 12 that encodes α_2-macroglobulin has been associated with AD. The ApoE alleles and the α_2-macroglobulin mutation predispose individuals to early onset of sporadic AD and even more to late-onset AD. The other mutations in APP, PS1, and PS2 are associated with early onset of the disease in the third through sixth decades.

Amyloid-beta precursor protein (AβPP) mutations may cause increased amyloid-beta (Aβ) production with subsequent aggregation in the neurons. This mutation changes the normal structure of the protein, altering its recognition by metabolizing enzymes like alpha-secretase and utilizing alternative pathways for degradation, leading to a progressive accumulation of the peptide. Other pathophysiologic mechanisms have been described, including inflammatory, oxidative, metabolic, nutritional, and immune mechanisms.

Clinical Manifestations

"Doctor, my mother is 75 years old and over the last 3 years I have noted that she is having more difficulty with her memory. She remembers her marriage 50 years ago but she does not remember that we were here yesterday. She asks the same questions constantly and forgets my answers. She is unable to balance her checkbook, and yesterday she could not find the way home from the drugstore." This history illustrates characteristic features of AD. At the beginning of the illness, the exam shows no difficulty with language, reasoning, or performance of normal social and personal behaviors. Only those close to the patient notice small slip-ups suggesting that something is wrong (becoming lost while driving, misplacement of objects, the kitchen left unattended, missed appointments, loss of social and interpersonal interactions). Later, the patient has more difficulty with activities of daily life.

As the disease progresses, other aspects of cognitive function are lost, including the ability to speak, understand, think, and make decisions. Characteristically, in contrast to patients with vascular dementia, elementary neurologic functions (motor, visual, somatosensory, and gait) remain normal until very late in the disease. Psychiatric manifestations are common at this time: personality changes (apathetic or impulsive), aggressive behavior (physical or verbal), paranoid thoughts and delusions (persecution, things being stolen), sleep disturbances (the word "sundowning" is used to describe worsening psychiatric manifestations during the evening and night), hallucinations (uncommon and in general a side effect of medications), and depression. The course is relentlessly progressive; the patient usually succumbs over 5 to 10 years due to a combination of neurologic and medical problems.

Diagnostic Evaluation

Except for brain biopsy, there are no tests that definitively establish the diagnosis of AD in living patients. The diagnosis is suggested by the clinical features and by the insidiously progressive course. Investigations are designed to exclude other causes of dementia (see Box 12-2). Elevated tau protein and low Aβ-42 levels in the CSF have been suggested as early diagnostic markers for AD. MRI-based volumetric measurements may show reduction of up to 40% in the size of the hippocampus, amygdala, and thalamus. Functional neuroimaging such as PET and SPECT (single-photon emission computed tomography), used to quantify cerebral metabolism and blood flow, may help to differentiate AD from other dementias. In Alzheimer disease, PET and SPECT scans show bilateral temporoparietal hypometabolism, but this is not specific enough to be diagnostic.

Pathology

The major pathologic features of AD are brain atrophy, senile plaques, and neurofibrillary tangles (NFTs), associated with substantial loss of neurons in the cerebral cortex and gliosis. NFTs represent intracellular accumulation of phosphorylated tau protein. Senile plaques are extracellular deposits of amyloid surrounded by dystrophic axons.

Treatment

At present there is no satisfactory treatment for patients with Alzheimer disease.

Therapy consists of the following:

- **Preventing associated symptoms:** Treatment of depression, agitation, sleep disorders, hallucinations, and delusions.

- **Preventing or delaying progression:** This includes therapy with acetylcholinesterase inhibitors such as donepezil or rivastigmine, as well as the newer agent memantine, an N-methyl-D-aspartate (NMDA) receptor antagonist.

- **Prophylaxis:** No data from randomized clinical trials are available. Use of vitamin E, NSAIDs, and estrogens has been proposed.

Table 12-1 provides information regarding therapy of AD and other dementias (not all of which have been proven effective).

TABLE 12-1 Dementia Therapy

	Dosage	Comments; rationale
Alzheimer disease		
Donepezil (Aricept)	5 to 10 mg po qid	Equal efficacy and fewer side effects than tacrine. Rare: hepatic toxicity. Common: diarrhea and abdominal cramps.
Rivastigmine (Exelon)	6 to 12 mg/day, given po bid; start 1.5 mg po bid	GI disturbances during dose adjustment. Rare: hepatic toxicity. Recently approved by FDA.
Tacrine	10 mg po qid	Hepatic toxicity. Check ALT every 2 weeks during dosage titration.
Ibuprofen	400 mg po tid	Targeting the anti-inflammatory theory of AD. Not proven different from placebo in recent studies.
Vitamin E	800 to 2,000 IU po daily	Mild anticoagulant effect, particularly with patients on warfarin. Not proven different from placebo in recent studies.
Conjugated estrogens	0.625 mg po daily	Women only. Not proven in recent clinical trials to alter the course of the disease.
Vascular dementia		
Antihypertensive medications	Any	Maintain systolic BP below 160 and diastolic between 85 and 95. Treatments that lower diastolic BP may worsen cognitive function.
Warfarin (Coumadin)	Variable	Check INR and maintain value between 2 and 3. Indicated in patient with atrial fibrillation and strokes.
Aspirin	81 to 325 po mg qD	Consider warfarin if atrial fibrillation is present.
Clopidogrel (Plavix)	75 mg po qD	Can produce TTP. Can be used in combination with aspirin.
Dipyridamole and aspirin (Aggrenox)	1 capsule (200 to 225 mg) po bid	Same indications as aspirin.
Vitamin E	800 to 2,000 IU daily	Mild anticoagulant effect, particularly with patients on warfarin.

ALT, alanine aminotransferase; bid; twice a day; BP, blood pressure; INR, international normalized ratio; po, by mouth; qid; four times a day; tid; three times a day; TTP, thrombotic thrombocytopenic purpura.

KEY POINTS

- AD is the most common neurodegenerative disease of the brain and accounts for 50% to 70% of all instances of dementia.
- Risk factors for developing AD include older age, female sex, head trauma, and family history.
- Potentially treatable causes of dementia should be excluded through laboratory testing and brain imaging.
- The average length of time from onset of symptoms until diagnosis is 2 to 3 years. The average duration from diagnosis to nursing home placement is 3 to 6 years. AD patients typically spend 3 years in nursing homes before death. Thus, the total duration of AD is roughly 9 to 12 years.

VASCULAR DEMENTIA

This dementia (previously referred to as multi-infarct dementia) may develop in patients with cerebrovascular disease. There are two recognized types: macrovascular, related to large infarcts, and microvascular, in which the pathophysiologic mechanism of brain injury is subcortical ischemia associated with cerebral small vessel disease (lacunes or deep white matter changes on MRI). Vascular dementia has the risk factors of cerebrovascular disease, including hypertension, diabetes, age, embolic sources, and extensive large artery atherosclerosis. It is not infrequent for vascular dementia and other diseases (AD, Lewy body disease) to coexist in the same patient. For this reason, it is unclear exactly how commonly dementia can arise from a purely vascular etiology.

Clinical Manifestations and Diagnostic Evaluation

The criteria for diagnosis of vascular dementia include presence of dementia and two or more of the following: focal neurologic signs on physical examination; onset that was abrupt, stepwise, or stroke-related; or brain imaging study showing multiple strokes, lacunes, or extensive deep white matter changes. Most patients with vascular dementia are hypertensive or diabetic. The diagnosis requires investigation of the cause of stroke. Cardiac and hypercoagulable workups should be considered in selected cases.

Treatment

The prevention and treatment of vascular dementia are essentially the same as prevention and treatment of stroke (see Table 12-1 and Chapter 14).

KEY POINTS

- Vascular dementia may be a common cause of dementia, but it often coexists with other causes.
- Vascular dementia is associated with Binswanger disease (microvascular disease), a lacunar state, and large strokes.

DEMENTIAS ASSOCIATED WITH EXTRAPYRAMIDAL FEATURES

This group of dementias includes dementia with Lewy bodies, progressive supranuclear palsy, corticobasal degeneration, striatonigral degeneration, Huntington disease, and Wilson disease.

DEMENTIA WITH LEWY BODIES

This is now thought by many to be the second most common cause of dementia after Alzheimer disease. The clinical picture is that of a parkinsonian dementia syndrome with visual hallucinations. Sometimes it is very difficult to differentiate this from the disease of a Parkinson disease patient who develops dementia.

Clinical Manifestations

The major features are cognitive impairment (severe problems of visuospatial perception and visual memory), marked fluctuations of alertness, prominent visual hallucinations (up to 80% of cases) and delusions, extrapyramidal symptoms, and an extraordinary sensitivity to neuroleptics (i.e., marked worsening with drugs like haloperidol).

Diagnostic Evaluation

The pathologic hallmark is the Lewy body (found in Parkinson disease in the substantia nigra), an eosinophilic intracellular inclusion of alpha synuclein. In dementia with Lewy bodies (unlike in Parkinson disease), the Lewy body is found in cortical neurons.

Other pathologic abnormalities can also be present, including varying degrees of AD-type abnormalities such as NFTs and senile plaques.

Treatment

Management of dementia with Lewy bodies can be complex, since treatment of the parkinsonian syndrome may worsen neuropsychiatric dysfunction, and treatment of the neuropsychiatric disorder may exacerbate the parkinsonian syndrome. Low doses of atypical neuroleptics such as risperidone and clozapine have been used to treat behavioral symptoms.

KEY POINTS

- Dementia with Lewy bodies may be the second most common type of dementia.
- Fluctuations of alertness, visual hallucinations, and an extraordinary sensitivity to neuroleptics are the three key distinguishing features of dementia with Lewy bodies.
- Death ensues after 10 to 15 years.

PROGRESSIVE SUPRANUCLEAR PALSY

Also known as the Steele-Richardson-Olszewski syndrome, progressive supranuclear palsy (PSP) may account for 2% to 3% of dementias. No clear predisposing or genetic factors have been identified.

Clinical Manifestations

The main features are supranuclear ocular palsy (mainly failure of vertical gaze), dysarthria, dysphagia, extrapyramidal rigidity, gait ataxia, and dementia. In the early stages of PSP, falls and gait abnormalities are prominent. Dementia may occur early or develop later. Frontal lobe abnormalities predominate. Patients become apathetic and talk and act less frequently. In early stages, PSP may be mistaken for AD.

Diagnostic Evaluation

The pathology shows atrophy of the dorsal midbrain, globus pallidus, and subthalamic nucleus. NFTs, neuronal loss, and gliosis in many subcortical structures are characteristic. The course is progressive, with a median survival of 6 to 10 years.

KEY POINTS

- PSP is a form of subcortical dementia with prominent extrapyramidal features.
- The characteristic clinical findings are palsy of vertical gaze, abnormal gait, and frequent falls.
- Median survival is 6 to 10 years.

HUNTINGTON DISEASE

Huntington disease (HD) is an autosomal dominant neurodegenerative disorder with predominant abnormalities of the basal ganglia.

Clinical Manifestations

Symptoms usually appear between the ages of 35 and 45 and include the triad of chorea, behavioral changes or personality disorder (frequently obsessive-compulsive disorder), and dementia. The three may occur together at onset, or one may precede the others by years.

Diagnostic Evaluation

Diagnosis is by family history, clinical signs, atrophy of the caudate on brain imaging, and the demonstration of more than 40 CAG repeats in chromosome 4.

Pathology

Pathologic examination shows severe destruction of the caudate and putamen (striatal and nigral GABA-ergic neurons) and loss of neurons in the cerebral cortex (layer 3). HD is linked to chromosome 4p16.3 on the HD gene, encoding for a protein named **huntingtin**. The mutation produces an unstable CAG repeat. This induces aberrant processing of cell proteins with formation of deposits in the nucleus and activation of intracellular mechanisms of cell death.

Treatment

Pharmacologic management of dementia and chorea often involves dopaminergic antagonists, including neuroleptic drugs, but it is far from adequate. Genetic counseling is fundamental.

KEY POINTS

- Huntington disease is characterized by chorea, dementia, and personality and behavioral changes.
- Death occurs 10 to 20 years after onset.
- Suicide is not rare in at-risk and early-onset HD patients.

PARKINSON DISEASE

Parkinson disease (PD) may produce subcortical dementia. Cognitive impairment develops in about 30% of patients with idiopathic PD. The distinction from other types of dementia is based on the natural history and the presence of associated symptoms. The clinical manifestations include those of subcortical-dementia, with marked psychomotor involvement.

FRONTOTEMPORAL DEMENTIA

Frontotemporal dementia (FTD) encompasses a group of degenerative disorders characterized by significant alterations in personality, social behavior, and language.

Clinical Manifestations

Unlike Alzheimer disease, FTD often presents initially with cognitive and behavioral deficits other than memory loss, because the frontal, temporal, or both cortices are affected early. For example, patients may neglect social and personal responsibilities, present failure in judgment, and show defective sequencing and organization. FTD includes Pick disease, primary progressive aphasia, and semantic dementia. In addition, there are forms of FTD associated with parkinsonism and with motor neuron disease.

Pick disease is a rare form of progressive dementia characterized by personality change, speech disturbance, inattentiveness, and sometimes extrapyramidal signs. The diagnosis is made by clinical history and the presence of circumscribed frontotemporal lobar atrophy. Argyrophilic round intraneuronal inclusions (Pick bodies) represent the characteristic pathologic change. Abnormal tau protein with tau-positive inclusions is found in neurons and glial cells.

Senile plaques are generally not present. Primary progressive aphasia is a form of FTD in which language deficits appear early.

KEY POINTS

- Frontotemporal dementia is uncommon.
- Anterior lobar atrophy is characteristic.
- Personality changes early in the disease are characteristic, in contrast to Alzheimer disease.

DEMENTIAS CAUSED BY INFECTIOUS AGENTS

PRION-RELATED DISEASES

Prion-related diseases include CJD (familial and sporadic), Gerstmann-Sträussler-Scheinker syndrome, and fatal familial insomnia.

These so-called spongiform encephalopathies are a group of disorders characterized by spongy degeneration, neuronal loss, gliosis, and astrocytic proliferation resulting from the accumulation in the brain of a mutated protease-resistant prion protein.

CJD is the most common of these disorders. It is characterized by a rapidly progressive dementia with pyramidal signs, myoclonus, cerebellar or extrapyramidal signs, and periodic sharp waves in the EEG. MRI with DWI (diffusion-weighted images) may show evolving cortical and basal ganglionic abnormalities during the course of the disease. CSF is typically normal, but the presence of protein 14-3-3 is relatively sensitive and specific for CJD. There is no therapy. This syndrome evolves over weeks to months, and death usually occurs within a year.

KEY POINTS

- CJD is rare.
- CJD presents as a rapidly progressive dementia with focal neurologic signs and myoclonus.
- EEG and MRI are not diagnostic, but they become more specific in the setting of the appropriate clinical history.

HIV-ASSOCIATED DEMENTIA COMPLEX

Most patients with human immunodeficiency virus (HIV) disease have CNS involvement. The virus can produce an encephalitis and also makes the individual susceptible to CNS infections such as toxoplasmosis, tuberculosis, and syphilis, which can cause dementia as well. HIV-associated dementia complex is a clinical entity recognized in HIV patients (usually with low CD4 cell counts) and is characterized by progressive deterioration of cognitive function.

Clinical Manifestations

Patients report memory problems, difficulty with concentration, and poor attention. The pathophysiologic bases for this cognitive impairment have not been clarified.

Diagnostic Evaluation

MRI usually shows cortical and subcortical atrophy.

Treatment

Zidovudine (AZT) treatment is controversial. Currently, selegiline and memantine (an NMDA antago-

nist) are being evaluated. High-dose antiretroviral therapy may be helpful in retarding cognitive loss.

KEY POINTS

- HIV-associated dementia is common in HIV patients with low CD4 cell counts.
- Therapy includes AZT, and possibly selegiline and memantine.

METABOLIC CAUSES OF DEMENTIA

Vitamin B_{12} deficiency may present as a progressive dementing illness. However, there are usually many other neurologic features, including dysfunction in the spinal cord (subacute combined degeneration) and peripheral nervous system, such that the diagnosis becomes clearer. The most common neurologic symptoms are those of neuropathy (paresthesias in hands and feet, sensory ataxia, visual loss, orthostatic hypotension) and memory loss. Systemic symptoms include anemia and sore tongue. Appropriate replacement of vitamin B_{12} should suffice in the treatment. Other metabolic causes of dementia are mentioned in Box 12-1.

Sleep Disorders

PHYSIOLOGY OF SLEEP

Sleep is a process necessary for life and is considered essential for restoration of energy, consolidation of memory and learning, and maintenance of the immune system. From a physiologic perspective, sleep can be divided into 5 stages: rapid eye movement (REM) sleep and 4 stages of nonrapid eye movement (nREM) sleep. REM sleep is distinguished not only by rapid eye movements as its name indicates, but also by atonia of all skeletal muscles other than the extraocular muscles and diaphragm. The 4 stages of nREM sleep are identified by characteristic electroencephalogram (EEG) patterns: 50% theta slow wave activity in stage 1, sleep spindles and K complexes in stage 2, 20% to 50% delta (still slower) activity in stage 3, and 50% or more delta activity in stage 4. The presence of delta EEG activity lends stages 3 and 4 the name "slow-wave sleep."

A typical night of sleep contains 4 to 6 cycles lasting approximately 90 minutes each, with an orderly progression between stages as shown in Figure 13-1. Note that stage 1 sleep is absent after the first sleep cycle and that both stage 3 and REM sleep follow stage 2. Infants spend approximately 50% of sleep in REM, with this percentage decreasing to the typical young adult value of 20% to 25% between ages 2 and 5. Healthy older healthy adults have a decrease in REM sleep to 15% to 20% of the night. As illustrated in Figure 13-1, REM sleep accounts for a greater percentage of sleep as the night progresses.

Certain drugs and toxins may alter the proportion of the night spent in the various stages of sleep. For example, benzodiazepines suppress stages 3 and 4, while antidepressants and alcohol suppress REM sleep.

KEY POINTS

- Sleep is divided into 5 stages: REM sleep and 4 stages of nREM sleep.
- Sleep spindles and K complexes characterize stage 2 sleep.
- Adults spend between 20% and 25% of their sleep in REM.

POLYSOMNOGRAPHY

Apart from the history and physical examination, polysomnography (PSG) is the most important step in the evaluation of a patient with a suspected sleep disorder. The PSG consists of a limited EEG montage which records brain activity and helps with the staging of sleep, electro-oculography (EOG) to monitor eye movements, surface EMG electrodes attached to the chin and legs to monitor skeletal muscle activity, transducers for measuring airflow and chest movements, pulse oximetry for measurement of oxygen saturation, and ECG to monitor cardiac activity. Modifications of standard PSG may also allow video monitoring to observe parasomnias such as REM sleep behavior disorder and somnambulism.

CIRCADIAN RHYTHMS AND SLEEP-PHASE DISORDERS

The body is governed by roughly 24-hour cycles of sleep and activity known as circadian rhythms. These rhythms are coordinated by the suprachiasmatic

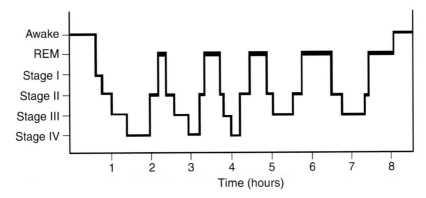

Figure 13-1 • Stages of sleep. Rapid-eye-movement (REM) sleep and the 4 stages of nonREM sleep alternate throughout the night in cycles that last approximately 90 minutes. There are typically four to six cycles each night in a healthy young adult.

nucleus of the hypothalamus, with important inputs from melatonin produced by the pineal gland. Pathological circadian rhythms include *advanced sleep-phase disorder* in which patients sleep or wake earlier than they desire, and *delayed sleep-phase disorder* in which sleep onset is delayed until early morning, with consequent awakening later than desired. Bright light therapy and melatonin can be used to treat sleep-phase disorders by resetting circadian rhythms.

RESTLESS LEGS SYNDROME/ PERIODIC LIMB MOVEMENTS OF SLEEP

Restless legs syndrome (RLS) is a common sleep disorder characterized by an urge to move the legs, usually during periods of rest or inactivity. Patients describe uncomfortable crawling sensations in the legs, with worsening discomfort if the legs remain still, and relief when they are moved. Typically, restless legs symptoms occur in the evening or at night. They are often accompanied by periodic limb movements of sleep, repetitive involuntary movements of the toe, ankle, knee, and hip that last 2 to 3 seconds and are followed by slow recovery of the normal leg position. These movements can awaken the patient or bed partner. RLS is more common in women, and in some families an autosomal dominant inheritance pattern is suggested.

Diagnosis of RLS is made by clinical history. PSG may help to confirm the diagnosis but is often not necessary. Laboratory evaluation of RLS should include measurement of ferritin levels, as many patients with RLS have iron deficiency.

Dopaminergic agents are the treatment of choice for RLS. Dopamine agonists such as ropinirole and pramipexole are preferred to levodopa, because levodopa is associated with a higher incidence of augmentation, i.e., progressive movement of symptoms toward an earlier time of day with continued therapy. Typically, these medications are given half an hour before the anticipated start of symptoms, and then every 2 to 3 hours afterward. Side effects of dopamine agonists include nausea, lightheadedness, and sometimes sleep attacks (falling asleep suddenly in the daytime).

If augmentation becomes a severe problem or RLS symptoms worsen despite treatment with dopaminergic agents, other treatment options include anticonvulsants (particularly gabapentin), opioids, and benzodiazepines. Iron deficiency should be corrected; this can help to relieve symptoms, although dopaminergic agents are often still required.

KEY POINTS

- RLS is associated with iron deficiency.
- Dopaminergic agonists such as ropinirole and pramipexole are the agents of choice in the treatment of RLS.
- Augmentation is the occurrence of RLS symptoms earlier in the day upon dopaminergic treatment.

NARCOLEPSY/CATAPLEXY

The four components of the narcolepsy/cataplexy syndrome are: excessive daytime sleepiness with narcolepsy, cataplexy, sleep paralysis, and hypnagogic hallucinations. All four components need not be present in an individual patient to make the diagnosis. Narcolepsy is the irresistible urge to sleep, often taking the form of sleep attacks, i.e., falling asleep suddenly in the daytime. Cataplexy is characterized by the sudden loss of muscle tone, often in the setting of laughter or other strong emotions. Hypnagogic hallucinations are those that occur immediately upon falling asleep. Patients usually experience the first symptoms of this syndrome in their teens or twenties.

The pathophysiology of narcolepsy/cataplexy is related to a loss of hypocretin-secreting neurons in the hypothalamus. Indeed, a CSF hypocretin level <110 pg/mL is diagnostic for the syndrome in the appropriate clinical setting. More typically, however, the diagnosis is established by performing a special type of PSG known as the multiple sleep latency test (MSLT). An MSLT involves several short naps and monitoring of the latency to sleep onset and latency to REM onset. Sleep latency less than or equal to 8 minutes, with more than two episodes of REM at sleep onset, are diagnostic for narcolepsy/cataplexy.

Treatment of narcolepsy has traditionally employed amphetamines such as methylphenidate and dextroamphetamine. Due to safety concerns and potential for abuse of these drugs, however, modafinil, a medication with an unknown mechanism of action, has become the agent of choice in the treatment of narcolepsy. Cataplexy is most often treated with tricyclic antidepressants such as clomipramine, with the newer agent sodium oxabate now being employed more frequently. Selective serotonin reuptake inhibitors and atypical antidepressants such as venlafaxine can also be effective.

KEY POINTS

- The clinical tetrad of narcolepsy/cataplexy is excessive daytime sleepiness with narcolepsy, cataplexy, sleep paralysis, and hypnagogic hallucinations.
- Shortened sleep onset latency and REM at sleep onset are multiple sleep latency test features in patients with narcolepsy/cataplexy.
- Modafinil has become the agent of choice for the treatment of narcolepsy.
- Tricyclic antidepressants and sodium oxabate are used to treat cataplexy.

PARASOMNIAS AND DYSSOMNIAS

Parasomnias are abnormal behaviors that occur during sleep or sleep-wake transition. There is a wide variety of these disorders, and only a few of the more common ones will be discussed here.

AROUSAL DISORDERS

These parasomnias are characterized, as their name suggests, by abnormal arousals from sleep. In confusional arousals, patients awaken with disorientation, slow speech, and incoordination. Sleep terrors involve rapid awakening from sleep with fearful behavior, often beginning with a scream, and are associated with autonomic hyperactivity such as facial flushing, diaphoresis, and tachycardia. Patients with sleep terrors may be difficult to console upon awakening. A lack of memory for the event helps to distinguish sleep terrors from nightmares. Somnambulism is characterized by interruption of sleep by a variety of complex motor activities, including not only walking, but also dressing, driving, or eating.

REM SLEEP-RELATED PARASOMNIAS

A variety of parasomnias may arise from REM sleep. Nightmares are frightening, vivid dreams that usually occur during the second half of the night and are remembered well by patients, unlike sleep terrors. Sleep paralysis is the perception of being unable to move, usually on awakening. REM behavior disorder is characterized by the loss of the normal skeletal muscle atonia during REM sleep, with the associated acting out of dreams. A wide range of behaviors including punching, kicking, jumping, and yelling may be observed. Injury to the patient or the bed partner may occur. Patients with this disorder are at increased risk of developing a synucleinopathy such as Parkinson disease, Lewy body dementia, or multiple system atrophy. Clonazepam administered at bedtime is the preferred treatment for REM behavior disorder.

SLEEP-WAKE TRANSITION DISORDERS

Nocturnal cramps are experienced as a painful tightness, most often in lower extremity muscles. They can be difficult to treat, with most success obtained from quinine. Somniloquy is unintelligble mumbling during sleep, which can be provoked by talking to the patient.

OTHER PARASOMNIAS

Sleep starts or hypnic jerks are commonly experienced myoclonic jerks that often occur with sleep onset. Enuresis is abnormal nocturnal bedwetting, defined as more than three episodes per week. Boys have enuresis more often than girls. Most cases of enuresis resolve spontaneously, although conditioning the child or use of imipramine may hasten this resolution. Bruxism is teeth grinding during sleep; treatment of underlying dental abnormalities or use of a biteplate is often helpful.

SLEEP APNEA

Obstructive sleep apnea (OSA) is produced by obstruction of the upper airway during sleep. Preservation of respiratory effort distinguishes OSA from central sleep apnea, which is derived from a central (nervous system) lack of ventilatory effort. Symptoms of OSA include excessive daytime sleepiness, snoring, cessation of breathing in the middle of the night, and morning headaches. Nonspecific cognitive complaints may also occur in patients with obstructive sleep apnea. Risk factors for the development of OSA include obesity (body mass index >30 kg/m^2 or neck circumference greater than 17 inches) and advanced age. Patients with OSA are at increased risk of developing cardiopulmonary disease.

PSG is the standard tool used to investigate OSA: a combination of more than 5 apneas, hypopneas, or respiratory event–related arousals are required to establish the diagnosis. Apneas are defined as respiratory pauses with cessation of airflow lasting 10 seconds or more, while hypopneas are defined as pauses with a reduction of 50% or more in airflow.

Continuous positive airway pressure (CPAP) is the standard treatment for OSA. This apparatus delivers air at a predetermined pressure through a tube connected to a facemask. Patients with a diagnosis of OSA may have a "split-night" PSG in which the first part of the night is spent in diagnosing and quantifying the severity of the disorder while the second part of the night is spent titrating the CPAP pressure to best prevent respiratory events. In addition to CPAP, patients with OSA benefit from weight loss, alcohol cessation, and sleeping on their sides rather than on the back. Surgical intervention may be indicated should CPAP and behavioral modification prove ineffective. The operation most commonly performed is uvulopalatopharyngoplasty to relieve upper airway obstruction.

 KEY POINTS

- Continuous positive airway pressure is the treatment of choice for obstructive sleep apnea.

14 Vascular Disease

A stroke is a brain injury caused by an abnormality of the blood vessels supplying the brain. In the United States, about 750,000 individuals have a stroke and 150,000 die from stroke annually. Every 45 seconds, someone in the United States has a stroke, and each 3 minutes, someone dies of stroke. Stroke is the third leading cause of death in the world, surpassed only by heart disease and cancer. Strokes are a very important cause of prolonged disability. Survivors of strokes often cannot return to work or assume their former effectiveness as spouses, friends, and parents. The economic, social, and psychological costs of stroke are huge.

Many general medical conditions and behaviors predispose to stroke. These include: hypertension, diabetes, obesity, hyperlipidemia, sedentary life style, smoking, cardiac disease, and heavy alcohol use. Prevention of stroke is very important and can be accomplished by physicians attending to these stroke risk factors and advising patients about their lifestyles and habits, and by prescribing appropriate medications. Prevention is primary in patients who have never had a stroke and secondary when preventing a stroke recurrence. Second and third strokes are most often due to the same stroke subtype as the initial stroke. Recognition of the cause of a stroke is the most important step in taking measures to avoid a recurrence.

VASCULAR ANATOMY

The nature of the neurologic symptoms and signs helps clinicians localize the findings to a particular location within the brain. In order to identify the abnormality within the blood vessel pathway that supplies that region of the brain, it is necessary for clinicians to have an intimate knowledge of vascular anatomy. They must also become familiar with the frequency of the various pathologies that affect blood vessels at various sites.

The anterior (carotid) circulation supplies the cerebral hemispheres except for the medial temporal lobes and a portion of the occipital lobes. The posterior (vertebro-basilar) circulation supplies the brainstem, thalami, cerebellum, and the posterior portions of the cerebral hemispheres (Fig. 14-1).

ANTERIOR CIRCULATION

The right common carotid artery (CCA) branches from the innominate artery. The left CCA arises directly from the aorta. The CCAs divide in the neck into the internal carotid artery (ICA) and the external carotid artery. The ICAs travel behind the pharynx, entering the skull where they form an S-shaped curve—the carotid siphon. This portion of the ICAs gives rise to ophthalmic artery branches to the eye. The ICAs then penetrate the dura and give off anterior choroidal and posterior communicating arteries before bifurcating into the anterior cerebral (ACAs), and middle cerebral arteries (MCAs).

The ACAs supply the anterior medial cerebral hemispheres and the caudate nuclei and basal frontal lobes. The anterior communicating artery connects the two ACAs. The MCAs course laterally, giving off lenticulostriate artery branches to the basal ganglia and internal capsule. The MCAs trifurcate into small anterior temporal branches and large superior and inferior divisions. The superior divisions supply the lateral cerebral hemispheres above the sylvian fissure, and the inferior divisions supply the temporal and inferior parietal lobes below the sylvian fissure.

The anterior choroidal arteries arise from the ICAs after the ophthalmic and posterior communicating

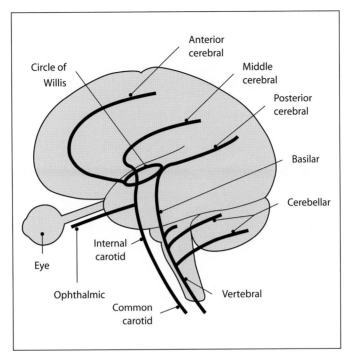

Figure 14-1 • Schematic diagram of the vessels of the brain, including the anterior and posterior circulation.
(Reproduced with permission from Wilkinson I, Lennox G. *Essential Neurology*, 4th ed. Oxford: Blackwell Publishing, 2005:27.)

arteries and course along the optic tract giving off branches to the globus pallidus and posterior limb of the internal capsule and then supply the medial temporal lobe and the lateral geniculate body.

POSTERIOR CIRCULATION

The first branch of each subclavian artery is the vertebral artery (VA). The VAs enter the transverse foramina of C6 or C5 and run within the intravertebral foramina, exiting to course behind the atlas before piercing the dura mater to enter the foramen magnum. The intracranial VAs end at the medullo-pontine junction, where they join to form the basilar artery.

The intracranial VAs give off posterior and anterior spinal artery branches, penetrating arteries to the medulla, and the large posterior inferior cerebellar arteries (PICAs). The basilar artery runs in the midline along the clivus giving off bilateral anterior inferior cerebellar artery (AICA) and superior cerebellar artery (SCA) branches before dividing at the pontomesencephalic junction into PCA branches. Small penetrating arteries arise at the basilar artery bifurcation to supply the medial portions of the midbrain and thalami.

The vascular supply of the brainstem includes large paramedian arteries and smaller, short circumferential arteries that penetrate through the basal portions of the brainstem into the tegmentum. Long circumferential arteries course around the brainstem giving off branches to the lateral tegmentum. The PCAs give off penetrating arteries to the midbrain and thalamus, course around the cerebral peduncles, and then supply the occipital lobes and inferior surface of the temporal lobes.

The circle of Willis allows for connections between the anterior circulations of each side, through the anterior communicating artery, and between the posterior and anterior circulations of each side through the posterior communicating artery (Fig. 14-2).

KEY POINTS

- Each carotid artery supplies two-fifths of the brain; the vertebro-basilar circulation, one-fifth.

- The anterior circulation supplies mainly the cerebrum, while the posterior circulation supplies the brainstem, cerebellum, and the visual cerebral cortex.

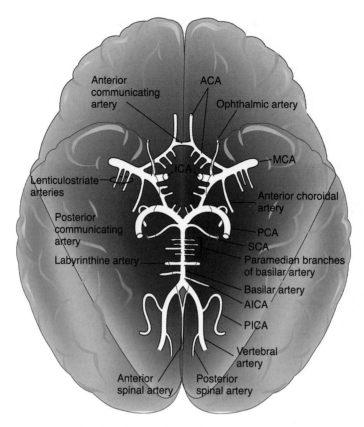

Figure 14-2 • Arteries of the circle of Willis.

BRAIN ISCHEMIA

About 80% of strokes are ischemic while 10% each are due to subarachnoid and intracerebral hemorrhages. Ischemia is traditionally divided into thrombotic, embolic, and systemic hypoperfusion mechanisms.

THROMBOSIS

Thrombosis refers to obstructed blood flow due to a localized occlusive process within one or more vessels. The vessel lumen is narrowed or occluded by an abnormal vessel wall or by superimposed clot. The most common vascular pathology is atherosclerosis, in which fibrous and muscular tissues and lipid materials form plaques that encroach on the lumen. Atherosclerosis affects mostly the large neck and intracranial arteries. Sometimes, a clot forms within the lumen because of a primary hematologic problem—polycythemia, thrombocytosis, or hypercoagulability. Less common occlusive vascular pathologies include: vasoconstriction, fibromuscular dysplasia, and arterial dissection.

The smaller, penetrating intracranial arteries are most often damaged by hypertension that causes hypertrophy of the media and deposition of fibrinoid material. Microatheromas can obstruct the penetrating artery origins.

EMBOLISM

In embolism, material formed elsewhere within the vascular system lodges in a vessel and blocks blood flow. The material arises proximally, mostly from the heart; from major arteries such as the aorta, ICAs, and VAs; and from systemic veins. Cardiac sources of embolism include the heart valves, endocardium, and clots or tumors within the atrial or ventricular cavities. Artery-to-artery emboli are composed of clot, platelet clumps, or fragments of plaques. Thrombi originating in systemic veins travel to the brain through cardiac defects such as an atrial septal defect or a patent foramen ovale, a process termed paradoxical embolism. Occasionally, air, fat, cholesterol crystals, bacteria, and foreign bodies enter the vascular system and embolize to brain vessels.

SYSTEMIC HYPOPERFUSION

Decreased flow to brain tissue can be caused by low systemic perfusion pressure. The most common causes are cardiac pump failure (most often due to myocardial infarction or arrhythmia) and systemic hypotension (due to blood loss or hypovolemia). The lack of perfusion is more generalized than in localized thrombosis or embolism and affects the brain diffusely and bilaterally. Poor perfusion is most critical in border zone or so-called watershed regions at the periphery of the major vascular supply territories.

 KEY POINTS

- Ischemia can be due to a localized process within an artery (thrombosis) or blockage of an artery by emboli arising proximally, or by a general decrease in blood flow (systemic hypoperfusion).
- Emboli most often come from the heart, aorta, and proximal portions of the neck or intracranial arteries.
- Atherosclerosis most often affects the large neck and intracranial arteries.

COMMON ISCHEMIC STROKE SYNDROMES

Clinical localization often involves pattern matching of the findings in individual patients with common stroke syndromes.

ANTERIOR CIRCULATION

1. Left cerebral hemisphere strokes lead to:
   a. Right hemiparesis: often arm, hand, and face > leg
   b. Right hemisensory loss
   c. Aphasia
   d. In deep lesions or large lesions, conjugate deviation of the eyes to the left; right hemianopia or hemi-inattention
   e. When caused by ICA occlusive disease, transient left monocular visual loss may also occur.
2. Right cerebral hemisphere strokes cause:
   a. Left hemiparesis: often arm, hand, and face > leg
      i. Left hemisensory loss
      ii. Poor drawing and copying
   b. Neglect of the left visual field
      i. In deep or large lesions, conjugate deviation of the eyes to the right, left hemianopia
      ii. When the signs are due to ICA occlusive disease, transient right monocular visual loss may accompany the brain signs.

These cerebral hemispheral lesions are most often caused by carotid artery occlusion, embolism to the MCA or its branches, or basal ganglionic intracerebral hemorrhages.

POSTERIOR CIRCULATION

1. Lateral medulla stroke (usually due to intracranial VA occlusion) causes:
   a. Ipsilateral facial pain, or reduced pain and temperature sensation on the ipsilateral face, or both
   b. Loss of pain and temperature in the contralateral limbs and body
   c. Ipsilateral Horner syndrome
   d. Nystagmus
   e. Incoordination of the ipsilateral arm
   f. Leaning and veering while sitting or walking, with gait ataxia
   g. In deep lesions, dysphagia and hoarseness
2. Bilateral pontine base and often medial tegmentum stroke (usually due to basilar artery occlusion, or pontine hemorrhage) causes:
   a. Quadriparesis
   b. Unilateral or bilateral conjugate gaze paresis; sometimes internuclear ophthalmoplegia, or VIth nerve palsy
   c. When the medial tegmentum is involved bilaterally, coma
3. Cerebellar infarction (usually due to embolism to the PICA or SCA, or cerebellar hemorrhage) causes:
   a. Gait ataxia; often inability to walk
   b. Dysarthria
   c. Ipsilateral arm dysmetria
4. Left PCA territory stroke causes:
   a. Right hemianopia
   b. At times, right hemisensory symptoms, dysmemory, and alexia without agraphia
5. Right PCA territory stroke causes:
   a. Left hemianopia
   b. At times, left hemisensory symptoms and left visual neglect
   PCA territory infarcts are most often caused by embolism to the PCAs arising from the heart, aorta, or VAs.

LACUNAR SYNDROMES

These smaller strokes also have clinical signs depending on their locations. They are most often due to occlusion of a penetrating artery. They may occur in either the anterior or the posterior circulation areas. Some lacunar stroke syndromes include:

Pure motor stroke: weakness of the arm, face, and leg on one side of the body without sensory, visual, or cognitive or behavioral signs.
Pure sensory stroke: paresthesiae on one side of the body and limbs and face, without motor, visual, or cognitive abnormalities.
Dysarthria—clumsy hand syndrome: slurred speech and clumsiness of one hand.
Ataxic hemiparesis: weakness and ataxia of the limbs on one side of the body.

DIAGNOSTIC EVALUATION

After taking a thorough history and performing a general examination emphasizing the heart and blood vessels, and a neurologic examination, the next step is usually a brain image. CT and MRI scans are used to separate brain infarction from hemorrhage. Figure

14-3 shows a deep brain hemorrhage. Figure 14-4 shows a brain infarction on CT scan. MRI with diffusion-weighted scanning can better show acute brain infarction (Fig. 14-5).

The symptoms and signs, and brain imaging, should allow localization to either the left or right anterior circulation, the posterior circulation, or a lacunar syndrome. In patients with transient or persistent brain ischemia, the heart, aorta, and neck and intracranial arteries and their branches should be imaged. This can be performed using echocardiography, extracranial and transcranial ultrasound, or CT or MR angiography. In patients in whom the signs localize to the anterior circulation, the ICAs are emphasized. The VAs and their intracranial branches are emphasized in posterior circulation cases. The blood should be checked for abnormalities of erythrocytes, leukocytes, and coagulation by ordering a complete blood count, platelet count, and prothrombin time reported as an International Normalized Ratio (INR). Some patients warrant more intensive investigation for coagulopathy.

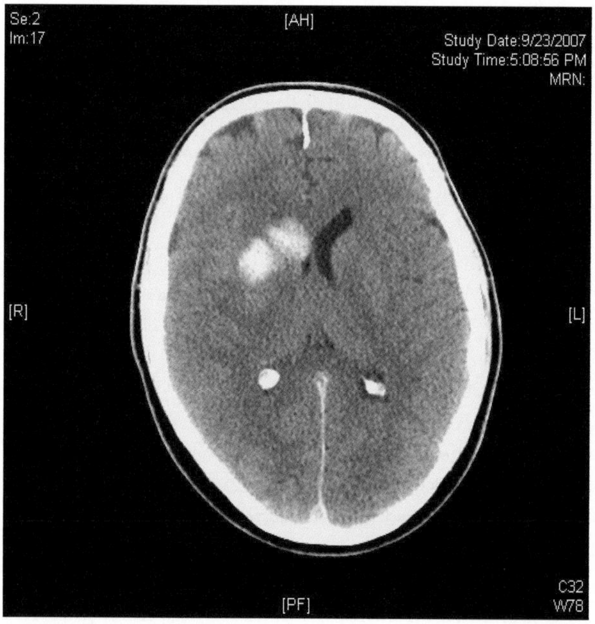

Figure 14-3 • Intracerebral hemorrhage. A CT scan showing a right basal ganglionic hemorrhage due to hypertension. The hemorrhage has extended into the right frontal horn of the lateral ventricle.

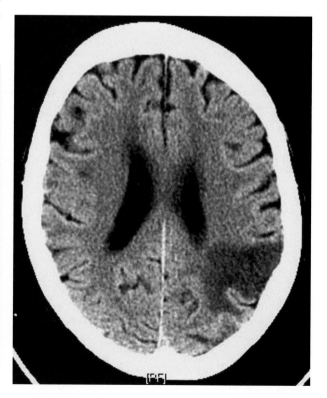

Figure 14-4 • CT scan of the head demonstrates a wedge-shaped hypodensity in the distribution of a branch of the left middle cerebral artery.

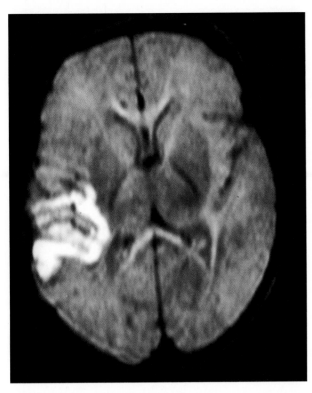

Figure 14-5 • Bright signal is seen on a diffusion-weighted MR image (DWI), indicating a recent infarction.

 KEY POINTS

- The course of development of symptoms and results of brain imaging should allow separation of ischemia from hemorrhage, and in case of ischemia, identification of the most likely stroke mechanism: thrombosis, embolism, or systemic hypoperfusion.
- Cardiac and brain and vascular imaging should identify the cause of the stroke.

TREATMENT

In patients seen soon after the onset of neurologic symptoms, an attempt should be made to reperfuse the ischemic brain if a brain-supplying large artery is occluded and if a large portion of the brain area supplied by that artery is not already infarcted. Brain and vascular imaging can show the location and extent of brain infarction and vascular occlusion. Reperfusion can be attempted using intravenous thrombolysis or by intra-arterial interventions using thrombolysis or mechanical means. Cerebral blood flow should be maximized by optimizing blood pressure and fluid volume.

Prevention of further brain ischemia often involves using an antithrombotic agent. Heparin, and later warfarin, is used in patients with cardiac origin embolization (mostly due to atrial fibrillation and myocardial infarction) and in some patients with arterial dissection and acute large artery occlusions. Antiplatelet drugs—aspirin, clopidogrel, a combination of aspirin and modified-release dipyridamole, or cilostazole—are given to patients with lacunar infarction and nonocclusive atherosclerotic lesions.

Control of stroke risk factors (hypertension, diabetes, obesity, hyperlipidemia, smoking) is accomplished by attention to lifestyle behavior, nutrition, and exercise, and by prescribing appropriate medications.

 KEY POINTS

- Acute and preventive treatments should be tailored to the individual patient.
- Maximizing cerebral blood flow to ischemic regions can be facilitated by opening blocked arteries chemically or mechanically, and by increasing blood flow in collateral vessels.

INTRACRANIAL HEMORRHAGE

Bleeding inside the skull can be divided into subarachnoid, intracerebral, epidural, and subdural hemorrhages. The latter two types of hemorrhages are almost always traumatic and are discussed in Chapter 17. Intracerebral hemorrhage (ICH) and subarachnoid hemorrhage (SAH) have different causes, clinical findings, and management.

SUBARACHNOID HEMORRHAGE

SAH is predominantly caused by bleeding from an aneurym located along the circle of Willis. The most common sites of cerebral aneurysms are shown in Figure 14-6. When blood under arterial pressure is suddenly released into the space around the brain, patients develop sudden headache, often vomit, and have a temporary interruption in behavior. If the resultant increase in intracranial pressure is severe, coma or death may ensue. An example of an SAH is shown in Figure 14-7.

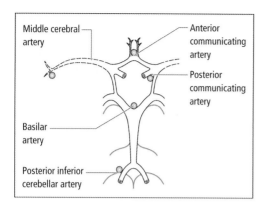

Figure 14-6 • Common sites of aneurysm in the circle of Willis. (Reproduced with permission from Ginsberg L. *Lecture Notes: Neurology*, 8th ed. Oxford: Blackwell Publishing, 2005:87.)

Treatment is aimed at prevention of rebleeding and vasoconstriction that often follows SAH. Aneurysms can be clipped surgically or "coiled" by interventional techniques. Calcium-channel blockers are often used to minimize vasoconstriction and delayed brain ischemia.

INTRACEREBRAL HEMORRHAGE

ICH describes bleeding directly into brain parenchyma. In contrast to SAH, the earliest symptoms

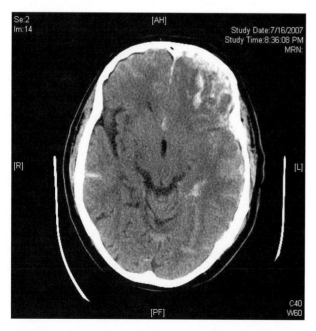

Figure 14-7 • Subarachnoid hemorrhage. A CT scan showing extensive subarachnoid blood within the sulci of the brain. The most bleeding is seen in the left frontal region.

are neurologic signs related to the region of the bleeding. Bleeding into the putamen-internal capsule region might cause early contralateral limb weakness, while cerebellar bleeding would cause gait instability. ICHs continue to grow until the pressure around the lesion equals that in the hematoma or the hematoma drains into the ventricular system or the pial surface.

Hypertension is the commonest cause of ICH. The commonest locations for hypertensive ICH are: basal ganglia-internal capsule, caudate nucleus, thalamus, pons, and cerebellum. Trauma, cerebral amyloid angiopathy, vascular malformations, and bleeding diatheses (especially with patients on anticoagulants) are other common causes.

VASCULAR MALFORMATIONS

There is a variety of congenital and acquired vascular anomalies (angiomas) that have the potential to bleed, either within the brain (ICH) or around it. **Arteriovenous malformations** (AVMs) contain arteries that empty into arterialized veins. These lesions contain no recognizable normal capillary bed, but abnormal gliotic parenchyma can be found between the component vessels. The most common brain vascular malformations are **developmental venous anomalies** (DVAs) that are composed of anomalous veins usually separated by morphologically normal brain parenchyma. One or more large central draining veins are usually conspicuous and may be dilated into a varix or varices. **Cavernous angiomas** consist of a relatively compact mass of sinusoidal vessels close together, without intervening brain parenchyma. The lesions are well encapsulated. **Telangiectasias** are dilated capillaries with intervening brain parenchyma. Brain and vascular imaging can distinguish between these subtypes.

KEY POINTS

- AVMs, DVAs, cavernous angiomas, and telangiectasis are different types of malformations, each with differing clinical findings and management.
- Medical therapy, surgery, interventional obliteration, and radiotherapy are all used in treating brain vascular malformations.

5 Seizures

Seizures are among the most common problems in neurology. Up to 10% of the population will have a seizure at some point in their lives. In addition, seizures can be among the most dramatic forms of nervous system dysfunction. Although seizures have many different causes and manifestations, by definition a seizure is an abnormal hypersynchronous electrical discharge of neurons. Epilepsy is defined as a condition in which there is a tendency toward recurrent unprovoked seizures. Practically, the diagnosis of epilepsy is often applied after a patient has had two unprovoked seizures.

CLASSIFICATION

Seizures can arise from one portion of the brain (**partial**) or from the entire brain at once (**generalized**). Those that arise from one portion of the brain can evolve and spread to involve the whole brain (**secondarily generalized**). Among partial seizures, those in which awareness is impaired are termed **complex**, whereas those in which awareness is preserved are termed **simple**.

SIMPLE PARTIAL SEIZURES

By definition, simple partial seizures begin in a focal area of the brain and do not impair awareness. In general, such seizures lead to positive rather than negative neurologic symptoms (e.g., tingling rather than numbness, hallucinations rather than blindness). The manifestations of simple partial seizures depend on their site of origin in the brain. Focal motor seizures, in which one part of the body may stiffen or jerk rhythmically, stem from the motor cortex in the frontal lobe. The classic jacksonian march occurs when the electrical discharge spreads along the motor strip, leading to rhythmic twitching that spreads along body parts following the organization of the motor homunculus. Simple partial seizures from other regions of the brain can cause sensory phenomena (parietal), visual phenomena (occipital), or gustatory, olfactory, and psychic phenomena (temporal). The latter may include déjà vu, jamais vu, or sensations of depersonalization ("out of body") or derealization.

COMPLEX PARTIAL SEIZURES

Complex partial seizures have a focal onset and involve an impairment of awareness. They commonly arise from the temporal lobe, although some may originate in the frontal lobe as well. Complex partial seizures may include automatisms (stereotyped motor actions without clear purpose) such as lip-smacking, chewing movements, or picking at clothing. The patient may have speech arrest or may speak in a nonsensical manner. By definition the patient does not respond normally to the environment or to questions or commands. Occasionally, patients may continue the activities they were participating in at the onset of the seizure, sometimes to remarkable lengths: patients may continue folding the laundry during a seizure or even finish driving home. Complex partial seizures of frontal lobe origin may involve bizarre bilateral movements, such as bicycling or kicking, or behavior such as running in circles.

GENERALIZED TONIC-CLONIC SEIZURES

Generalized tonic-clonic (GTC) seizures were formerly called **grand mal** seizures and are the seizure type with which the lay public is most familiar. They typically begin with a tonic phase, lasting several seconds, in which the entire body becomes stiff (including the pharyngeal muscles, sometimes leading to a vocalization known as the epileptic cry). This is followed by the clonic phase, in which the extremities jerk rhythmically, more or less symmetrically, typically for less than 1 to 2 minutes. Toward the end of the clonic phase, the frequency of the jerking may peter out until the body finally becomes flaccid. The patient may bite his tongue and become incontinent of urine during a GTC seizure. There is typically a postictal state after the seizure, lasting minutes to hours, during which the patient may be tired or confused, before returning slowly back to normal.

ABSENCE SEIZURE

An absence seizure is a generalized seizure that most commonly occurs in children and is characterized primarily by an unresponsive period of staring that lasts for several seconds, with immediate recovery afterward. Absence seizures can occur tens or even hundreds of times a day and may first be diagnosed by schoolteachers as daydreaming or difficulty concentrating. A classic 3-Hz spike-and-wave EEG pattern accompanies absence seizures (Fig. 15-1). Hyperventilation is a common trigger.

OTHER SEIZURE TYPES

Rarer seizure types include atonic, tonic, and myoclonic seizures, all of which are generalized in onset.

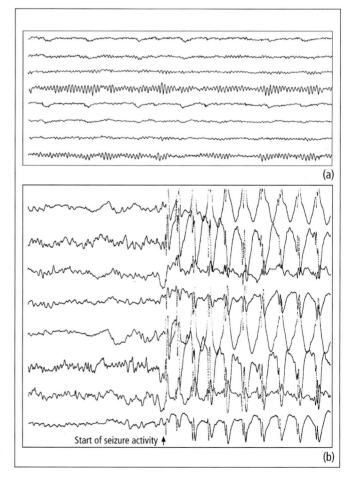

Figure 15-1 • Characteristic EEG findings in the absence seizures. **(A)** This tracing demonstrates a normal EEG recording in an awake adult. The top four channels are derived from electrodes over the left side of the head, from front to back, while the bottom four are derived from the right side of the head. A normal sinusoidal alpha rhythm is seen most prominently over the posterior head regions bilaterally (fourth and eighth channels). **(B)** Midway through the tracing, rhythmic 3-Hz generalized spike-and-slow-wave discharges appear. This is the typical EEG pattern of an absence seizure; during these discharges, the patient may stare and be unresponsive.

(Reproduced with permission from Ginsberg L. *Lecture Notes: Neurology,* 8th ed. Oxford: Blackwell Publishing, 2005:75.)

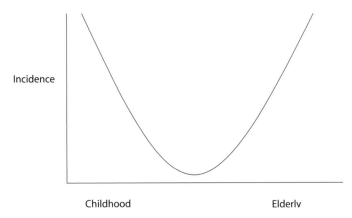

Figure 15-2 • Incidence of new-onset seizures by age.

 KEY POINTS

- A seizure is an abnormal hypersynchronous electrical discharge involving neurons in the brain.
- Epilepsy is a tendency to have recurrent unprovoked seizures.
- Seizures may manifest with motor, sensory, or psychic phenomena and are usually characterized by positive rather than negative neurologic symptoms.
- Partial seizures originate in a focal area of the brain but may become secondarily generalized; awareness is preserved during simple partial seizures and impaired during complex partial seizures.
- Generalized seizures originate in the entire brain at once; tonic-clonic and absence seizures are examples of such seizures.

EPIDEMIOLOGY AND ETIOLOGIES

Seizures often have their onset in the very young and the very old (Fig. 15-2). Etiologies vary depending on age of onset. In infants, a variety of neonatal infections, hypoxic-ischemic insults, and genetic syndromes are common causes of seizures.

Febrile seizures are a special case. They are the most common cause of seizures in children, affecting up to 3% to 9% of this age group. They occur between 6 months and 5 years of age in the setting of a febrile illness without evidence of intracranial infection and are usually generalized in onset. The risk of future epilepsy is small unless the seizures are prolonged or partial in onset or if other neurologic abnormalities or a family history of epilepsy is present.

Older children may also develop seizures related to head injury or meningitis; genetic syndromes continue to be a significant etiology in this age group. Among young adults, head injury and alcohol are common causes of new-onset seizures, but brain tumors become one of the most common etiologies by middle age. Finally, in the elderly, strokes become the most common etiology, and metabolic disturbances from systemic problems such as hepatic or renal failure are a frequent cause as well.

Frequently, seizures occur in children (and sometimes adults) as part of a syndrome that may include specific seizure types, EEG patterns, and associated neurologic abnormalities. The diagnosis of a specific syndrome may have implications both for genetic testing and for the proper choice of pharmacologic treatments. Examples of epilepsy syndromes are outlined in Table 15-1.

 KEY POINTS

- The incidence of new-onset seizures is highest among the very young and the very old.
- Common etiologies of new-onset seizures differ depending on age of onset.
- Febrile seizures in children are common and generally carry a benign prognosis.
- Seizures may occur as part of specific epilepsy syndromes characterized by distinctive seizure types, EEG patterns, or associated neurologic abnormalities.

TABLE 15-1 Selected Epilepsy Syndromes

	Age of Onset	Seizure Types	Associated Findings	EEG Findings	Treatment
Lennox-Gastaut syndrome	Childhood	Tonic, atonic, myoclonic, generalized tonic-clonic, absence	Mental retardation	Slow (1 to 2 Hz) spike-and-wave	Valproic acid, lamotrigine, felbamate
Benign rolandic epilepsy	Childhood	Simple partial involving mouth and face, generalized tonic-clonic	Nocturnal preponderance of seizures	Centrotemporal spikes	Carbamazepine; sometimes no treatment
Absence epilepsy	Childhood and adolescence	Absence, generalized tonic-clonic	Hyperventilation as trigger	3-Hz spike-and-wave	Ethosuximide, valproic acid
Juvenile myoclonic epilepsy	Adolescence and young adulthood	Myoclonic, absence, generalized tonic-clonic	Early morning preponderance of seizures	4- to 6-Hz polyspike-and-wave	Valproic acid, lamotrigine

CLINICAL MANIFESTATIONS

HISTORY

The diagnosis of seizures is a clinical one. Most commonly the patient will be seen after an event has occurred and the diagnosis will have to be made on the history alone. In these cases the patient (and, more importantly, witnesses, if the seizure was not simple partial) must be pressed for an exact description of the event itself, any premonitory symptoms, and the character of the recovery period in order for the clinician to decide whether the event was a seizure, and, if so, what type of seizure it was. It is these clinical details that should allow for the differentiation of seizures from other paroxysmal neurologic events (Table 15-2).

TABLE 15-2 Characteristics of Partial Seizures and Other Paroxysmal Neurologic Events

	Partial Seizures	Transient Ischemic Attacks (TIAs)	Migraines
Onset	Progression of symptoms over seconds	Sudden onset of symptoms	Progression of symptoms over 15 to 20 minutes
Neurologic symptoms	Positive motor or sensory symptoms, "psychic" symptoms such as déjà vu	Negative motor, sensory, or visual symptoms	Positive sensory or especially visual symptoms, such as scintillating scotomata
Duration	Usually less than a few minutes	Usually less than 30 minutes, always less than 24 hours	Symptoms for 15 to 20 minutes, followed by headache for up to hours
Consciousness	Impaired (if complex)	Preserved	Preserved
Headache	Occasionally postictal	None	Throbbing pain following progression of symptoms
Recovery	Postictal confusion, sleepiness	Immediate	Fatigue common
Risk factors	Structural brain lesion, family history of seizures	Hypertension, hyperlipidemia, smoking, diabetes	Family history of migraines

PHYSICAL EXAMINATION

Examination will be of diagnostic benefit in the rare instances in which the patient is seen during the event or shortly thereafter. In the latter case, a postictal hemiparesis, or Todd paralysis, may be detected after a secondarily generalized seizure. Such a finding indicates that the seizure was of partial onset, even if that was not apparent to onlookers at the time. Other abnormalities on neurologic exam may also suggest the presence of a focal brain lesion. Of course, the general physical exam may yield findings suggestive of infection or other systemic disease that might explain a new-onset seizure. In particular, signs of meningitis should be sought in any patient who has had a seizure.

DIAGNOSTIC EVALUATION

LABORATORY STUDIES

Laboratory testing may reveal an underlying metabolic abnormality that might explain a new-onset seizure, such as hyponatremia or hypocalcemia. There is commonly a lactic acidosis, resulting in decreased serum bicarbonate, after a GTC seizure. In cases where infection is suspected, an LP should always be performed.

RADIOGRAPHIC IMAGING

An uncomplicated seizure in a patient with known epilepsy does not generally warrant head imaging. However, with rare exceptions, neuroimaging should usually be performed in patients with new-onset seizures. For seizures of probable partial onset, an MRI is typically a necessary part of the diagnostic workup, so as to look for a structural abnormality that may serve as a focus for a partial seizure. A head CT may suffice in the urgent setting, however.

ELECTROENCEPHALOGRAPHY

An EEG may be useful for several reasons: It may identify a potential focus of seizure onset, it may reveal characteristic findings that are diagnostic of a specific epilepsy syndrome, and it may establish whether a patient who has had a seizure and is still not waking up is merely postictal or is having continuous nonconvulsive seizures. However, the diagnosis of whether a particular paroxysmal event was a seizure or not must rest primarily on clinical grounds, because up to 50% of EEGs performed on known epilepsy patients may be normal.

KEY POINTS

- The diagnosis of seizure is a clinical one and usually rests primarily on the history.
- Certain elements of the history may help to differentiate seizures from other paroxysmal events.
- Physical exam, laboratory studies, and neuroimaging may help to identify the cause of a new-onset seizure.
- EEG may help to refine the diagnosis of seizures in particular settings.

TREATMENT

DRUGS

The mainstay of epilepsy treatment is medical therapy. The number of available antiepileptic drugs (AEDs) has more than doubled in recent years, and there is now a large selection of agents from which to choose, each with its own set of indications and adverse effects (Table 15-3).

An AED is typically not started after a single seizure. This applies especially to symptomatic seizures, namely those that are due to a treatable or reversible condition, such as meningitis, alcohol withdrawal, or hyponatremia. Most neurologists would also not start an AED after a single seizure for which no underlying cause is found.

AED treatment is usually begun after two seizures that are not symptomatic or provoked. The primary goal of AED usage is monotherapy—that is, control of seizures using a single drug. Most neurologists increase the dosage of a single drug until either seizure control is achieved or adverse effects become intolerable. If the latter occurs, the dose is lowered and a second drug added if necessary. If seizure control is achieved, an attempt is then made to taper the first drug, leaving the second as monotherapy. For about 70% of epilepsy patients, seizures will be well controlled on monotherapy. For the remainder, two or more AEDs may be

■ TABLE 15-3 Selected Antiepileptic Drugs

	Site of Action	Seizure Types Treated*	Characteristic Side Effects
Phenytoin (Dilantin)	Na⁺ channel	Partial	Gingival hyperplasia, coarsening of facial features, ataxia
Carbamazepine (Tegretol)	Na⁺ channel	Partial	Hyponatremia, agranulocytosis, diplopia
Valproic acid (Depakote)	Na⁺ channel, GABA receptor	Partial, generalized, absence	GI symptoms, tremor, weight gain, hair loss, hepatotoxicity, thrombocytopenia
Phenobarbital	GABA receptor	Partial, generalized	Sedation
Ethosuximide (Zarontin)	T-type Ca^{2+} channel	Absence	GI symptoms
Gabapentin (Neurontin)	Unknown	Partial	Sedation, ataxia
Lamotrigine (Lamictal)	Na⁺ channel, glutamate receptor	Partial, generalized	Rash, Stevens-Johnson syndrome
Topiramate (Topamax)	Na⁺ channel, GABA activity	Partial, generalized	Word-finding difficulty, renal stones, weight loss
Tiagabine (Gabitril)	GABA reuptake	Partial	Sedation
Levetiracetam (Keppra)	Unknown	Partial, generalized	Insomnia, anxiety, irritability
Oxcarbazepine (Trileptal)	Na⁺ channel	Partial	Sedation, hyponatremia
Zonisamide (Zonegran)	Unknown	Partial, generalized	Sedation, renal stones, weight loss

*Drugs effective against partial seizures can also be used against seizures that are secondarily generalized.

required, or the seizures may remain refractory to all medical therapy.

 KEY POINTS

- Most neurologists begin drug therapy after two unprovoked seizures.
- Each drug has its own set of indications and adverse effects.
- Monotherapy is the primary goal of antiepileptic therapy; most patients' seizures are well controlled on one medication.

VAGUS NERVE STIMULATION

The vagus nerve stimulator is a novel treatment device that has recently become available; it has been shown to be effective in the treatment of partial seizures. The device is implanted subcutaneously in the chest and stimulates the left vagus nerve through programmed electrical impulses delivered through leads placed in the neck.

SURGERY

Patients refractory to medical management may be treated with epilepsy surgery. (Exactly what constitutes being medically refractory will depend on an individual patient's circumstances; contributing factors typically include seizure type and frequency, tolerance of AED therapy, number of AEDs tried, and effect on patient's quality of life.) The most common surgical procedure is resection of the epileptogenic area, typically following a presurgical evaluation in which continuous video-EEG monitoring combined with neuroimaging and other tests is used to identify the focus of seizure onset. For seizures of medial temporal lobe origin, the rate of seizure freedom following resective surgery may be as high as 90%. Other less commonly used surgical procedures include corpus callosotomy, hemispherectomy, or multiple subpial transection.

STATUS EPILEPTICUS

Status epilepticus (SE) is an abnormal state in which either seizure activity is continuous for a prolonged period or seizures are so frequent that there is no recovery of consciousness between them. There are several types of SE, including the generalized convulsive form (ongoing clonic movements of the extremities) and more subtle forms in which the patient may appear merely comatose or have subtle motor signs such as eyelid twitching or nystagmus. Potential etiologies of SE include acute metabolic disturbances, toxic or infectious insults, hypoxic-ischemic damage to the brain, and underlying epilepsy. Morbidity from SE can be high; outcome depends largely on etiology and duration. SE is a medical emergency, the management of which centers on stopping the seizure activity and preventing the occurrence of systemic complications (Fig. 15-3). It is important to note that a cluster of frequent seizures may warrant similarly aggressive management, particularly because this condition may evolve to SE quickly.

SPECIAL TOPICS

FIRST AID FOR SEIZURES

All physicians should be familiar with first aid measures for those having a seizure. In general, the goal is to prevent the patient from becoming injured and to prevent well-meaning bystanders from intervening unwisely. The patient with complex partial seizures may wander or make semipurposeful movements; if necessary, he or she should be gently guided out of harm's way. More aggressive attempts at restraint may provoke a violent reaction. The patient with GTC seizures should be laid on his or her side, if possible, so that vomiting does not lead to aspiration. Tight clothing should be loosened. **Nothing should be placed in the mouth.** Most GTC seizures stop within 1 to 2 minutes; immediate medical attention should be sought if a seizure becomes more prolonged.

SEIZURES AND DRIVING

Each state has its own licensing requirements for those with epilepsy; physicians who care for seizure patients should be aware of these. Most states require a specific seizure-free interval before a patient may

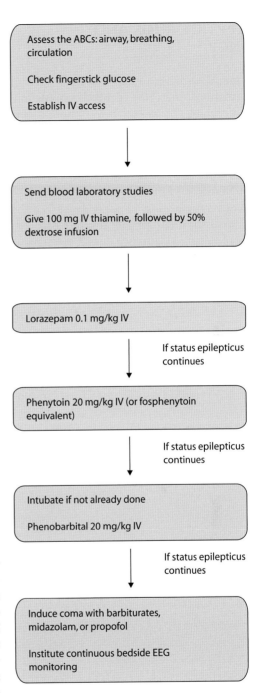

Figure 15-3 • Neurologic emergency: status epilepticus.

drive; exceptions can sometimes be made for purely nocturnal seizures or those with a prolonged simple partial onset that provides the patient with a warning without impaired awareness. A few states require physicians to report patients with seizures to the department of motor vehicles.

ANTIEPILEPTIC DRUGS AND PREGNANCY

Women taking AEDs have a somewhat higher risk of fetal malformations than the general population, though the absolute risk is still low. Valproic acid specifically has been associated with a higher rate of neural tube defects. All women with epilepsy who are considering becoming pregnant should take folic acid (1 mg or more per day). It is reasonable to consider modifying a woman's AED regimen prior to conception depending on the severity of her epilepsy, but the risk of anticonvulsant teratogenicity must be balanced with the risk of seizure occurrence during pregnancy.

PSYCHOGENIC NONEPILEPTIC SEIZURES

A reported 10% to 30% of patients evaluated at tertiary referral centers for medically refractory epilepsy actually have events resembling seizures that have no EEG correlate and are felt to be psychogenic in nature. Some of these patients may also have true epileptic seizures at other times. Many patients with psychogenic events have comorbid psychiatric illnesses or a history of abuse. Continuous video-EEG monitoring to record the typical events may be the most reliable method of differentiating psychogenic events from epileptic seizures.

16 Movement Disorders

IDIOPATHIC PARKINSON DISEASE

Idiopathic Parkinson disease (PD) is a chronic degenerative disorder with characteristic clinical findings, response to L-dopa replacement therapy, and pathologic changes in the brain. **Parkinsonism** is a term used to describe a heterogeneous group of conditions that share some of the clinical features of idiopathic PD but differ partially in their clinical expression, response to L-dopa therapy, and underlying pathologic substrates.

EPIDEMIOLOGY

PD is a common neurodegenerative condition. Most instances are sporadic, although several genes have been implicated in familial forms of PD in which mutations in the α-synuclein, parkin, DJ-1, PINK1 (PTEN-induced kinase), UCH-L1 (ubiquitin carboxy-terminal esterase L1), and LRRK2 (leucine rich repeat kinase 2) genes have been described.

PATHOLOGY

PD is characterized by the progressive death of selected neuronal populations, notably the ventral tier of the neuromelanin-containing dopaminergic neurons of the substantia nigra pars compacta. The pathologic hallmark of PD is the Lewy body.

CLINICAL MANIFESTATIONS

The four cardinal clinical features of idiopathic PD are tremor, rigidity, bradykinesia, and postural instability. Features that may be useful in distinguishing idiopathic PD from other parkinsonian syndromes are summarized in Table 16-1.

The tremor is slow (3 to 5 Hz) and most prominent when the limb is at rest. It affects the distal arm more often than the leg and is described as "pill rolling." It may also affect the lips, chin, and tongue. Rigidity typically affects the distal limbs more than the axial musculature and is described as "lead pipe" or "cogwheel." Slowness of movement (bradykinesia) and thought (bradyphrenia) are common features in idiopathic PD. Postural instability is the result of impaired postural reflexes and is largely responsible for falls. Dementia is increasingly recognized as an important feature of PD and occurs in 25% to 30% of patients as the disease advances.

TREATMENT

Replacement of the deficient dopamine with its precursor L-dopa is the mainstay of treatment. L-Dopa is administered because dopamine does not cross the blood-brain barrier. It is given together with a peripheral decarboxylase inhibitor (e.g., carbidopa) in a combined formulation (e.g., Sinemet). Carbidopa prevents the peripheral conversion of L-dopa to dopamine and thus reduces the incidence of peripheral dopaminergic side effects such as nausea, vomiting, and hypertension.

Dopaminergic agonists have been proposed as alternative initial agents for symptomatic treatment, but the evidence that early therapy with dopami-

■ **TABLE 16-1** Parkinsonian Syndromes

Parkinsonian Syndrome	Distinguishing Clinical Features
Progressive supranuclear palsy	Supranuclear ophthalmoplegia, with limitation of vertical more than horizontal gaze; axial rigidity and neck extension; early falls as a consequence of impaired postural reflexes, neck extension, and inability to look down
Corticobasal ganglionic degeneration	Apraxia, cortical sensory impairment and alien-limb phenomenon; severe unilateral rigidity; stimulus-sensitive myoclonus
Diffuse Lewy body disease	Early dementia; prominent visual hallucinations; extreme sensitivity to extrapyramidal side effects of antidopaminergic neuroleptic drugs
Vascular parkinsonism	"Lower-half" parkinsonism with rigidity in the legs and marked gait impairment; other evidence of diffuse vascular disease (corticospinal tract dysfunction, pseudobulbar palsy)
Multiple system atrophy	Early and prominent features of autonomic dysfunction; evidence of corticospinal tract dysfunction; cerebellar signs; stimulus-sensitive myoclonus; vocal cord paresis

nergic agonists (e.g., ropinirole) may reduce the subsequent risk of dopa-induced dyskinesias is controversial.

Several other agents have been used in early PD. The anticholinergics may be particularly useful in the treatment of tremor-predominant disease. Amantadine may be helpful for the early treatment of bradykinesia, rigidity, and gait disturbance. The selective mono-amine oxidase B inhibitor selegiline may also provide early symptomatic benefit. The catechol-O-methyl transferase inhibitors are the most recent addition to the antiparkinsonian armamentarium. They decrease removal of L-dopa and thereby augment its effects. The pharmacologic agents used in the treatment of PD are summarized in Table 16-2, and an approach to commonly encountered clinical scenarios is outlined in Table 16-3.

There has been a recent resurgence in lesioning and deep brain stimulation for the treatment of PD. These procedures target the motor thalamus, the internal segment of the globus pallidus, or the subthalamic nucleus.

KEY POINTS

- Idiopathic PD results from loss of dopaminergic neurons in the substantia nigra.
- The pathologic hallmark is the Lewy body.
- Tremor, rigidity, bradykinesia, and postural instability are the four cardinal symptoms.

DRUG-INDUCED MOVEMENT DISORDERS

Drugs with dopamine receptor–blocking activity have a particular propensity for inducing a variety of movement disorders, including akathisia, acute dystonic reactions, parkinsonism, tardive dyskinesia, and the neuroleptic malignant syndrome.

Neuroleptic malignant syndrome (NMS) is an uncommon disorder characterized by muscular rigidity, fever, autonomic lability, altered level of consciousness, elevated creatine kinase level, and leukocytosis. Treatment involves discontinuation of the offending agent, antipyretics, rehydration, and occasionally the use of bromocriptine or dantrolene.

Akathisia is a dysphoric state characterized by the subjective desire to be in constant motion and is often associated with an inability to sit or stand still. Anticholinergics and beta blockers have been used with the most success in the treatment of this disorder.

Tardive dyskinesia is an orolinguomasticatory dyskinesia that occurs as the most common (late and persistent) movement disorder complicating neuroleptic use. Commonly observed are chewing movements, lip smacking, and rolling of the tongue inside the mouth and up against the inside of the cheek. The limbs and trunk may also be affected. A history of the use of dopamine receptor–blocking drugs is essential to the diagnosis. The offending drug should be discontinued when possible; further therapeutic benefit may be obtained from dopamine-depleting agents such as reserpine and tetrabenazine. Some tardive dyskinesias remain unresponsive to any treatment.

■ TABLE 16-2 Pharmacologic Treatment of Parkinson Disease

Drug	Mechanism of Action	Dosing	Side Effects
Levodopa/carbidopa	Dopamine precursor/dopa decarboxylase inhibitor	Start with a half of a 25/100 tablet bid; increase dosage as needed; typically dosed 3 to 5 times a day	Anorexia, nausea, psychosis, hallucinations, orthostatic hypotension, dyskinesia
Trihexyphenidyl	Anticholinergic	Start with 1 mg at mealtime; increase to 2 mg tid as needed	Dry mouth, constipation, urinary retention, confusion, hallucinations, narrow-angle glaucoma
Benztropine	Anticholinergic	Start with 0.5 to 1 mg at bedtime; increase to 2 mg qid as needed	As above
Amantadine	NMDA antagonist	100 mg bid	Hallucinations, leg edema, livedo reticularis
Bromocriptine	Dopamine agonist	Start with a half 2.5-mg tablet bid; titrate gradually to 5 to 7.5 mg/day	Nausea, orthostatic hypotension, psychosis, hallucinations, dyskinesia
Pergolide	Dopamine agonist	Start with 0.05 mg/day; titrate gradually to 0.75 to 3 mg/day divided into three doses	As above
Pramipexole	Dopamine agonist	Start with 0.125 mg tid; titrate gradually to 1.5 mg tid	As above
Ropinirole	Dopamine agonist	Start with 0.25 mg tid; titrate gradually to 1 mg tid	As above
Tolcapone	COMT inhibitor	100 to 200 mg tid	Nausea, vomiting, insomnia, orthostatic hypotension, confusion, dyskinesia
Entacapone	COMT inhibitor	200 mg with each L-dopa dose	As above

bid, twice a day; quid, four times a day; tid, three times a day.

KEY POINTS

- Antipsychotics (haloperidol as well as the newer atypical agents) are the most common cause of drug-induced movement disorders.
- The propensity of a drug to cause these movement disorders is related to its D_2-receptor–blocking activity.

STIFF-PERSON SYNDROME

Stiff-person (or stiff-man) syndrome is a rare disorder characterized by fluctuating and progressive muscle rigidity with spasms. It may occur as an autoimmune or paraneoplastic process. Symptoms usually begin with stiffness of the axial and trunk muscles, with spread to the proximal limb muscles over time. Patients develop a lumbar

■ **TABLE 16-3** Therapeutic Strategies in Parkinson Disease	
Scenario/Problem	**Therapeutic Approach**
Initial treatment	Levodopa/decarboxylase inhibitor or dopamine agonist
Poor or no response to initial treatment	Increase dose and consider alternative diagnoses
Tremor-predominant disease	Anticholinergic or amantadine
Early-morning stiffness	Consider overnight controlled-release preparation of L-dopa
L-dopa–induced hallucinations	Discontinue concurrent therapy with anticholinergics, amantadine, selegiline, or dopamine agonists
	Decrease dose of levodopa
	Low-dose atypical antipsychotic
"Wearing off"	Combine levodopa and dopamine agonist
	Switch dopamine agonist
	Smaller doses, more frequent dosing
	Add anticholinergic
	Add COMT inhibitor
Dyskinesia	Reduce dose of levodopa
	Add or increase dose of dopamine agonist
	Change dopamine agonist
	Discontinue selegiline
	Add amantadine
	Consider surgery

hyperlordosis with restricted movements of the hip and spine that leads to the description of the gait as like that of a tin man. Superimposed on this background rigidity, they develop paroxysmal painful muscle spasms, often provoked by sudden movement or startle.

Diagnosis rests on the characteristic clinical profile and the demonstration of continuous motor unit activity without evidence of neuromyotonia, pyramidal or extrapyramidal dysfunction, or structural spinal cord disease. CSF is usually normal, and antibodies directed against glutamic acid decarboxylase (GAD) may be present.

Benzodiazepines and baclofen are the most useful antispasticity agents. The presence of anti-GAD antibodies and the occurrence of the stiff-man syndrome as a paraneoplastic syndrome have led some to use immunosuppressive therapy (steroids, plasmapheresis, or intravenous immunoglobulins), with varying success.

KEY POINTS

- Stiff-person syndrome is characterized by chronic axial muscle rigidity and stiffness with superimposed painful muscle spasms.
- Stiff-person syndrome may be associated with anti-GAD antibodies.

TREMOR

Tremor is an involuntary rhythmic oscillation of a body part (arm, leg, head, jaw, lips, or palate). Tremor is described as **resting** (present while the body part is not moving), **postural** (emerges during sustained maintenance of a posture), or **action** (appears during a voluntary movement). Action tremor may increase as the target is approached (**intention** tremor). Common

■ **BOX 16-1** Tremor
Resting
Idiopathic Parkinson disease
Other parkinsonian syndromes
Postural
Essential tremor
Physiological tremor
Drugs (e.g., theophylline, β-agonists)
Alcohol
Action
Cerebellum and cerebellar outflow tract dysfunction (e.g., infarction, multiple sclerosis, tumor, Wilson disease, drugs)

causes of the various types of tremors are summarized in Box 16-1.

Essential tremor (ET) is a condition in which postural tremor is the only symptom. It may begin at any age, develops insidiously, and progresses gradually. A family history is common but not invariable. ET almost always affects the hands but may also affect the head, face, voice, trunk, or legs. It is almost always bilateral. Improvement of the tremor with small quantities of alcohol is a characteristic feature. Primidone and propranolol are of proven benefit in the treatment of ET. Topiramate and gabapentin have also been used with some success.

KEY POINTS

- Tremor is an involuntary rhythmic oscillation of a body part.
- PD causes a resting tremor.
- Essential tremor is the most common cause of postural tremor.
- Action or intention tremor suggests disease of the cerebellum or its connections.

CHOREA

Chorea is defined as involuntary, abrupt, and irregular movements that flow as if randomly from one body part to another. Patients are often unaware of even severe chorea. One of the earliest symptoms may be clumsiness or incoordination. Involvement of bulbar muscles may cause dysarthria and dysphagia. Chorea is usually accompanied by an inability to maintain a sustained muscle contraction (motor impersistence). Classic examples include an inability to keep the tongue protruded (serpentine tongue) and the inability to maintain a tight handgrip (milkmaid grip).

There are many causes of chorea, and it is impossible to determine the etiology based simply on the phenomenology of the abnormal movements. It is necessary to consider the age and relative acuity of onset, the presence or absence of a family history, the presence of associated symptoms, and the distribution of the movements. The different causes are summarized in Box 16-2.

For treatment, haloperidol has been used with greatest success.

■ **BOX 16-2** Chorea
Hereditary
Huntington disease
Neuro-acanthocytosis
Wilson disease
Drugs
Neuroleptics
Antiparkinsonian medications
Toxins
Alcohol
Anoxia
Carbon monoxide
Metabolic
Hyperthyroidism
Hyperglycemia and hypoglycemia
Hepatocerebral degeneration
Pregnancy
Immunologic
Systemic lupus erythematosus
Poststreptococcal (Sydenham chorea)
Vascular
Caudate infarction or hemorrhage

KEY POINTS

- Chorea comprises involuntary, abrupt, and irregular movements that flow randomly from one body part to another.
- Huntington disease, poststreptococcal infection, systemic lupus erythematosus, thyrotoxicosis, and pregnancy are among the more common causes of chorea.

BALLISM

Ballism is defined as large-amplitude and poorly patterned flinging or flailing movements of a limb that are frequently unilateral (**hemiballismus**). It usually results from a contralateral lesion in the caudate, putamen, or subthalamic nucleus. Stroke is the most common cause. Hyperglycemia may also cause hemiballismus.

Dopamine-depleting and blocking agents are the most useful treatment. When ballism is severe, contralateral thalamotomy or pallidotomy may be beneficial.

DYSTONIA

Dystonia is sustained muscle contraction leading to repetitive twisting movements or abnormal postures. The dystonias are classified as idiopathic or symptomatic. Recognition of secondary or symptomatic causes of dystonia is important because this may influence treatment.

A characteristic feature of dystonic movements is that they may be diminished by sensory tricks such as gently touching the affected body part (**geste antagoniste**). Dystonic movements tend to be exacerbated by fatigue, stress, and emotional states and may be suppressed by relaxation and sleep. Dystonia typically worsens during voluntary movement. At the time of onset, dystonia may be present only during a specific movement (action dystonia). With progression, however, the dystonia may emerge with other movements and eventually may be present at rest. Thus, dystonia at rest usually represents a more severe form than a pure action dystonia. Early onset of dystonia at rest should raise suspicion of an underlying cause ("secondary"). Other clinical features suggesting that the dystonia is symptomatic include the presence of associated neurologic abnormalities or involvement of one side of the body only (hemidystonia).

Idiopathic torsion dystonia is a primary dystonia and may occur as a familial condition. The spectrum of the disorder is broad and includes focal (blepharospasm, torticollis, spasmodic dysphonia, writer's cramp), segmental, and generalized forms. The gene for the autosomal dominant familial form has been located on chromosome 9q, and mutations have been identified in the ATP-binding protein designated *torsin A*. Botulinum toxin is the treatment of choice.

Secondary causes of dystonia include metabolic disorders (e.g., Wilson disease), degenerative diseases (PD, progressive supranuclear palsy, corticobasal ganglionic degeneration, Huntington disease, multiple-system atrophy), and nondegenerative CNS disorders (anoxia, head or peripheral trauma, prior stroke, multiple sclerosis, or drug-induced).

KEY POINTS

- Dystonia is a sustained muscle contraction leading to repetitive twisting movements or abnormal postures.
- Idiopathic torsion dystonia is a familial condition that may manifest as torticollis, writer's cramp, blepharospasm, or spasmodic dysphonia.

MYOCLONUS

Myoclonus is a sudden lightning-like movement produced by abrupt and brief muscle contraction (positive myoclonus) or inhibition (negative myoclonus or asterixis).

The four etiologic categories are physiologic, essential, epileptic, and symptomatic. **Essential** myoclonus is a nonphysiologic variety that occurs in isolation without evidence of other neurologic symptoms or signs. It may occur in familial and sporadic forms. Some patients may note a striking improvement with small quantities of alcohol. The causes of the other varieties of myoclonus are summarized in Box 16-3.

Clonazepam and valproate are used with greatest success in the management of myoclonus.

■ BOX 16-3 Myoclonus

Physiologic
Hypnic jerks
Anxiety and exercise induced
Hiccups
Essential
Epileptic
Primary generalized epilepsies (e.g., juvenile myoclonic epilepsy)
Myoclonic epilepsies (often associated with encephalopathy or ataxia)
Symptomatic
Metabolic encephalopathy (uremia, liver failure, hypercapnia)
Wilson disease
Creutzfeldt-Jakob disease
Hypoxic brain injury

KEY POINTS

- Myoclonus is a sudden, lightning-like movement produced by abrupt and brief muscle contraction.
- Clonazepam is the most effective treatment for many patients.

TICS

Tics are abrupt, stereotyped, coordinated movements or vocalizations. They may vary in intensity and be repeated at irregular intervals. The individual will frequently describe an inner urge to move, may be able to suppress the movement temporarily at the expense of mounting inner tension, and then obtain relief from the performance of the movement or vocalization. Tics may be exacerbated by stress and relieved by distraction.

Tics may be motor or vocal and are classified as being either simple or complex. Examples of simple motor tics include eye blinking, shoulder shrugging, and toe curling. Spitting and finger cracking are examples of complex motor tics. Simple vocal tics may take the form of sniffing, throat clearing, snorting, or coughing. The best-recognized example of a complex vocal tic is coprolalia (involuntary obscene utterances). Tics may also be classified as idiopathic (the majority) or secondary. Secondary causes include head trauma, encephalitis, stroke, and various drugs.

Gille de la Tourette syndrome is a genetic disorder characterized by motor and vocal tics with onset in childhood. Boys are affected more than girls, although there is some suggestion that obsessive-compulsive disorder (OCD) may represent the phenotypic expression of the same genetic defect in girls. The motor and vocal tics may change over time. There is a trend toward periodic remission and exacerbation. In general, the disease is most active in adolescence and tends to diminish in severity during adulthood. There is an association with learning disability and OCD.

Pediatric autoimmune neurologic disorders associated with streptococcal infection (PANDAS) is a relatively recently described syndrome in which children develop exacerbation of tics, OCD, or both following a group A β-hemolytic streptococcal infection. The proposed, although unproved, etiology is that the streptococcal infection triggers an autoantibody response that cross-reacts with components of the basal ganglia in susceptible individuals.

For treatment of tics, dopamine antagonists (haloperidol or the atypical antipsychotics) are most effective. Because of the adverse effect profile of these agents, however, less potent drugs such as clonazepam and clonidine should be tried first.

KEY POINTS

- Tics are abrupt, stereotyped, coordinated movements or vocalizations.
- Gilles de la Tourette syndrome is a common genetic disorder with onset of motor and vocal tics in childhood.
- Dopamine antagonists are often the most effective therapy for tics.

WILSON DISEASE

Wilson disease (WD) is an autosomal recessive disorder of copper metabolism. The clinical presentation is usually with liver dysfunction and neuropsychiatric symptoms.

WD results from mutation of a copper-binding protein, dysfunction of which results in impaired conjugation of copper to ceruloplasmin and entry of copper into the biliary excretory pathway. This results in accumulation of copper within the liver and spillover into the systemic circulation, with deposition in the kidney, cornea, and CNS.

Neurologic manifestations of WD include tremor, ataxia, dysarthria, dyskinesia, parkinsonism, and cognitive dysfunction as well as disturbances of mood and personality. The Kayser-Fleischer ring is a golden brown or greenish discoloration in the limbic region of the cornea that results from copper deposition in Descemet's membrane. Kayser-Fleischer rings are almost invariably present in untreated patients with neurologic involvement.

In diagnosing WD, increased serum copper and decreased serum ceruloplasmin levels are expected but not always present. Increased 24-hour urinary copper excretion is the most sensitive screening test. Diagnosis may be confirmed by demonstrating increased copper staining on liver biopsy. Examination by an ophthalmologist for Kayser-Fleischer rings can be very helpful.

Copper chelation with D-penicillamine has been the traditional therapy for WD. More recently, there has been a trend toward using a less toxic chelator, trientine, in conjunction with zinc. Therapy is lifelong. Given the inherited nature of this disorder, family members of an affected individual should be screened.

PAROXYSMAL DYSKINESIAS

The paroxysmal dyskinesias are a rare group of movement disorders characterized by recurrent attacks of hyperkinesis with preserved consciousness. In paroxysmal kinesogenic choreoathetosis (PKC), episodes of chorea, athetosis, or dystonia are triggered by sudden movements and last for seconds to minutes. Attacks of paroxysmal (nonkinesogenic) dystonic choreoathetosis (PDC) are longer, lasting minutes to hours, and are triggered by alcohol, fatigue, and stress. In paroxysmal exercise-induced dystonia, episodes of dystonia are induced by sustained exercise and may persist for a number of hours. PKC is most effectively treated with agents such as carbamazepine.

 KEY POINTS

- Wilson disease is a disorder of copper metabolism.
- Hyperkinetic and hypokinetic movement disorders as well as cognitive, personality, and mood disturbances are the most common neurologic manifestations of WD.
- Kayser-Fleischer rings represent copper deposition in the cornea.
- Elevated serum copper levels, low ceruloplasmin levels, and elevated 24-hour urinary copper are useful screening tests.

Head Trauma

EPIDEMIOLOGY

Estimates of the annual number of head injuries in the United States range from 500,000 to 1.5 million, with the large majority being mild in severity. In young adults, motor vehicle accidents are the most common cause of head trauma, while in the elderly, falls are the most common cause. Men are more often the victims of head trauma than are women by a ratio of at least 2:1.

TYPES OF HEAD TRAUMAS

EPIDURAL HEMATOMA

An epidural hematoma is an accumulation of blood between the skull and dura mater. It is usually the result of a severe head injury with a temporal bone fracture and resulting laceration of the middle meningeal artery. Less frequently, laceration of the middle meningeal vein or a dural venous sinus may produce an epidural hematoma. The classical presentation of epidural hematoma is a "lucid interval" in which the patient has preserved consciousness immediately after the precipitating event, followed by a decline in the level of consciousness, with often rapid progression to coma as the hematoma enlarges. Brain herniation, especially uncal herniation (see later discussion), may develop as a result of this hematoma expansion. The characteristic CT appearance of an epidural hematoma is a lens-shaped hyperdense lesion between the skull and dura (see Fig. 17-1).

Surgical evacuation is required and, if performed in a timely fashion, can be lifesaving.

SUBDURAL HEMATOMA

A subdural hematoma is an accumulation of blood between the dura mater and brain. It results from tearing of bridging veins which connect the surface of the brain and the dural sinuses. Subdural hematoma may have both acute and chronic presentations. Acute subdural hematoma develops immediately after head trauma and can be life-threatening. Headache is the most common symptom, with contralateral hemiparesis, seizures, and a wide variety of cortical dysfunction also common. If sufficiently large, a subdural hematoma can produce increased intracranial pressure with a resulting alteration in the level of consciousness. The CT scan in Figure 17-2 shows a crescent-shaped hyperdensity overlying the brain surface and underlying the skull. Subdural hematoma can be distinguished from an epidural hematoma by its ability to cross suture lines. Acute subdural hematoma may require treatment with surgical drainage depending on the severity and progression of the clinical deficit.

Chronic subdural hematoma typically develops after mild head trauma, and is more common in the elderly, particularly those who are anticoagulated. Like the acute variety, chronic subdural hematoma results in a variety of neurologic symptoms, including hemiparesis, seizures, and behavioral changes. A chronic subdural hematoma may resolve on its own; indications for operation include rapidly expanding

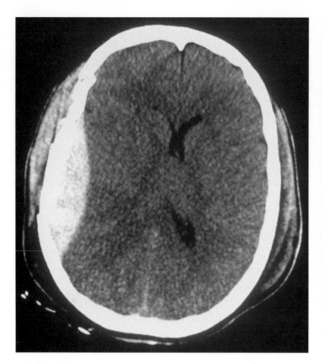

Figure 17-1 • CT scan of the head demonstrating the typical hyperdense lens-shaped appearance of an epidural hematoma.
(Courtesy of David M. Dawson, MD, Brigham and Women's Hospital, Boston, MA.)

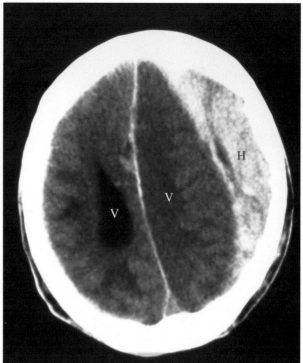

Figure 17-2 • Typical CT scan appearance of a large subdural hematoma (H) on the left cerebral hemisphere with compression of the lateral ventricle (V) and shift of the midline.
(Reproduced with permission from Armstrong P, Wastie M, Rockall A. *Diagnostic Imaging*, 5th ed. Oxford: Blackwell Publishing, 2004:416.)

lesions and progressive clinical deficits. Anticoagulation should be discontinued to offer the best chance of resolution.

CONCUSSION

A concussion is an alteration or loss of consciousness produced by head trauma. The symptoms of a concussion are the result of a functional rather than a structural change, and brain imaging studies are typically normal. Patients usually have short periods of amnesia for events that occurred before the injury (retrograde amnesia) and for learning new material after the incident (anterograde amnesia). The severity of a concussion can be gauged by the duration of the loss of consciousness and amnesia. Other consequences of concussion include headache, disorientation, dizziness and vertigo, nausea, and cortical blindness. Concussions are frequent in sporting events, particularly in children. Guidelines have been established by the American Academy of Neurology to determine the severity of a concussion and to determine when an athlete can return to competition:

- Children with no loss of consciousness and concussion symptoms for less than 15 minutes may return to play.
- Children with no loss of consciousness and concussion symptoms for more than 15 minutes may return to play in 1 week.
- Children with loss of consciousness should be transported to a hospital for overnight observation; they may return to play in 1 week if loss of consciousness was brief (seconds), or in 2 weeks if loss of consciousness was longer in duration.

DIFFUSE AXONAL INJURY

Diffuse axonal injury is associated with severe head trauma and may be seen on CT as multiple areas of punctate hemorrhage in the deep white matter and corpus callosum (Fig. 17-3). The presence of diffuse axonal injury is usually associated with poor prognosis.

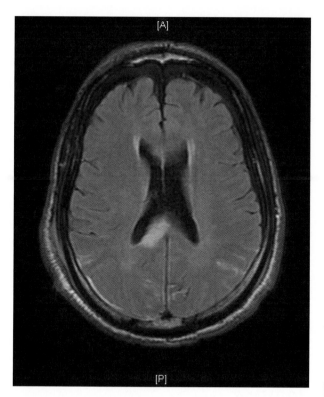

Figure 17-3 • Diffuse axonal injury on CT.

POSTCONCUSSION SYNDROME

Postconcussion syndrome is usually the consequence of mild traumatic brain injury. The source of the syndrome is unclear, but structural, biochemical, and psychogenic components have been implicated. Features of the syndrome include headache, dizziness, sleep disturbance, cognitive impairment, and behavioral abnormalities such as irritability. Most patients with the syndrome have normal neuroimaging studies. Pending litigation or workers' compensation issues and depression are associated with prolonged postconcussion syndrome. Treatment should address the individual components of the syndrome: headache, sleep disturbance, and psychological problems, including with mood.

POSTTRAUMATIC SEIZURES AND EPILEPSY

Seizures after head trauma can be divided into early (within 1 week of head trauma) and late (beginning 1 week or more later). Approximately 25% of patients

with acute severe head injury (characterized by intracranial hematoma or depressed skull fracture, without regard to the duration of loss of consciousness or posttraumatic amnesia) will have early posttraumatic seizures, most often generalized tonic-clonic seizures. Of these, 25% go on to develop epilepsy (recurrent unprovoked seizures). Antiepileptic drugs reduce the incidence of early seizures, but will not change the overall risk for the later development of epilepsy.

Overall, posttraumatic epilepsy occurs in about 2% of patients with head trauma, with higher frequencies in patients with severe head injuries. Approximately 50% of patients who develop posttraumatic epilepsy will do so within 1 year. Patients who have a single late seizure (defined as a seizure with onset more than 1 week after head trauma) usually require treatment with anticonvulsants, as they are at high risk for the development of posttraumatic epilepsy.

KEY POINTS

- Epidural hematoma is usually caused by laceration of the middle meningeal artery, and is often clinically associated with a "lucid interval."
- Subdural hematoma is usually caused by tearing of bridging veins, and can be associated with a variety of neurologic deficits.
- Concussion is a loss or alteration of consciousness produced by head injury, and usually has normal neuroimaging.
- The components of the postconcussion syndrome include headache, dizziness, cognitive impairment, and behavioral abnormalities.
- Treatment of early posttraumatic seizures does not alter the long-term chance of developing epilepsy.

HERNIATION SYNDROMES

Brain herniation is a life-threatening condition which occurs when increased intracranial pressure causes a shift of brain contents, resulting in compression of brain parenchyma and ventricles, and, compromise of cerebral blood vessels.

CENTRAL (TRANSTENTORIAL) HERNIATION

Diffuse cerebral edema or a large intracranial mass may cause downward herniation of the diencephalon through the tentorial notch. The first stage of the central herniation syndrome is heralded by a decrease in the level of alertness. This change in alertness is accompanied or shortly followed by small, reactive pupils, due to disruption of sympathetic pathways from the hypothalamus. As central herniation proceeds, the patient often assumes a decorticate posture upon stimulation. Progressive herniation leads to midbrain compression, with fixed midposition pupils and decerebrate posturing. In the final stage, the patient becomes motionless to stimulation, with eventual progression to death.

UNCAL HERNIATION

Uncal herniation is most often produced by the expansion of a mass located laterally within the brain, resulting in a medial shift of the uncus of the temporal lobe. Uncal herniation may be preceded by neurologic deficits, particularly hemiparesis, related to the mass itself. As the brain begins to shift away from the mass, the first clinical deficit is often an ipsilateral third nerve palsy. This may be accompanied or followed in short order by an impairment of consciousness. Continued uncal herniation produces compression of the contralateral cerebral peduncle against the free edge of the tentorium with a resulting hemiplegia *ipsilateral* to the herniating uncus, the Kernohan's notch phenomenon. Alternatively, compression of the posterior cerebral artery may produce medial temporal lobe or occipital lobe ischemia or infarction. As signs of herniation appear, neurologic deterioration may be rapid and often irreversible.

SUBFALCINE HERNIATION

Expansile frontal lobe masses may produce herniation of the cingulate gyrus beneath the falx cerebri. Most often, the patient has been symptomatic from the frontal lobe mass, and subfalcine herniation may not alter the clinical picture appreciably, though compression of the anterior cerebral arteries may result in leg weakness.

KEY POINTS

- A dilated pupil ipsilateral to the side of a mass region is an early sign of uncal herniation.
- Uncal herniation is also associated with an ipsilateral hemiplegia due to compression of the contralateral cerebral peduncle against the free edge of the tentorium.

INITIAL ASSESSMENT OF HEAD TRAUMA

Head trauma may be life-threatening, and careful attention to the patient's airway, breathing, and circulation are essential to its initial management. Once life support is assured, the neurologic aspects of head trauma can be addressed by clinical examination and CT scan. One tool for grading the severity of traumatic brain injury is the Glasgow Coma Scale (Table 17-1). Scores of 13 to 15 are classified as mild head injury, 8 to 12 moderate, and 3 to 7 severe. Limitations of the Glasgow Coma Scale include inaccuracy in assessment of patients who are already intubated and sedated, and a lack of utility in tracking serial changes. Also, while the GCS assesses the severity of coma, it does not assist with diagnosis of the cause of coma.

■ **TABLE 17-1** Glasgow Coma Scale			
Points	**Best Eye Opening**	**Best Verbal**	**Best Motor**
6	—	—	Obeys commands
5	—	Oriented	Localizes pain
4	Spontaneous	Confused	Withdraws to pain
3	To speech	Inappropriate	Decorticate posturing
2	To pain	Incomprehensible	Decerebrate posturing
1	None	None	None

MANAGEMENT OF INCREASED INTRACRANIAL PRESSURE

In adults, normal intracranial pressure (ICP) is <15 mm Hg. Because the skull is a rigid container, the total volume of its three components (brain, blood vessels, and cerebrospinal fluid) is fixed and does not leave room for expansion. Change in the volume of one of these compartments can compromise the status of the other two. In patients with head trauma, intracranial masses, or other causes of cerebral edema, ICP monitoring may be necessary to determine whether cerebral perfusion pressure (CPP) is adequate. CPP is defined as the difference between the mean arterial pressure and ICP. A goal CPP is between 60 and 75 mm Hg: excessively high CPP can cause hypertensive encephalopathy and cerebral edema, while lower pressures may result in diffuse cerebral ischemia. ICP monitoring, usually in the form of an intraventricular pressure monitor, should be considered in any head injury patient with a Glasgow Coma Score of <9 and an abnormal head CT.

Correction of the proximate cause of increased ICP, whether by resection of a tumor or drainage of a hematoma, is the most effective therapy. There are situations, however, in which this is not possible, and other treatments for increased ICP must be employed. The first and easiest step to reduce ICP is to elevate the head of the bed, usually to 30 degrees, in order to improve venous drainage. Hyperventilation to a PCO_2 between 25 and 30 mm Hg can be useful in the short term: low PCO_2 results in vasoconstriction, reducing cerebral blood volume and ICP, but prolonged hyperventilation (and therefore low PCO_2) increases the risk for cerebral infarction. Mannitol, an osmotic diuretic, or hypertonic saline, may be used to lower ICP. Sedation with barbiturates may be used to reduce cerebral metabolism, but prolonged use can have complications. Drainage of CSF with a ventricular drain may be employed to reduce ICP. Hypothermia for elevated ICP is employed in clinical trials, but cannot be recommended in a routine clinical setting, as the complications of therapeutic hypothermia can outweigh the established benefits. As stated earlier, correction of the cause of increased ICP is the definitive therapy, and in some cases, this may require hemicraniectomy to expand the volume available for the intracranial contents.

KEY POINTS

- Cerebral perfusion pressure is defined as the difference between mean arterial pressure and intracranial pressure.
- Increased intracranial pressure is best treated by addressing its proximate cause.
- Elevation of the head of the bed, hyperventilation, and use of mannitol or hypertonic saline are short-term measures that may be helpful in the treatment of increased intracranial pressure.

Systemic and Metabolic Disorders

The CNS and peripheral nervous system may be affected by a range of systemic and metabolic diseases. A few of these disorders have been selected for more detailed description in this chapter. Table 18-1 summarizes the more common neurologic manifestations of some systemic disorders that are not discussed below.

HEPATIC ENCEPHALOPATHY

"Hepatic encephalopathy" is a general term used to describe the altered mental state that accompanies liver failure. It encompasses two entities: the encephalopathy of fulminant hepatic failure and the portosystemic encephalopathy that is associated with cirrhosis and portal hypertension or that may develop following portacaval shunting.

CLINICAL MANIFESTATIONS

The encephalopathy of fulminant hepatic failure progresses rapidly, within days, from mild inattention to stupor and coma. The essential feature of portosystemic encephalopathy is the presence of waxing and waning cerebral dysfunction in the setting of liver failure. Traditionally, hepatic encephalopathy is graded in severity on a scale from 0 (normal) to 4 (coma). The intermediate stages are characterized by impaired attention and concentration, altered sleep patterns, abnormal visuospatial perception, and subtle personality changes. Asterixis (negative myoclonus) is usually present. Other neurologic findings may include increased muscle tone, hyperreflexia, and extensor plantar responses.

PATHOGENESIS

The pathophysiology of hepatic encephalopathy is incompletely understood but is thought to result from the accumulation of neurotoxic substances (e.g., ammonia), leading to increased brain glutamine concentrations, depressed glutamatergic neurotransmission, and increased expression of the peripheral-type benzodiazepine receptors. Manganese deposition in the basal ganglia may also play a pathogenic role.

PATHOLOGY

The Alzheimer type II astrocyte is the pathologic hallmark of this disorder. These astrocytes appear to be metabolically hyperactive, which has led to the suggestion that hepatic encephalopathy is a primary astrocytopathy.

DIAGNOSTIC EVALUATION

The diagnosis is usually suspected clinically on the basis of the encephalopathy in the context of liver failure. Hepatic synthetic function is impaired, with low serum albumin and prolonged prothrombin time (PT) and partial thromboplastin time (PTT). The EEG usually shows background slowing and may demonstrate triphasic waves, and MRI may reveal increased T1 signal in the basal ganglia, but these findings are not specific. In a patient with known liver disease who develops encephalopathy, it is important to identify underlying precipitating factors such as gastrointestinal hemorrhage, infection, increased dietary protein intake, drugs, constipation, or hypokalemia.

■ **TABLE 18-1** Neurologic Manifestations of Systemic Disease	
Disease	**Manifestations**
Polyarteritis nodosa	Mononeuropathy multiplex, seizures, stroke
Churg-Strauss	Mononeuropathy multiplex, encephalopathy, stroke, chorea
Giant cell arteritis	Headache, blindness, polyneuropathy, stroke
Wegener granulomatosis	Mononeuropathy multiplex, cranial neuropathy, basal meningitis
Rheumatoid arthritis	Myelopathy
Sjögren syndrome	Sensory polyneuropathy
Behçet disease	Aseptic meningoencephalitis
Cryoglobulinemia	Transient ischemic attack, stroke, peripheral neuropathy
Disseminated intravascular coagulation	Encephalopathy
Thrombotic thrombocytopenic purpura	Encephalopathy, seizures, stroke
Whipple disease	Dementia, seizures, myoclonus, ataxia, supranuclear ophthalmoplegia, oculomasticatory myorhythmia

TREATMENT

Treatment should be directed toward the underlying cause of the liver disease when possible and to the alleviation of precipitating factors. Lactulose, titrated to produce two to three stools per day, is the mainstay of symptomatic therapy.

KEY POINTS

- The essential feature of portosystemic encephalopathy is the presence of waxing and waning cerebral dysfunction in the setting of liver failure.
- Asterixis is frequently present.
- Hepatic encephalopathy is thought to be a primary astrocytopathy.
- Lactulose and the treatment of precipitating factors are the mainstays of therapy.

NEUROSARCOIDOSIS

Sarcoidosis is a multisystem granulomatous disorder of unknown etiology. Pulmonary disease is most common, and involvement of the nervous system occurs in around 5% of cases. It is very uncommon for sarcoidosis to involve the nervous system in the absence of other systemic disease.

CLINICAL MANIFESTATIONS

Sarcoidosis may involve almost any part of the CNS or the peripheral nervous system. Cranial neuropathy due to chronic basal meningitis is the most common presentation of neurosarcoidosis, with the facial and optic nerves most frequently affected. Facial neuropathy may also occur due to parotid inflammation. Visual changes are common and may be due to direct involvement of the optic nerve or its meningeal covering or to uveitis. Raised intracranial pressure with papilledema may result from a space-occupying lesion, diffuse meningeal involvement, or hydrocephalus. Meningoencephalitis may manifest itself with cognitive and affective symptoms, and hypothalamic involvement may cause hypopituitarism, diabetes insipidus, sleep disturbance, obesity, and thermoregulatory disturbance. Space-occupying lesions may become apparent because of seizures or focal deficits. Myelopathy may result from an infiltrating or focal granulomatous process. Peripheral nerve involvement may become manifest as a symmetric distal polyneuropathy or mononeuropathy multiplex.

PATHOLOGY

The typical pathology is that of noncaseating granulomata.

DIAGNOSTIC EVALUATION

Definitive diagnosis of neurosarcoidosis requires positive histology from affected tissue. Since there is often reluctance to obtain brain parenchymal or meningeal biopsy, the diagnosis is often presumptive, based on a consistent clinical presentation and histology from an alternative site. CSF is frequently abnormal, with elevated protein and lymphocytic pleocytosis, but it may be normal in the context of focal parenchymal disease. Serum angiotensin converting enzyme (ACE) concentration may be elevated. CSF ACE levels are often difficult to interpret in the context of elevated CSF protein. MRI may demonstrate white matter lesions, hydrocephalus, parenchymal mass lesion, nodular meningeal enhancement, or involvement of the optic nerve or spinal cord.

TREATMENT

Steroids are the mainstay of therapy. Although used often, there are limited data regarding the use of steroid-sparing agents such as methotrexate and azathioprine.

KEY POINTS

- Sarcoidosis is a multisystem granulomatous disorder.
- The nervous system is mostly affected in conjunction with systemic disease, but it may be affected in isolation.
- Cranial neuropathy and basal meningitis are common.

DIABETES MELLITUS

Diabetes mellitus is common in patients with neurologic disease, primarily because the nervous system is susceptible to the damaging effects of impaired glycemic control. However, there are also a number of disorders that are characterized by both diabetes and neurologic symptoms. These include mitochondrial diseases, myotonic dystrophy, Friedreich ataxia, and the stiff-man syndrome.

Peripheral neuropathy is the most common complication of diabetes mellitus and takes many forms (Box 18-1). Distal symmetric sensory polyneuropathy

BOX 18-1 Diabetic Neuropathies
Hyperglycemic neuropathy
Generalized neuropathies
Distal symmetric predominantly sensory polyneuropathy
Autonomic neuropathy
Chronic inflammatory demyelinating polyradiculoneuropathy (CIDP)
Focal neuropathies
Cranial neuropathies (especially III, IV, and VI)
Thoracolumbar radiculopathy
Focal compression and entrapment neuropathies
Proximal diabetic neuropathy (diabetic amyotrophy)
Mononeuropathy multiplex

is the most common. Onset of this neuropathy is insidious, and it may often be asymptomatic. There is a predilection for involvement of small myelinated and unmyelinated fibers, with the result that loss of temperature and pinprick sensation are the most commonly reported symptoms. There may be associated distal motor neuropathy, but it is invariably minor. Once established, this neuropathy is largely irreversible. The incidence of this complication is reduced in type 1 diabetic patients by strict glycemic control. There is frequently an associated autonomic neuropathy, the common symptoms of which include gustatory sweating, orthostatic hypotension, diarrhea, and impotence. Neurogenic bladder and gastroparesis occur less frequently.

Focal peripheral neuropathies also occur more commonly in diabetic patients. These include cranial neuropathies (most commonly affecting cranial nerves III, IV, and VI) and focal compression neuropathies, such as distal median neuropathies (carpal tunnel) and meralgia paresthetica (compression of the lateral cutaneous nerve of the thigh). Radiculopathy, especially thoracic, occurs with greater frequency in diabetic patients. Typically, these radiculopathies manifest with nonradicular pain, truncal sensory loss, and focal weakness of the muscles of the anterior abdominal wall. Spontaneous recovery usually occurs within a few months.

The entity of proximal diabetic neuropathy is well recognized but poorly understood. Another term that has been used to describe at least some of the patients with this disorder is **diabetic amyotrophy**. At least

■ **TABLE 18-2** Effects of Alcohol on the Nervous System	
Condition	**Manifestations**
Peripheral neuropathy	Distal sensorimotor axonal neuropathy; recovery with abstinence is slow and incomplete
Cerebellar degeneration	Gait ataxia greater than limb ataxia, dysarthria, no nystagmus
Tobacco-alcohol amblyopia	Insidious and painless loss of vision; centrocecal scotoma
Marchiafava-Bignami syndrome	Frontal-type dementia, seizures, and pyramidal signs; focal demyelination and necrosis of corpus callosum
Acute intoxication	Impaired cognition, ataxia, dysarthria, nystagmus, diplopia
Acute withdrawal	Agitation, insomnia, tremulousness, hallucinations, seizures
Wernicke's encephalopathy	Confusion, ataxia, ophthalmoplegia
Korsakoff's syndrome	Isolated memory disturbance with confabulation

some of these proximal neuropathies are immune-mediated, perhaps involving a vasculitis, and respond to treatment with steroids and other immunosuppressive therapies. Finally, chronic inflammatory demyelinating polyradiculoneuropathy (CIDP) occurs more commonly in patients with diabetes.

Hyperglycemia may affect both the peripheral nervous system and the CNS. There is a syndrome of an acute distal sensory neuropathy that presents with dysesthesias and pain in the feet. This typically resolves with establishment of the euglycemic state. Nonketotic hyperglycemia (common in type 2 diabetes mellitus) may produce lethargy and drowsiness as well as focal or generalized seizures. An uncommon manifestation of nonketotic hyperglycemia is a syndrome of dystonia and chorea associated with reversible T1 signal hyperintensity in the basal ganglia. Finally, cerebral edema may complicate diabetic ketoacidosis. Children are particularly susceptible to this potentially fatal complication.

Many of the symptoms of hypoglycemia are referable to the nervous system, including headache, blurred vision, dysarthria, confusion, seizures, and coma. Repeated episodes of hypoglycemia may produce injury to the anterior horn cells of the spinal cord and result in a syndrome similar to amyotrophic lateral sclerosis. Recurrent and prolonged hypoglycemia may also lead to the development of permanent cognitive deficits.

Cerebrovascular disease (TIAs and stroke) is more common in diabetic patients, with hypertension being the main risk factor for stroke among patients with diabetes. Most ischemic strokes in diabetic patients are due to intracranial small vessel disease (lacunar stroke).

 KEY POINTS

- Distal, primarily sensory polyneuropathy is the most common neurologic complication of diabetes.
- Hyperglycemia may cause seizures, focal neurologic deficit, transient painful peripheral neuropathy, and occasionally chorea.
- Stroke occurs more commonly in diabetic patients.

ALCOHOL AND NUTRITIONAL DISORDERS

Alcohol may affect the nervous system adversely in many ways (Table 18-2), and the manifestations of vitamin deficiency (Table 18-3) are frequently associated with alcoholism. Two of the better-known syndromes that result from alcohol abuse and

■ **TABLE 18-3** Vitamin Deficiency Syndromes	
Symptom	**Deficient Vitamin**
Confusion and encephalopathy	Thiamine, niacin
Dementia	Vitamin B_{12}, folate, niacin
Seizures	Pyridoxine, niacin
Ataxia	Vitamin E, niacin
Myelopathy	Vitamins B_{12} and E, niacin
Peripheral neuropathy	Thiamine, pyridoxine, vitamins B_{12}, and E, niacin

vitamin deficiency are presented in more detail below.

WERNICKE'S ENCEPHALOPATHY AND KORSAKOFF'S SYNDROME

Wernicke's encephalopathy and Korsakoff's syndrome are related conditions that represent different stages of the same pathologic process. Wernicke's encephalopathy is characterized by the clinical triad of ophthalmoplegia, (truncal) ataxia, and confusion developing over a period of days to weeks. Associated signs and symptoms include impaired pupillary light response, hypothermia, postural hypotension, and other evidence of nutritional deficiency. The syndrome results from a deficiency of thiamine and may be precipitated by the administration of intravenous glucose. It is a clinical diagnosis and warrants immediate therapy with intravenous thiamine. Untreated, the condition is progressive and the mortality is high. Following the administration of thiamine, the ocular signs can resolve within hours and the confusion over days to weeks. The gait ataxia may persist. Once the global confusion has receded, isolated memory deficits may persist (Korsakoff's syndrome).

SUBACUTE COMBINED DEGENERATION OF THE SPINAL CORD

Subacute combined degeneration of the spinal cord results from vitamin B_{12} deficiency and derives its name from the degeneration of the posterior and lateral white matter tracts of the spinal cord. The clinical manifestations reflect disease within the dorsal columns and the lateral corticospinal tracts. The presentation is usually with insidious onset of paresthesias in the hands and feet. With time, weakness and spasticity may develop in the legs. Frequently, there is an associated large-fiber peripheral neuropathy (also due to the B_{12} deficiency, but typically, hematologic abdormalities occur without neurologic deficits). Hematologic abnormalities (macrocytic anemia) are variably present. Normal serum B_{12} levels do not preclude the diagnosis, and it may be necessary to measure levels of serum homocysteine and methylmalonic acid, the precursors of B_{12} (which are elevated when B_{12} is deficient). With B_{12} replacement therapy, partial improvement may be expected. Since folate is a necessary component to

the B_{12} synthetic pathway, its deficiency (theoretically) may cause the same deficits as B_{12} deficiency, but typically, hematologic abnormalities occur without neurologic deficits.

KEY POINTS

- Wernicke's encephalopathy is characterized by the triad of confusion, ataxia, and ophthalmoplegia.
- Subacute combined degeneration of the spinal cord refers to the damaging effects of vitamin B_{12} deficiency on the posterior and lateral columns of the spinal cord.

SYSTEMIC LUPUS ERYTHEMATOSUS

Systemic lupus erythematosus (SLE) is an inflammatory connective tissue disorder of unknown etiology. It occurs predominantly in young women, and neurologic involvement is common.

CLINICAL MANIFESTATIONS

The neurologic manifestations of SLE are diverse, with both the peripheral nervous system and CNS affected. Neuropsychiatric manifestations, including psychosis and affective disorders, are most common, although their pathophysiology remains uncertain. Stroke, both venous and arterial, may result from the hypercoagulable state associated with antiphospholipid antibodies. Chorea and transverse myelitis may occur similarly in association with antiphospholipid antibodies. Headaches and seizures are other important symptoms of CNS dysfunction in SLE. The most common manifestation of peripheral nervous system involvement is a distal symmetric sensory polyneuropathy, although a mononeuropathy multiplex due to vasculitis may also occur.

DIAGNOSTIC EVALUATION

The recognition that neurologic dysfunction is due to SLE is greatly facilitated by the presence of concurrent systemic manifestations (including but not limited to symmetric small joint arthritis, characteristic malar rash, proteinuria, etc.). Antinuclear antibody (ANA) titers are elevated in most patients with SLE. Isolated CNS lupus, manifesting with psychosis or depression, can be extremely difficult to recognize, as there is no diagnostic test.

TREATMENT

Treatment may be symptomatic (e.g., anticonvulsants for seizures) or directed at the underlying immune/inflammatory process. The decision to use immunosuppressant therapy depends on the severity of the disease but is usually warranted for neurologic manifestations. Corticosteroids, often in conjunction with cyclophosphamide, are the mainstay of therapy.

KEY POINTS

- Neuropsychiatric manifestations of SLE, including psychosis and depression, are most common.
- Other manifestations of CNS involvement include seizures, stroke, headache, chorea, and transverse myelitis.
- Distal sensory polyneuropathy is the most common manifestation of peripheral nervous system involvement.

ANTIPHOSPHOLIPID SYNDROME

The antiphospholipid syndrome (APS) is a disorder in which venous or arterial thrombosis, recurrent fetal loss, and thrombocytopenia are associated with elevated titers of antibodies directed against phospholipids. The presence of these antibodies may be demonstrated by solid-phase immunoassay (e.g., anticardiolipin antibody) or by the in vitro prolongation of the partial thromboplastin time (lupus anticoagulant). The APS may occur in isolation (primary APS) or in association with an underlying autoimmune disorder, most commonly systemic lupus erythematosus (secondary APS). Involvement of the nervous system is not uncommon in the antiphospholipid syndrome.

CLINICAL MANIFESTATIONS

Most thrombotic episodes in patients with antiphospholipid antibodies are venous, but when thrombosis does occur in the arterial circulation, the brain is most commonly affected. Both small- and large-vessel stroke have been reported, and cardiac embolism may result in embolic stroke. In Sneddon syndrome, cerebral ischemia and livedo reticularis are associated.

DIAGNOSTIC EVALUATION

Antiphospholipid antibodies should be sought in young patients with stroke or in those with otherwise unexplained stroke, especially if any of the other features of the antiphospholipid syndrome are present. Diagnosis requires the demonstration of high-titer IgG antiphospholipid antibodies on two occasions at least 6 weeks apart.

TREATMENT

Long-term anticoagulation with warfarin to achieve an international normalized ratio (INR) of three to four is the recommended therapy.

KEY POINTS

- Venous and arterial thrombosis, recurrent fetal loss, and thrombocytopenia are the major features of the antiphospholipid syndrome.
- "Antiphospholipid antibody" is a general term that encompasses the lupus anticoagulant, anticardiolipin antibodies, and antibodies directed against a mixture of various phospholipids.
- Anticoagulation is the treatment of choice for antiphospholipid-associated stroke.

THYROID DISEASE AND THE NERVOUS SYSTEM

The nervous system is more commonly affected by hypothyroidism than by hyperthyroidism.

■ **BOX 18-2** Neurologic Manifestations of Hypothyroidism

Mental state: Poor concentration and memory, dementia, psychosis, coma
Seizures
Headaches: Pseudotumor cerebri
Cranial nerves: Papilledema, ptosis, tonic pupil, trigeminal neuralgia, facial palsy, tinnitus, hearing loss
Cerebellar ataxia: Truncal and gait ataxia more than limb ataxia; dysarthria; nystagmus
Muscles: Cramps, pain and stiffness; proximal more than distal; creatine kinase level may be markedly increased
Neuromuscular junction: Worsening of myasthenia gravis
Nerves: Entrapment neuropathy (e.g., carpal tunnel), axonal polyneuropathy (improves with thyroxine replacement); delayed relaxation of deep tendon reflexes
Sleep apnea: Obstructive and central

Neurologic signs and symptoms are very rarely the only manifestations of thyroid disease. The periodic paralyses and proximal myopathy associated with the hyperthyroid state are discussed in Chapter 24. Seizures, chorea, and dysthyroid eye disease may also result from hyperthyroidism, and there is an association with myasthenia gravis. The range of neurologic manifestations of hypothyroidism is summarized in Box 18-2.

CENTRAL PONTINE MYELINOLYSIS

Central pontine myelinolysis is a rare demyelinating disorder that occurs most often in alcoholic patients and may be precipitated by too rapid correction of hyponatremia. As the name indicates, the pons is most commonly affected, but the basal ganglia, thalamus, and subcortical white matter may also be involved. The clinical presentation includes an acute confusional state, spastic quadriparesis, locked-in syndrome, dysarthria, and dysphagia.

Central Nervous System Tumors

The most common tumors in the central nervous system (CNS) are metastases from distant neoplasms. Primary brain tumors (PBT) are a heterogeneous group of neoplasms originating from CNS tissue and meninges and range from benign to aggressive. They can occur anywhere in the intracranial space and are named according to their cellular origin and histologic appearance. In adults, 70% of PBT are supratentorial, and of those, 80% to 90% are gliomas and meningiomas. The remaining 30% of PBT are infratentorial: medulloblastoma, cerebellar astrocytoma, brainstem glioma, and ependymoma in children, and schwannoma, hemangioblastoma, and meningioma in adults. In children, approximately 70% of PBT are infratentorial. Table 19-1 is a condensed version of the World Health Organization classification of PBT.

EPIDEMIOLOGY

About 18,000 new cases of PBT are reported in the United States every year—the most common solid malignancy in childhood, the second leading cause of cancer death in children, and the fifth in adults. Metastatic lesions occur in 100,000 to 200,000 cases per year and account for 20% of cancer deaths annually. PBT are more common in males than in females (ratio 1.5:1), except for meningioma (1:1.8). Tumors of cranial and spinal nerves have a similar gender distribution to those of PBT. Survival depends on the age of the patient, histologic subtype of the tumor, Karnofsky performance status (a measure of functional independence) and presenting symptoms.

CAUSES AND GENETICS

Primary brain tumors generally originate from genetic disruptions in cells, causing them to bypass normal growth regulatory mechanisms, with simultaneous evasion of the immune system. Some brain tumors have a strong hereditary component (Table 19-2).

Ionizing radiation use in therapeutic dosages has been associated with an increased risk of meningiomas, astrocytomas, and sarcomas. The use of mobile phones, low-frequency electromagnetic fields, specific infections (various viruses, *Toxoplasma gondii*, etc.), diet (nitrates, aspartame), tobacco, alcohol, and history of head trauma have not been validated in epidemiologic studies as risk factors for CNS tumors.

CLINICAL FEATURES

There are no specific clinical symptoms or signs of brain tumors. The clinical presentation depends on the location of the tumor, the rate of growth, and the degree of invasion of surrounding structures. Tumors can mimic many other CNS disorders and should be considered part of the differential diagnosis of almost any neurologic dysfunction. In general, tumor symptoms tend to present as progressive nonremitting neurologic symptoms. Nonetheless, a tumor can present as an acute, subacute, or chronic neurologic problem. The most common symptoms include *headaches* as the result of traction of pain-sensitive structures (arteries and veins) or from increased intracranial pressure; focal or generalized *seizures*, particularly when tumors infiltrate the cortex; and *altered mental status* such as

■ TABLE 19-1 World Health Organization Brain Tumor Classification (1993)

Neuroepithelial Tumors of the CNS

1. Astrocytic tumors
   1. Astrocytoma (WHO grade II)
   2. Anaplastic (malignant) astrocytoma (WHO grade III)
   3. Glioblastoma multiforme (WHO grade IV)
   4. Pilocytic astrocytoma (noninvasive, WHO grade I)
   5. Subependymal giant cell astrocytoma (noninvasive, WHO grade I)
2. Oligodendroglial tumors
   1. Oligodendroglioma (WHO grade II)
   2. Anaplastic (malignant) oligodendroglioma (WHO grade III)
3. Ependymal cell tumors
   1. Ependymoma (WHO grade II)
   2. Anaplastic ependymoma (WHO grade III)
   3. Myxopapillary ependymoma
   4. Subependymoma (WHO grade I)
4. Mixed gliomas
   1. Mixed oligoastrocytoma (WHO grade II)
   2. Anaplastic (malignant) oligoastrocytoma (WHO grade III)
   3. Others (e.g., ependymo-astrocytomas)
5. Tumors of the choroid plexus
   1. Choroid plexus papilloma
   2. Choroid plexus carcinoma
6. Neuronal and mixed neuronal-glial tumors
   1. Gangliocytoma
   2. Ganglioglioma
   3. Anaplastic (malignant) ganglioglioma

7. Pineal parenchymal tumors
   1. Pineocytoma
   2. Pineoblastoma
   3. Mixed pineocytoma/pineoblastoma
8. Tumors with neuroblastic or glioblastic elements (embryonal tumors)
   1. Medulloepithelioma
   2. Medulloblastoma
   3. Neuroblastoma
   4. Retinoblastoma
   5. Ependymoblastoma

Other CNS Neoplasms

1. Tumors of the sellar region
   1. Pituitary adenoma
   2. Craniopharyngioma
2. Hematopoietic tumors
   1. Primary malignant lymphomas
   2. Plasmacytoma
3. Germ cell tumors
   1. Germinoma
   2. Choriocarcinoma
   3. Teratoma
4. Tumors of the meninges
   1. Meningioma
   2. Anaplastic (malignant) meningioma
5. Tumors of cranial and spinal nerves
   1. Schwannoma (neurinoma, neurilemoma)
   2. Neurofibroma
6. Metastatic tumors

■ TABLE 19-2 Hereditary Syndromes Associated with Primary Brain Tumors

Syndrome	Chromosome	Tumors
Neurofibromatosis 1	17	Glioma (optic nerve) and ependymoma
Neurofibromatosis 2	22q12	Meningioma and glioma
VonHippel-Lindau	3p25	Hemangioblastoma
Li-Fraumeni cancer family syndrome	17p13.1 (inherited p53 mutation)	Glioma and medulloblastoma

memory loss, lack of concentration, changes in personality, and apathy. In children, the predilection of tumors for the posterior fossa may lead to presentation with a decreased appetite and weight loss, reduced school performance, dizziness, ataxia (especially of gait), neck pain, bulbar weakness, gaze palsy, or opisthotonos. Clinical findings depend on the location of the tumor and can include cognitive, motor, sensory, and coordination abnormalities on exam.

DIAGNOSTIC EVALUATION

Imaging studies (MRI and CT) play a central role in the diagnosis of brain tumors. Blood work, EEG, and plain x-rays are of limited use. MRI with contrast may show a ring-enhancing mass due to disruption of the blood-brain barrier by the infiltrating neoplasm, but a ring-enhancing lesion can also be seen with an abscess, subacute infarction, resolving hematoma, multiple sclerosis plaques, thrombosed aneurysms, AVMs, and radiation necrosis. Depending on the size and location of the tumor, MRI features can include hydrocephalus, midline shift, hemorrhages, large areas of edema surrounding the lesion, meningeal enhancement, etc. MR spectroscopy can detect changes in brain tissue that are associated with the type and grade of the tumor (including a decreased peak of N-acetyl aspartate (NAA) associated with neuronal loss), but these studies need further validation. The definitive diagnosis of brain tumors requires histologic examination of samples obtained either by brain biopsy or open surgery.

KEY POINTS

- The two most important prognostic factors for brain tumors are histologic type and patient age.
- Brain tumors tend to present as progressive non-remitting neurologic symptoms.
- The most common type of brain tumor is metastatic. The most common primary brain tumors are gliomas and meningiomas.
- Headache and seizures are among the most common presenting symptoms.

PRIMARY BRAIN TUMORS

GLIOMAS

Gliomas are a group of tumors that originate from glial cells, the supportive nonneuronal cells of the CNS. Glioma is a generic histologic term used for four different CNS tumors: astrocytoma, oligodendroglioma, ependymoma, and choroid plexus papilloma.

GLIOBLASTOMA MULTIFORME (GRADE IV ASTROCYTOMA)

- Origin: arises from astrocytes.
- Epidemiology: 15% of all intracranial tumors, and 50% to 60% of PBT in adults. Peak onset at age 40 to 60.
- Pathology: highly malignant tumors with anaplasia, high cellularity, round and pleomorphic cells, nuclear atypia, vascular proliferation, and necrosis. Necrosis and neovascular proliferation help to differentiate between anaplastic astrocytoma (grade III) and glioblastoma (grade IV). On occasion it is multifocal or infiltrates the entire brain (gliomatosis cerebri). Mitotic activity is very high.
- Presentation: headaches 30% to 50%, seizures 30% to 60%, focal neurologic deficits 40% to 60%, mental status changes 20% to 40% at the time of diagnosis. Symptoms may start when the tumor has grown substantially.
- Imaging: CT or MRI demonstrates a solitary brain lesion (commonly in the deep white matter, basal ganglia and thalamus; rarely infratentorial) with contrast enhancement and surrounding edema. About 4% to 10% of GBM do not enhance. Commonly, the tumor infiltrates white matter tracts involving the corpus callosum, producing the typical "butterfly" pattern (Fig. 19-1).
- Treatment: surgical debulking of tumor (if the location allows), followed by radiation and chemotherapy, often including temozolamide and BCNU (Gliadel wafers) implanted in the cavity to slow the delivery of the nitrosourea drug. Stereotactic radiosurgery can be used for local recurrences.
- Prognosis: poor 3- and 5-year survival.

LOW-GRADE GLIOMAS (GRADE I AND II ASTROCYTOMA)

- Origin: astrocytes (glial cells) or ependymal cells.
- Epidemiology: up to 10% of PBT; can occur throughout the brain; in children, more common in the cerebellar hemispheres.
- More common in the fourth decade of life.

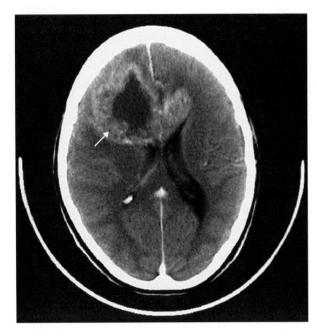

Figure 19-1 • Contrast-enhanced CT scan of the brain showing glioblastoma multiforme (*arrow*). Note the irregular enhancement pattern with a central area of necrosis. The tumor has also crossed the corpus callosum.
(Reproduced with permission from Patel P. *Lecture Notes: Radiology.* Oxford: Blackwell Publishing, 2005:268.)

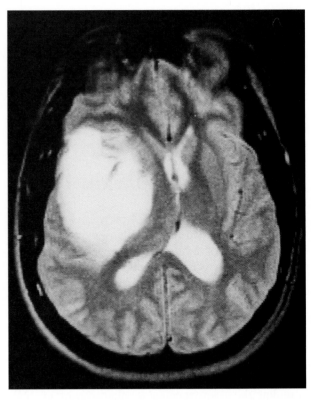

Figure 19-2 • T2-weighted MRI scan of the brain showing a large glioma characterized by high-intensity signal in the right hemisphere. The tumor is displacing and compressing the ventricular system.
(Reproduced with permission from Armstrong P, Wastie M, Rockall A. *Diagnostic Imaging*, 5th ed. Oxford: Blackwell Publishing, 2004:401.)

- Pathology: histologic features define the tumor grade. More benign grade I is without infiltration of surrounding brain.
- Presentation: seizure is a typical presentation of slow growing tumors.
- Imaging: MRI with contrast is the study of choice. Most lesions are bright on T2 and FLAIR, usually without enhancement (Fig. 19-2).
- Treatment: close observation with serial neuroimaging may be the first approach, depending on prognostic factors. Surgical removal can be curative for grade I astrocytomas; it can be considered for grade II tumors if a "gross total" resection is possible, but is often not curative. Radiation or chemotherapy can be used depending on other prognostic factors.
- Prognosis: median survival around 7 years.

OLIGODENDROGLIOMA

- Origin: arises from oligodendrocytes.
- Epidemiology: 10% of all gliomas; 2% to 4% of PBT; peak incidence at age 35 to 45. Common in the frontal lobes, but can appear in the basal ganglia and thalamus. Typically very slow growth.

- Pathology: calcifications are common. Most distinctive microscopic feature is the "fried egg" appearance (perinuclear halos with swollen cytoplasm).
- Presentation: seizures in up to 70%.
- Imaging: MRI shows low intensity on T1, high intensity on T2; vasogenic edema uncommon. Contrast enhancement is a negative prognostic factor, usually seen with anaplastic oligodendroglioma. CT scan better to visualize intratumoral calcifications.
- Treatment: total resection if possible, local radiation and PCV (procarbazine, lomustine, and vincristine) chemotherapy. Temozolamide is used increasingly and is less marrow-toxic.
- Prognosis: better survival with surgery plus radiation; can be decades. Tends to recur locally and progress into a malignant form.

EPENDYMOMA

- Origin: arises from ependymal lining of the ventricles.

- Epidemiology: 6% to 9% of PBT; 30% of PBT in children under age 3. In children, 90% are intracranial (often in the fourth ventricle) with ready subarachnoid spread. In adults, 75% arise within the spinal canal as intramedullary tumors of the spine.
- Pathology: perivascular pseudorosettes (a halo of cells surrounding a central vascular lumen) are the histologic hallmark.
- Presentation: intraventricular location can produce obstructive hydrocephalus with raised intracranial pressure (papilledema, cranial nerve palsies, cerebellar dysfunction, etc.). Myxopapillary ependymoma of the conus and cauda equina can produce conus medullaris or cauda equina syndromes.
- Imaging: MRI enhancement is variable.
- Treatment: surgery to decrease tumor burden, followed by radiation and chemotherapy. Recurrence rates are high; close MRI follow-up is necessary.
- Prognosis: overall 10-year survival 45% to 55%, depending on tumor grade.

MENINGIOMA

- Origin: arises from meningothelial (mesodermal) cells of the dura mater. Almost always benign. Can occur intracranially (with predilection for cerebral convexities, falx cerebri, and the sphenoid wing) or within the spinal canal.
- Epidemiology: second most common PBT after GBM; 15% to 20% of all PBT. More common in women at ages 40 to 60. Incidence increases with age. Some genetic conditions are associated with increased susceptibility to develop meningiomas, as with NF-2 (see Table 19-2), associated with abnormalities on chromosome 22.
- Pathology: histology shows sheets of plump, uniform meningothelial cells with the tendency to form whorls. Progesterone receptors found frequently.
- Presentation: low growth; symptoms produced by local impingement on brain (seizures) and nerves (weakness) or compression of nearby structures (weakness, headache, apathy).
- Imaging: MRI usually shows a rounded extra-axial mass adjacent to dura. In general, isointense on T1 and T2, with intense contrast enhancement and associated "dural tail" of enhancement (Fig. 19-3).
- Calcification seen on CT. Angiography can show rich vascularization. Also noted on CT or plain x-rays is "hyperostosis" (osteoblastic reaction) which may represent tumor invasion of the bone.

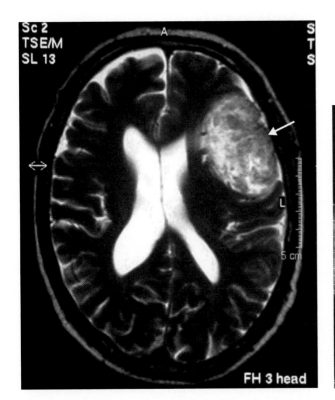
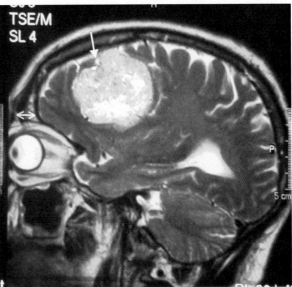

Figure 19-3 • Axial and sagittal MRI scans of the brain showing a brightly enhancing meningioma (*arrows*). On the sagittal view, the arrow tip is also pointing to the dural tail at the margin of the tumor.
(Reproduced with permission from Patel P. *Lecture Notes: Radiology.* Oxford: Blackwell Publishing, 2005:269.)

- Treatment: surgical removal, often preceded by endovascular embolization of the feeding vessels, but many lesions <4 cm are treated with radiosurgery, with good control rates. Stereotactic radiosurgery such as gamma knife radiosurgery is an option when resection or other radiation is difficult or dangerous. Recurrent meningiomas are difficult to treat.
- Prognosis: 5-year survival 70% to 95%; malignant transformation very rare.

MEDULLOBLASTOMA

- Origin: primarily at the medullary velum of the fourth ventricle (Fig. 19-4); up to 30% from the cerebellar hemispheres. Among the primitive neuroectodermal tumors (PNET).
- Epidemiology: almost 8% of PBT, and 30% of pediatric brain tumors.
- Pathology: small round cells with a high mitotic index.

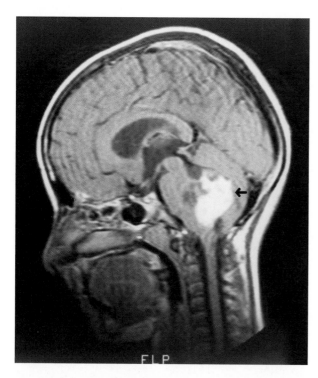

Figure 19-4 • Medulloblastoma (*arrow*) in a child as shown by sagittal MRI scan with contrast enhancement. Note that the fourth ventricle and middle portion of the cerebral aqueduct are obliterated, resulting in hydrocephalus, as illustrated by the dilated third and lateral ventricles.
(Reproduced with permission from Patel P. *Lecture Notes: Radiology*. Oxford: Blackwell Publishing, 2005:271.)

- Presentation: fast growing tumor that infiltrates surrounding tissue and extends toward the fourth ventricle, producing hydrocephalus (with headache, unsteadiness, and vomiting); may spread via the CSF intracranially, and to the spinal cord. Can also spread extracranially to bone and bone marrow.
- Imaging: MRI of the brain and the spinal cord, with contrast, to evaluate subarachnoid metastasis. CSF studies for malignancy (if no contraindication). Bone scan and bone marrow aspiration are indicated due to the possible extracranial extension of the tumor.
- Treatment: surgery plus radiation and chemotherapy. Children <3 years old are more susceptible to adverse effect of radiation on brain development. In those cases, chemotherapy may allow the delay of radiation treatment. High recurrence rate.
- Prognosis: poor in children <3 years, or with metastatic disease or subtotal resection. Good prognostic factors include radical resection and radiation dose above 50 Gy to the entire neuroaxis. Under these conditions, recurrence-free survival is about 50% at 5 years.

SCHWANNOMA

- Origin: arises from Schwann cells.
- Epidemiology: ~7% of all intracranial tumors. More common in middle-aged women. More common in the vestibular (VIII) cranial nerve (acoustic neuromas) where they can occupy the cerebellopontine angle, followed by the trigeminal and facial nerves. Bilateral schwannomas can be associated with NF (neurofibromatosis)-2.
- Pathology: tumor is made up of sheets of uniform spindle cells, forming palisades called "Verocay bodies."
- Presentation: can be asymptomatic, or present with loss of function of the affected cranial nerve (hearing loss, vestibular symptoms, facial paresthesias or pain, etc.).
- Imaging: MRI with contrast.
- Treatment: if symptomatic, stereotactic radiosurgery (i.e., gamma knife) is the first choice, particularly when the lesion does not compress the brainstem and is smaller than 3 cm. Surgery (microsurgical approach) is an alternative but can produce facial nerve lesions.
- Prognosis: good.

OTHER LESS COMMON PRIMARY BRAIN TUMORS

GANGLIOGLIOMA

These infrequent PBT are commonly seen in children and young adults, and include a mixture of neurons and glial cells. They are usually located in the cerebral hemisphere and characterized by a slow growth, with long duration of symptoms (e.g., seizures). MRI shows increased T2 signal with characteristic swollen gyri. Surgical removal leads to excellent outcome. Radiation is reserved for those with frankly malignant features, or inoperable or recurrent tumors.

HEMANGIOBLASTOMA

These uncommon cerebellar cystic lesions represent less than 1% of intracranial tumors. They are often associated with von Hippel-Lindau disease (hereditary retinal angiomas, pancreatic cysts, and kidney tumors).

PRIMARY CNS LYMPHOMA

Lymphoma involving the CNS can be primary or metastatic from systemic non-Hodgkin's lymphoma.

Primary CNS lymphoma (PCNSL) accounts for less than 2% of PBT, affecting men more than women (2:1) and with higher incidence in AIDS patients. They are almost exclusively intermediate to high-grade non-Hodgkin lymphomas of B cell origin. The clinical presentation is usually insidious, with progressive neurologic dysfunction (change in mental status, seizures, focal deficits, etc.). MRI appearance varies, with single or multiple lesions, a butterfly appearance, enhancing lesions, etc.

The role of surgery is limited to biopsy. Methotrexate-based chemotherapies are the treatment of choice. PCNSL are radiosensitive, but radiation is used as palliation. PCNSL can show a dramatic response to steroids, but the tumor invariably recurs within months. Recurrence is very common (median time to recurrence: 4 to 5 years). The tumor can then be retreated with chemotherapy with good response.

SELLAR AND SUPRASELLAR TUMORS

Pituitary tumors originate in the pituitary gland in the sellar region (Fig. 19-5). They can be classified as microadenomas (<1 mm) and macroadenomas (>1 mm). Their histologic cell of origin is responsible for the initial symptoms, usually related to the production of a pituitary hormone. When tumors

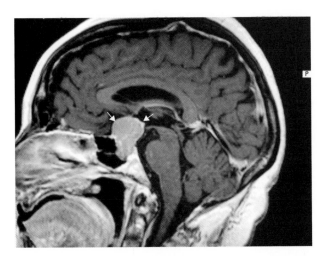
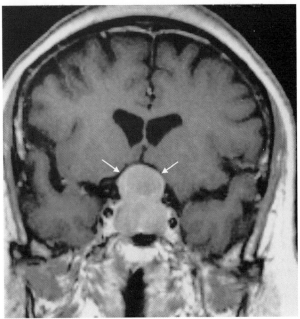

Figure 19-5 • Sagittal and coronal postcontrast MRI scans of the brain demonstrating a pituitary adenoma (*arrows*). Note that the tumor is anterior to the brainstem and extends upward, compressing the optic chiasm.
(Reproduced with permission from Armstrong P, Wastie M, Rockall A. *Diagnostic Imaging*, 5th ed. Oxford: Blackwell Publishing, 2004:406.)

become large enough, they can compress neighboring structures (optic chiasm, cavernous sinus, etc.), producing focal symptoms. In general, diagnosis is by imaging studies and laboratory evaluation of hormonal status. Surgical removal may be through a trans-sphenoidal approach.

Suprasellar craniopharyngioma is a slow-growing tumor characterized by the benign nature of its cells but malignant behavior of its growth. It accounts for 1% to 3% of intracranial tumors and 13% of suprasellar tumors in adults and 50% in children. It tends to invade neighboring structures, complicating treatment. Tumors present with headache, visual disturbance, and endocrine dysfunction. The radiologic hallmark is the appearance of a suprasellar calcified cyst. Treatment can entail full surgical resection, or minimal resection with radiation or radiosurgery.

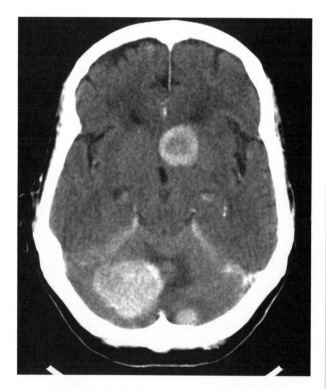

Figure 19-6 • Contrast-enhanced CT scan of the brain showing several metastatic lesions characterized by rounded areas of hyperdensity.
(Reproduced with permission from Armstrong P, Wastie M, Rockall A. *Diagnostic Imaging*, 5th ed. Oxford: Blackwell Publishing, 2004:402.)

SECONDARY (METASTATIC) BRAIN TUMORS

Metastases are the most common brain tumors and originate from malignant neoplasms outside the CNS. The most frequent metastatic brain tumors originate in the lung, skin (melanoma), kidney (renal cell carcinoma), breast, and colon. Malignant cells reach the brain via the bloodstream (crossing the blood-brain barrier) or through Batson's plexus (pelvic and GI tumors). In general, metastatic lesions are located at the junction of white and gray matter and tend to be solitary, but multiple metastases are not unusual. MRI with contrast is the preferred diagnostic study (see Fig. 19-6). Treatment depends on the number of metastases, the immediate mass effect of the lesion, and the general status of the patient. Single lesions can be resected, followed by whole brain radiation or radiosurgery. Radiosurgery is used more often for three or fewer lesions, especially if the systemic disease is under good control—to prevent the long-term side effects of whole brain radiation, chemotherapy, or both. The prognosis is poor because metastases usually represent a more advanced stage and extension of the primary cancer.

KEY POINTS

• "Drop metastases" are intradural extramedullary spinal metastases that arise from intracranial lesions. The most frequent source is ependymomas and medulloblastomas, but they can also be seen with choroid plexus papilloma and other PBT.

• Medulloblastoma: avoid lumbar puncture unless CT shows no obstructive lesion—to prevent cerebellar tonsillar herniation due to increased intracranial pressure.

• NF (neurofibromatosis)-2–associated tumors: bilateral vestibular schwannomas, meningiomas, and intramedullary ependymomas.

• In primary CNS lymphoma remember to evaluate the patient's immune status.

• Metastases that bleed easily include melanoma, renal carcinoma, and choriocarcinoma.

Demyelinating Diseases of the Central Nervous System

MULTIPLE SCLEROSIS

Demyelinating diseases of the CNS are characterized by the pathologic hallmark of acquired loss of myelin with relative preservation of axons. The most common and best known of the CNS demyelinating diseases is multiple sclerosis (MS). For many reasons MS is also one of the most feared diagnoses in Neurology: it strikes young, healthy people in the prime of their lives, its course is marked by unpredictable relapses, almost any aspect of neurologic function may be affected, and the specter of lifelong disability requiring a wheelchair is a devastating one.

However, MS has a wide range of presentations and an equally wide range of prognoses; effective treatments aimed at both the underlying disease process and some specific complications are available. For the student, the study of demyelinating diseases provides an excellent opportunity to learn about dysfunction of different parts of the CNS and to master the wide variety of neurologic exam abnormalities that accompany these disorders.

EPIDEMIOLOGY

MS is a chronic neurologic disease that begins most commonly in young adulthood. The peak incidence of MS is between 20 and 30 years of age. Women are affected twice as often as men. Its prevalence in the northern United States is about 60 per 100,000. As discussed below, there are epidemiologic patterns to suggest both environmental and genetic influences.

Geographically, MS is more common in northern latitudes. The incidence in Scandinavian countries is higher than that in Italy, and the incidence in the northern United States is higher than that in the South. However, there are racial differences as well (with a higher prevalence in white populations), and the implication of the geographic disparities is unclear. Interestingly, those who move from a low-risk to a high-risk geographic region or vice versa before the age of 15 adopt the risk of MS associated with their new home, while those who migrate after age 15 retain the risk associated with their childhood home. This supports the theory that a latent viral infection acquired in childhood may play a role in the pathogenesis of the disease.

There is strong evidence supporting a genetic predisposition to MS as well. For example, there is a greater incidence of MS in monozygotic as compared to dizygotic twins of patients with MS, as well as an increased incidence in association with particular HLA alleles.

KEY POINTS

- The peak incidence of MS occurs in young adulthood, between 20 and 30 years of age.
- MS is more common in women and more common in whites.
- The epidemiology of MS supports both environmental and genetic influences.

CLINICAL MANIFESTATIONS

The neurologist's classic definition of MS is a disease marked by multiple white matter lesions separated in space and time. This means that multiple distinct areas of the CNS must be involved (rather than one area recurrently, for example), and that the disease must not be just a monophasic illness (with multiple areas affected only once simultaneously).

The clinical features are defined, as might be expected, by the location of the lesions. Thus, a right occipital lesion could result in a left homonymous hemianopia, while a right cervical spinal cord lesion may lead to an ipsilateral hemiparesis and loss of joint position sense with contralateral loss of pain and temperature sensation. Almost any neurologic symptom, in fact, can be produced by an MS lesion.

Common clinical features (Table 20-1) include corticospinal tract signs such as weakness and spasticity, cerebellar problems such as intention tremor and ataxia, sensory abnormalities such as paresthesias and loss of vibration and proprioception, and bladder dysfunction. Commonly, patients complain of fatigue. In later stages, cognitive and behavioral abnormalities and seizures may occur. A few particular syndromes characteristic of MS warrant further description.

Optic neuritis (ON) is a common initial presenting symptom of MS. (This fact reminds us that the optic nerve is actually an extension of the CNS rather than a true peripheral nerve.) ON is characterized by a painful loss of visual acuity in one eye. The vision may be blurry and there may be loss of color discrimination; severe episodes may lead to actual blindness. Pain may be predominant when the eye moves (i.e., when looking around). On exam there is loss of acuity and color vision, and the optic disc may be swollen, with indistinct margins (papilledema). A past history of ON is suggested by the presence of red desaturation (subtle loss of color appreciation), optic disc pallor or atrophy, and an RAPD (see Chapter 4).

Transverse myelitis describes an area of inflammatory demyelination in the spinal cord. Most commonly this is a partial lesion and does not mimic a complete spinal cord transection; rather, particular tracts may be interrupted at the level of the lesion in a patchy way. Thus there may be unilateral or bilateral weakness or sensory loss below the lesion. Bowel and bladder function may be lost. Reflexes may be exaggerated below the lesion, and Babinski signs may be present. Patients may report a band of tingling or pain around the torso at the level of the lesion.

TABLE 20-1 Common Clinical Features of Multiple Sclerosis

Neurologic System	Clinical Sign or Symptom
Cranial nerves	Optic nerve dysfunction
	Visual acuity loss
	Red desaturation
	Papilledema or optic disc pallor
	Relative afferent pupillary defect (RAPD)
	Eye movement disorders
	Internuclear ophthalmoplegia
	Nystagmus
Motor system	Weakness
	Spasticity
	Reflex abnormalities
	Increased muscle stretch reflexes
	Babinski signs
	Clonus
Sensory system	Paresthesias
	Vibratory loss
	Joint position sense loss
	Lhermitte's sign
Cerebellar function	Ataxia
	Intention tremor
	Dysarthria
Autonomic system	Bladder dysfunction
Other	Fatigue
	Depression
	Uhthoff's phenomenon

Internuclear ophthalmoplegia (INO) is not a common finding in MS patients, but it is quite characteristic. The presence of an INO in a young person suggests few other diagnostic possibilities. An INO results from dysfunction of the MLF and leads to an inability to adduct one eye when looking toward the opposite side, with associated nystagmus of the abducting eye. Adduction of both eyes when observing a near target (convergence) is preserved.

Other clinical features characteristic of MS include **Lhermitte's sign**, a tingling, electric sensation down the spine when the patient flexes the neck, and a worsening of symptoms and signs in the heat, termed **Uhthoff's phenomenon**.

KEY POINTS

- MS is characterized by multiple lesions separated in space and time.
- Almost any neurologic symptom can occur, depending on the location and burden of lesions.
- Features characteristic of MS include ON, transverse myelitis, INO, Lhermitte's sign, and a worsening of symptoms in the heat.

CLINICAL COURSE AND PROGNOSIS

Most MS patients begin with a relapsing-remitting course (Fig. 20-1), in which there are discrete episodes of neurologic dysfunction (relapses or "flares") that resolve after a period of time (usually weeks to months). Unfortunately, such a course usually evolves into one in which recovery from each relapse is incomplete and baseline functioning deteriorates (secondary progressive). Rarely, patients may have a relentlessly progressive course from the onset, either with superimposed relapses (progressive-relapsing) or without (primary progressive).

To put the prognosis in broad terms, about one-third of MS patients lead lives of minimal disability and continue to work, about one-third have disability significant enough to prevent them from continuing at their jobs, and about one-third have severe disability, typically becoming wheelchair-bound. Features predicting a good prognosis include young age at onset, female sex, rapid remission of initial symptoms, mild relapses that leave little or no residual deficits, and a presentation with sensory symptoms or optic neuritis rather than motor symptoms.

KEY POINTS

- Most MS patients have a relapsing-remitting course, which frequently evolves into a secondary progressive course.
- Prognosis is quite variable and ranges from minimal to severe disability.

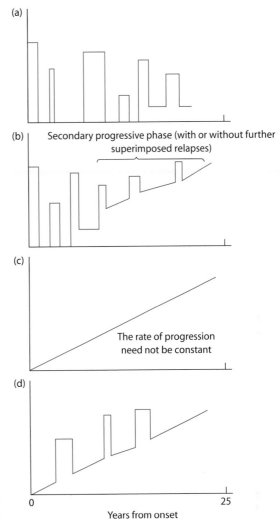

Figure 20-1 • Clinical course of multiple sclerosis: **(A)** relapsing-remitting, **(B)** secondary progressive, **(C)** primary progressive, **(D)** progressive-relapsing.
(Reproduced with permission from Ginsberg L. *Lecture Notes: Neurology*, 8th ed. Oxford: Blackwell Publishing, 2005:131.)

DIAGNOSTIC EVALUATION

The diagnosis of MS begins with a thorough history and examination. In particular, patients often present with what appears to be a single episode of neurologic dysfunction, but upon further questioning may recall past episodes of seemingly unrelated neurologic symptoms that may in fact represent prior lesions separated in space and time. It is important to inquire specifically about past neurologic symptoms, particularly those that suggest optic neuritis, transverse myelitis, or other typical MS features. On

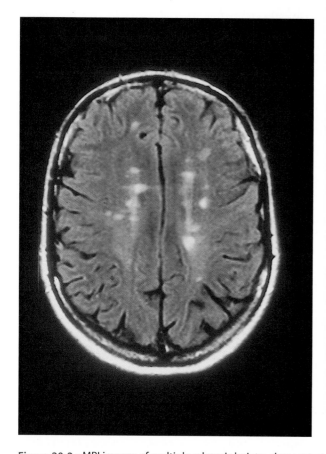

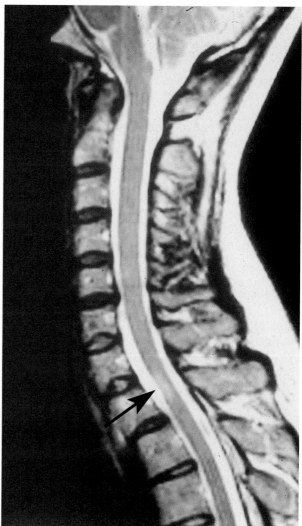

Figure 20-2 • MRI images of multiple sclerosis lesions, demonstrated on FLAIR sequences.
(Reproduced with permission from Ginsberg L. *Lecture Notes: Neurology,* 8th ed. Oxford: Blackwell Publishing, 2005:133.)

exam, as well, evidence of old optic nerve or other neurologic lesions should be sought.

The two most useful laboratory studies are MRI and CSF analysis. On MRI, new MS lesions appear as discrete T2-hyperintense areas in the white matter of the brain or spinal cord. Ovoid lesions are classic. Fluid-attenuated inversion recovery (FLAIR) sequences also show these lesions particularly well (Fig. 20-2). Acute lesions may not be evident on T1-weighted images but may enhance with gadolinium. Old, chronic MS lesions may become T1-hypointense, with a "black hole" appearance. MS lesions have a predilection for particular areas, including the periventricular white matter, juxtacortical regions, corpus callosum, and cerebellar peduncles. Sagittal images may demonstrate foci of demyelination spreading upward from the corpus callosum, termed **Dawson's fingers.**

The characteristic CSF finding is oligoclonal bands, found in more than 90% of MS patients at some point during their illness. These reflect intrathecal production of IgG antibodies by plasma cell clones. Although highly suggestive of MS, they can also be found in other neurologic disorders. CSF studies during an acute relapse may show a moderate pleocytosis and elevated protein. Calculation of the IgG index, based on relative levels of IgG and albumin in the CSF and serum, can also suggest intrathecal antibody production.

Finally, visual evoked potentials can be used in suspected MS to document evidence of old optic neuritis. There is often an increased latency of the P100 wave on the affected side.

KEY POINTS

- The diagnosis of MS begins with a thorough history and examination, particularly directed toward identifying past episodes of neurologic dysfunction.
- MRI is the best imaging modality to detect both new and old MS lesions.
- The characteristic CSF abnormality is the presence of oligoclonal bands.
- Visual evoked potentials may provide evidence of old optic neuritis.

PATHOLOGY

The histologic appearance of an acute MS lesion is a sharply defined area of myelin loss with relative preservation of axons and associated signs of perivascular inflammation, including the presence of macrophages, lymphocytes, and plasma cells. Reactive astrocytes may be present. Chronic MS lesions are hypocellular and have extensive glial proliferation.

TREATMENT

Treatment for MS falls into three categories: acute therapies for relapses, chronic therapies that treat the underlying disease process, and symptomatic therapies that address the various complications of the disease.

Acute relapses of MS are most commonly treated with corticosteroids. A course of intravenous methylprednisolone followed by an oral prednisone taper is a common protocol. Although the effect of steroids on the long-term outcome is unclear, the duration of acute relapses is often shortened. A well-publicized trial demonstrated that intravenous steroids used to treat optic neuritis delayed but did not prevent the subsequent development of MS.

The therapies used in the chronic treatment of MS are immune-modulating agents (Table 20-2). These include beta-1a interferon and beta-1b interferon, which are available in injection form and have been shown to decrease the rate of relapses, the burden of lesions seen on MRI, and the rate of accumulated disability. Both are currently used in relapsing-remitting and some secondary progressive patients. Side effects can include flu-like symptoms, depression, and injection-site reactions. It is important to check a CBC and liver function test routinely; interferons may cause leukopenia and reversible transaminitis. Patients who are doing poorly on interferons may have developed neutralizing antibodies to the interferons that reduce their effectiveness.

Glatiramer acetate is a polypeptide formulation injected subcutaneously that is also used in relapsing-remitting patients. Mitoxantrone, a chemotherapeutic agent that may be useful in patients with worsening MS, has dose-limiting cardiotoxicity as a potential drawback.

In patients who no longer respond to the above therapies, other immunosuppressive agents may be used, including azathioprine, cyclophosphamide, and methotrexate. Some use periodic pulses of corticosteroids. Of course these agents have a wide range of accompanying toxicities.

Several of the symptomatic complications that accompany MS have specific treatments. Spasticity can be managed with baclofen, diazepam, or tizanidine. Bladder dysfunction can be managed with

■ TABLE 20-2 Immune-Modulating Agents Used in the Treatment of Multiple Sclerosis		
Drug	**Administration**	**Side Effects**
Interferon beta-1a (Avonex)	30 µg IM every week	Flu-like symptoms, anemia, depression, development of neutralizing antibodies
Interferon beta-1b (Betaseron)	250 µg SC every other day	Injection-site reactions, flu-like symptoms, depression, hematologic/liver abnormalities, development of neutralizing antibodies
Interferon beta-1b (Rebif)	44 µg SC three times a week	Flu-like symptoms, anemia, depression, development of neutralizing antibodies
Glatiramer acetate (Copaxone)	20 mg SC daily	Injection-site reactions, injection-related chest pain and shortness of breath

anticholinergic agents (for urinary urgency) as well as intermittent self-catheterization. It is particularly important to address urinary problems so as to prevent recurrent infections, which can trigger MS relapses and lead to chronic renal disease. Unfortunately there are no effective treatments for tremor and ataxia, which are common disabling symptoms.

KEY POINTS

- Acute MS relapses are treated with intravenous corticosteroids.
- Interferons and glatiramer acetate are immune-modulating agents used to treat relapsing- remitting MS.
- More toxic immunosuppressants are often used in refractory cases.
- Symptomatic therapies include those for spasticity and bladder dysfunction.

ACUTE DISSEMINATED ENCEPHALOMYELITIS

Acute disseminated encephalomyelitis (ADEM) is a monophasic illness leading to areas of demyelination within the CNS, commonly following an antecedent viral infection or vaccination. ADEM may be difficult to distinguish from the initial presentation of MS.

CLINICAL AND RADIOLOGIC MANIFESTATIONS

As in MS, almost any neurologic symptom or sign can occur, depending on the location of the demyelinating lesions. In ADEM, the lesions are multiple and are frequently more patchy, bilateral, and confluent than in MS, where the lesions may be more discrete. ADEM lesions have a predilection for the posterior cerebral hemispheric white matter. Clinically, behavioral and cognitive abnormalities are often seen in ADEM, whereas they are uncommon until the late stages of MS. Radiologically, all areas of demyelination in ADEM appear acute and may enhance with gadolinium.

DIAGNOSTIC EVALUATION

The diagnosis of ADEM may be suspected based on the clinical presentation and radiologic findings.

CSF typically will show a lymphocytic pleocytosis (usually with more cells than seen in MS) and an elevated protein. Oligoclonal bands are rarely present. When the illness is indistinguishable clinically or radiologically from the initial episode of MS, definitive diagnosis of MS may not be possible unless or until a second episode of neurologic dysfunction occurs.

PROGNOSIS AND TREATMENT

By definition ADEM is a monophasic illness, and neurologic recovery is typically nearly complete. A course of intravenous corticosteroids is often administered to shorten the duration of the episode and lessen the severity of the symptoms.

LEUKOENCEPHALOPATHIES

Progressive multifocal leukoencephalopathy (PML) is characterized by dementia, focal cortical dysfunction, and cerebellar abnormalities. It is seen almost exclusively in patients with AIDS, leukemia, lymphoma, and other immunocompromised states. The JC virus is the causative agent and leads to demyelination by infecting oligodendrocytes. MRI characteristically shows multiple foci of white matter abnormalities, particularly in posterior regions. CSF analysis is usually normal. There are no effective treatments, and the prognosis is uniformly fatal.

Immunosuppressants such as tacrolimus and cyclosporine may cause a post–organ transplant leukoencephalopathy. Most commonly, these drugs produce an acute confusional state and cortical visual loss (blindness with preserved pupillary reactivity). MRI shows posterior white matter hyperintensities on T2-weighted images. The posterior leukoencephalopathy associated with these immunosuppressants can often be reversed by discontinuing or lowering the dose of the offending agent.

A sudden increase in blood pressure can cause hypertensive leukoencephalopathy. Patients present with an acute confusional state, seizures, headaches, and vomiting. Funduscopic examination shows papilledema with retinal hemorrhages and hard exudates. This syndrome may be accompanied by cardiac ischemia and hematuria. MRI shows T2-hyperintensities, usually in the parietal and occipital regions. Although completely reversible with appropriate antihypertensive treatment, hypertensive leukoencephalopathy can progress to coma or death.

Infections of the Nervous System

It is important for physicians to be familiar with the common types and manifestations of nervous system infections for several reasons. First, this category of neurologic illness can be quite acute in presentation. Additionally, nervous system infections can have devastating and potentially life-threatening consequences in some cases. Finally, for many of them, specific therapies are tailored to the identified etiologic organism.

BACTERIAL INFECTIONS

Three common and important forms of bacterial nervous system infection are acute bacterial meningitis, brain abscess, and spinal epidural abscess.

ACUTE BACTERIAL MENINGITIS

Clinical Findings

Acute bacterial meningitis is a medical emergency. It is critical for all physicians to know its presentation, its initial diagnostic evaluation, and the urgency with which a potential case of bacterial meningitis needs to be addressed. The cardinal findings include headache, fever, and neck stiffness. Patients can also be confused or have a depressed level of consciousness, develop seizures, or have other focal neurologic symptoms or signs, depending on the extent to which the meningeal infectious or inflammatory process also affects the brain parenchyma (causing **meningoencephalitis**). Two classically described physical signs associated with meningitis, though not specific to the bacterial form, are **Kernig's sign** (pain upon attempted passive extension at the knee when the hip is flexed) and **Brudzinski's sign** (an involuntary flexion at the hip[s] when the neck is flexed).

Etiology

The most common organisms causing bacterial meningitis vary depending on age of presentation. The introduction of vaccines against *Streptococcus pneumoniae* ("pneumococcus"), *Neisseria meningitides* ("meningococcus"), and *Haemophilus influenzae* has successfully reduced the incidence of acute bacterial meningitis among children in the United States. In most cases, bacteria reach the subarachnoid space through hematogenous spread from the respiratory tract, although bacterial meningitis may also be a direct sequela of traumatic or mechanical invasion into the subarachnoid space, such as after neurosurgical procedures or open head injury. It is also possible to have direct infiltration of the subarachnoid space from parameningeal foci, such as the sinuses.

Diagnostic Workup

The critical test in the diagnosis of acute bacterial meningitis is cerebrospinal fluid (CSF) analysis from lumbar puncture (LP). Because of the concern that LP may precipitate brain herniation in the presence of a focal intracranial mass with increased intracranial pressure, it is generally accepted that head imaging (usually with CT, because it is available more readily) should be performed before LP when papilledema is present on fundoscopic examination or if there are any focal signs on neurologic examination suggesting the possibility of an intracranial lesion. Some physicians advocate head imaging prior to LP under any circumstances of an acute presentation, but this is controversial.

The characteristic CSF profile in acute bacterial meningitis includes an elevated white blood cell count, with a predominance of polymorphonuclear leukocytes (generally never acceptable in a CSF sample), elevated protein, and low glucose (less than 40 mg/dL or less than two-thirds of a simultaneously measured serum glucose level). CSF Gram stain can demonstrate the bacteria and narrow down the differential diagnosis of etiologic organisms. CSF cultures in acute bacterial meningitis can often identify the specific organism, which can then be tested for antibiotic sensitivity.

Because of the potentially life-threatening nature of acute bacterial meningitis, a prolonged delay in being able to obtain a CSF sample may require the institution of empiric antibiotic coverage prior to LP—using antibiotics that are effective against the most likely organisms at dosages that ensure adequate penetration into the subarachnoid space, or "meningitis doses." In this case, CSF cultures may not grow organisms if they were not obtained until well after antibiotic therapy was begun, and it may be necessary to complete an entire course of empiric therapy.

Treatment

Appropriate antibiotic therapy needs to be administered promptly upon the diagnosis of acute bacterial meningitis, with specific drugs initially chosen based on most likely organisms and subsequently modified based on Gram stain or culture results. In addition to the direct anti-infective therapy, some adjunctive therapies may also be helpful in certain situations. Corticosteroids are often used in children in an attempt to prevent some of the long-term complications of acute bacterial meningitis, such as deafness.

KEY POINTS

- Acute bacterial meningitis is a medical emergency.
- The typical clinical presentation consists of headache, fever, neck pain or stiffness, and/or altered consciousness.
- The classic cerebrospinal fluid profile demonstrates a high white blood cell count (mostly polymorphonuclear leukocytes), high protein, and low glucose.
- Antibiotic treatment can be tailored based on identification of responsible organisms and penetration into the subarachnoid space.

BRAIN ABSCESS

Clinical Findings

Brain abscesses typically present much like any other focal intracranial lesions, with headache, focal neurologic signs (that depend on the exact intracranial location of the abscess), seizures, and potentially, signs of increased intracranial pressure. Sometimes fever is present, but this is not invariable.

Etiology

Solitary brain abscesses often arise from invasion of the intracranial space from neighboring sites of infection, such as the sinuses, or from direct open trauma or mechanical instrumentation. Multiple brain abscesses are seen typically as a result of hematogenous dissemination, such as from infective bacterial endocarditis, or with immunocompromised states. Responsible organisms depend on the etiology; respiratory pathogens invade from the sinuses; abscesses from trauma or instrumentation are often skin flora; and multiple abscesses are often caused by organisms that cause infective bacterial endocarditis. In general, most abscesses contain multiple organisms, often a mixture of aerobic and anaerobic pathogens.

Diagnostic Workup

The diagnosis of brain abscess is typically made upon neuroimaging. CT or MRI with intravenous contrast agents will usually demonstrate a mass lesion, often rounded with ring enhancement and signs of central necrosis, within the brain parenchyma (Fig. 21-1). At the top of the radiologic differential diagnosis are malignant neoplastic lesions, which can often have a similar ring-enhancing mass appearance. Sometimes single photon emission computed tomography (SPECT) scanning can help differentiate a neoplastic process from an abscess. Depending on the source of the infection, blood cultures can sometimes identify the responsible organisms, although neurosurgical drainage is often necessary for definitive pathogen identification.

Treatment

Prolonged courses of intravenous antibiotics, either chosen empirically for broad-spectrum coverage of aerobic and anaerobic organisms or tailored specifically based on culture results, are the mainstay of treatment for brain abscesses.

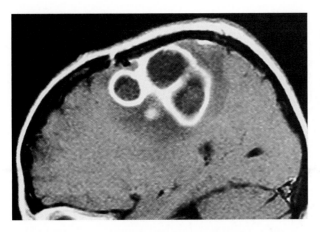

Figure 21-1 • Parasagittal MRI showing a multilocular brain abscess. The MRI was performed with a gadolinium and shows ring enhancement of the lesion with surrounding edema. (Reproduced with permission from Ginsberg L. *Lecture Notes: Neurology.* 8th ed, Oxford: Blackwell Publishing, 2005:113.)

SPINAL EPIDURAL ABSCESS

Clinical Findings

Spinal epidural abscesses typically present with the combination of neck or back pain and focal neurologic signs consistent with spinal cord compression or cauda equina involvement, depending on the level of the abscess. For thoracic or lumbar abscesses, these signs may include lower extremity weakness, sensory loss with a detectable sensory "level" on examination, and urinary and sexual dysfunction, while for cervical abscesses the upper extremities may be involved as well. Fever is not necessarily present. Symptoms may come on acutely or more insidiously; an acute presentation often suggests associated spinal cord infarction.

Etiology

Spinal epidural abscesses can be sequelae of spinal instrumentation, including epidural or spinal anesthetic introduction and spine surgery. In these cases the responsible organisms are often skin pathogens such as staphylococcal species. Abscesses can also be the result of spread from more anterior infections, including vertebral body osteomyelitis or diskitis.

Diagnostic Workup

Spine imaging is generally indicated when there is clinical suspicion based on history and physical examination of an intraspinal lesion such as an epidural abscess. In general, the administration of contrast (with either

CT or MRI) can help to demonstrate the enhancing nature of spinal epidural abscesses. Lumbar puncture is contraindicated in most situations before the anatomic extent of the lesion is defined clearly by imaging, because there is a theoretical possibility of seeding the subarachnoid space with bacteria using the spinal needle. As with intracranial abscesses, blood cultures can sometimes reveal the responsible organisms, but in many cases radiologically guided biopsy or surgical drainage for microbiological studies may be necessary.

Treatment

Prolonged courses of intravenous antibiotics are the mainstay of treatment for spinal epidural abscesses, although in some cases neurosurgical drainage is necessary. When a clinical syndrome of acute cord compression or cauda equina involvement is present, surgical decompression may be required urgently.

KEY POINTS

- Abscesses affecting the central nervous system are mass lesions that are often ring-enhancing on radiologic studies with contrast.
- They present with focal neurologic signs that are dependent on their intracranial or spinal location.
- Prolonged courses of intravenous antibiotics are the mainstay of treatment, but surgical drainage is necessary sometimes.

TUBERCULOUS INFECTION

Tuberculosis, though less common in the United States, is a prevalent infection throughout much of the world. *Mycobacterium tuberculosis* affects the nervous system in a number of recognized ways: tuberculous meningitis, intracranial tuberculomas, and Pott disease (tuberculoma of the spine).

Tuberculous Meningitis

Tuberculous meningitis arises from hematogenous dissemination of mycobacteria from a pulmonary source. A number of features distinguish tuberculous meningitis from acute pyogenic bacterial meningitis (described previously). First, meningitis caused by

Mycobacterium tuberculosis has a predilection for affecting the basal meninges (those at the base of the brain) and thus can present with cranial nerve palsies in addition to the usual features of acute bacterial meningitis. Also, a basal meningitis more commonly leads to hydrocephalus or brain infarcts from inflammation affecting cerebral vessels. Second, tuberculous meningitis tends to have a more subacute or chronic, insidious presentation than acute bacterial meningitis, so a prolonged prodrome of malaise and fairly nonspecific constitutional symptoms may precede the appearance of frank neck pain or stiffness. Finally, the cerebrospinal fluid profile in tuberculous meningitis typically demonstrates a leukocytosis with lymphocytic predominance, rather than polymorphonuclear predominance (except initially), and the CSF glucose is often very low. Acid-fast bacilli staining of the CSF can identify mycobacterial infection, but cultures of this organism can take weeks to grow and may never actually become positive. Polymerase chain reaction (PCR) testing of mycobacterial antigens is available, however. Treatment of tuberculous meningitis requires a regimen of multiple antituberculous drugs that penetrate the intrathecal space effectively.

Intracranial Tuberculoma

Tuberculomas are mass lesions caused by *M. tuberculosis* infection. Although uncommon in the United States, tuberculomas are one of the most common focal brain lesions in the developing world. Typically, they present with features that would be expected for any inflammatory mass lesion within the brain, including headache, focal neurologic symptoms and signs, and seizures. They can calcify, be variably enhancing on radiologic studies with contrast, and are sometimes associated with hydrocephalus. Radiologic differential diagnosis typically includes brain tumor, bacterial abscess, or cysticercosis (see below). Appropriate treatment includes prolonged courses of antituberculous therapy and neurosurgical intervention if needed.

Pott's Disease

Pott's disease, or tuberculosis of the spine, typically presents with neurologic symptoms and signs when vertebral body infection extends into the epidural space, leading to subacute spinal cord or cauda equina compression, depending on the level of involvement. Fever and back pain are common. Spread to adjacent vertebral bodies often suggests this diagnosis rather than metastatic cancer. Treatment includes antituberculous drugs and spine stabilization procedures if necessary.

KEY POINTS

- Tuberculosis affects the nervous system in several different ways, including meningitis, focal brain lesions, or focal spine lesions.
- Tuberculous meningitis has a predilection for the basal meninges, is typically insidious, can present with cranial nerve palsies, and has a different CSF profile from bacterial meningitis.
- Pott's disease, or tuberculosis of the spine, affects the nervous system when there is direct invasion into the epidural space.

LYME DISEASE

Lyme disease, caused by the spirochete *Borrelia burgdorferi* and transmitted by the deer tick, is a common infection in the northern United States and in Europe. Lyme disease affects the nervous system in several recognizable ways, including Lyme-associated meningitis, cranial nerve palsies, and a syndrome of polyradiculopathy.

Clinical Findings

While the typical rash of *erythema chronicum migrans* can occur within the first week after a bite from an infected tick, neurologic manifestations typically do not appear until the more disseminated stage of Lyme disease, several weeks after the bite. Headache, neck stiffness, and myalgias may develop into more frank signs of meningismus along with cranial nerve palsies (most commonly affecting the facial nerve, either unilaterally or bilaterally). In the persistent stage of systemic disease, several months after the initial bite, polyradiculopathy (often with significant pain), polyneuropathy, and/or encephalopathy (with signs of white matter signal change) may occur.

Diagnostic Workup

Serologic tests of the blood or CSF can be diagnostic, but sometimes not until late in the course of the disease. The routine CSF profile typically demonstrates a lymphocytic pleocytosis with elevated protein and normal glucose. A PCR assay of the CSF is available for spirochetal antigen. In cases of encephalopathy, MRI of the brain can sometimes show patchy foci of signal change in the white matter, while in cases of peripheral nervous system involvement EMG/nerve conduction studies may be useful.

Treatment

Patients with isolated facial palsy and negative CSF studies can often be treated with oral antibiotics, while signs of more disseminated neurologic infection suggest the need for intravenous antibiotics at dosages that can penetrate the subarachnoid space.

KEY POINTS

- Lyme disease, caused by the spirochete *Borrelia burgdorferi*, is a common infection in the northern United States and in Europe.
- Early neurologic manifestations of Lyme disease include an aseptic meningitis, facial nerve palsy, or both, within weeks after infection.
- Later neurologic manifestations include leukoencephalopathy, painful polyradiculopathy, or both, sometimes months after infection.

VIRAL INFECTIONS

Most viral infections of the nervous system present as one of several clinically recognized syndromes. Viral meningitis and encephalitis are discussed below.

VIRAL MENINGITIS

Viral meningitis is commonly caused by enteroviruses, such as coxsackievirus, or arboviruses, such as West Nile virus. Clinically, the presentation may be very similar to that of acute bacterial meningitis, and it is mainly the latter entity that needs to be considered and ruled out immediately, even if viral meningitis is suspected to be the more likely diagnosis. The CSF profile differs from that of acute bacterial meningitis, as viral meningitis usually features a lymphocytic predominance of white blood cells (except initially, when polymorphonuclear leukocytes can be present) and an elevated protein without a concomitant lowering of CSF glucose. Gram stain and culture of CSF, of

course, are unrevealing. Testing the blood and CSF for virus-specific serologies and PCR assays can be useful in identifying the responsible virus. Treatment generally involves just supportive care, unless HSV1 is suspected (see below).

ENCEPHALITIS

Viral encephalitis, which affects the brain parenchyma itself, usually presents with headache, fever, altered level of consciousness, seizures, and focal neurologic abnormalities. While most etiologies of viral encephalitis have no specific anti-infective therapy available, **encephalitis caused by herpes simplex virus (HSV) 1 leads to some distinct clinical features and warrants specific therapy.** HSV1 encephalitis has a predilection for the base of the brain, specifically including the medial temporal lobes and orbitofrontal regions of cortex. Limbic dysfunction, including complex partial seizures of mesial temporal lobe origin, olfactory hallucinations, and memory disturbances (including sometimes profound anterograde amnesia and some degree of retrograde amnesia), is a common part of the clinical presentation. The CSF in HSV1 encephalitis often demonstrates an elevated red blood cell count in addition to leukocytosis (and thus needs to be distinguished from traumatic tap results), and a CSF PCR test is available for HSV1. EEG recording may demonstrate periodic epileptiform discharges over one or both temporal regions, particularly after several days of infection. HSV1 encephalitis is treated with a prolonged intravenous course of acyclovir. This drug can be started empirically if there is initial clinical or laboratory-based suspicion for HSV1 encephalitis, while awaiting results of the more definitive CSF PCR test to return, which can take several days. Other cases of viral encephalitis are managed with supportive care, including analgesics for headache and anticonvulsants for seizures, as appropriate.

KEY POINTS

- Viral meningitis may resemble acute bacterial meningitis but has a different CSF profile, and specific anti-infective therapy is generally not available.
- Viral encephalitis can be caused by a number of different agents, but HSV1 encephalitis is associated with some distinct clinical features and is treated with intravenous acyclovir.

FUNGAL INFECTIONS

There are several fungi that cause nervous system infection, including *Cryptococcus neoformans*, *Coccidioides immitis*, *Histoplasma capsulatum*, and various *Candida* species. *Cryptococcus* is the most common form of fungal meningitis and is discussed here.

CRYPTOCOCCAL MENINGITIS

Cryptococcal meningitis is typically an infection that affects those who are immunocompromised, such as patients with AIDS, although it sometimes infects immunocompetent hosts. The infection is acquired by inhalation of the fungus (which is present in soil and pigeon droppings) and then disseminated hematogenously. Cryptococcal meningitis often presents insidiously with headache, neck pain, and confusion; fever is variably present. The CSF profile demonstrates a lymphocytic predominance of white blood cells (except initially), elevated protein, and low glucose, which is a pattern seen across most fungal infections. Although India ink staining of CSF was historically a time-honored way of detecting the presence of *Cryptococcus* organisms, a rapid latex agglutination assay for cryptococcal antigen is the standard means of testing now. Treatment for cryptococcal infections involves the use of antifungal agents such as amphotericin.

KEY POINTS

- Cryptococcal meningitis typically occurs in immunocompromised individuals.
- It usually has an insidious presentation and, like other fungal meningitides, has a CSF profile distinct from most bacterial and viral infections.

PARASITIC INFECTIONS OF THE NERVOUS SYSTEM

Two important parasitic infections of the nervous system are discussed here, one that commonly affects those who are immunocompromised and another that is endemic in much of the developing world.

TOXOPLASMOSIS

Toxoplasma gondii is an intracellular parasite that most commonly affects humans either as a congenital infection (it is one of the TORCH infections, the others being "other," rubella, cytomegalovirus, and herpes simplex) or as an intracranial infection in patients with AIDS. Humans are exposed through cat feces or ingestion of undercooked meat. Clinically, toxoplasmosis in the AIDS patient presents as expected for any intracranial mass lesion, with headache, mental status changes, and focal neurologic signs and symptoms that depend on the lesion location. Fever can be present. Radiologic studies typically show multiple ring-enhancing lesions in the basal ganglia or at the gray matter–white matter junction. Serologies and CSF PCR assays can help to confirm the diagnosis. Primary CNS lymphoma is often in the radiologic differential diagnosis in AIDS patients with such intracranial lesions. In some cases, brain biopsy may be necessary to make a definitive diagnosis, particularly if empiric antitoxoplasmosis therapy has not led to any improvement.

NEUROCYSTICERCOSIS

Neurocysticercosis, an infection caused by the pork tapeworm *Taenia solium*, is the most common parasitic infection of the central nervous system and one of the most common causes of new-onset focal seizures in much of the developing world. It is endemic in, among other places, Central and South America, and thus is commonly seen in immigrant populations in the United States. Clinically, nervous system infection presents with seizures, headache, and signs of increased intracranial pressure. Radiologic studies demonstrate multiple cystic lesions which can be ring-enhancing or calcified, and often have surrounding edema. Anti-infective treatment includes albendazole, and steroids are often used to control the inflammation and edema that accompany the initial treatment and can actually lead to increased symptoms. Anticonvulsant medications are used to control the seizures.

KEY POINTS

- Toxoplasmosis, acquired from cat feces or undercooked meat, is a common cause of intracranial mass lesions in AIDS patients.
- Congenital toxoplasmosis is one of the TORCH infections.
- Cysticercosis, caused by a pork tapeworm, is the most common parasitic infection of the CNS and one of the most common causes of new-onset focal seizures in much of the world.

NERVOUS SYSTEM COMPLICATIONS OF HIV INFECTION

The retrovirus human immunodeficiency virus (HIV) is associated with a variety of nervous system syndromes, some of which appear to be late complications of direct HIV infection and prolonged immunosuppression (**HIV-associated dementia, vacuolar myelopathy**), some of which are due to opportunistic infections (**toxoplasmosis, cryptococcal meningitis, progressive multifocal leukoencephalopathy**), some of which reflect peripheral nervous system involvement (discussed in Chapter 23), and some of which are neurologic complications of antiretroviral therapy.

HIV-associated dementia is a late complication of HIV infection, generally occurring after prolonged periods of immunosuppression. Its incidence has declined in recent years with the widespread use of highly active antiretroviral therapy (HAART). Clinically, this syndrome presents as a subcortical dementia, with cognitive impairment and psychomotor slowing. MRI can show patchy T2 hyperintensity in the white matter as well as cerebral atrophy. There is no specific treatment other than aggressive antiretroviral therapy and supportive therapies. Prior to HAART, the development of HIV-associated dementia was often seen as one of the final stages of terminal illness due to HIV.

Vacuolar myelopathy is also a late complication of HIV infection that occurs with severe immunosuppression. Clinically, this disorder resembles the subacute combined degeneration syndrome associated with vitamin B_{12} deficiency, in that patients develop posterior column signs and symptoms (loss of vibration and joint position sense, with sensory ataxia) and signs of corticospinal tract dysfunction (spasticity and hyperreflexia) bilaterally. Urinary and sexual dysfunction may also occur. Treatment involves HAART and supportive therapy.

Progressive multifocal leukoencephalopathy (PML) is a demyelinating disease of the central nervous system caused by infection of oligodendrocytes by JC virus, a ubiquitous virus to which most individuals have been exposed early in life. PML can occur in the context of immunosuppression from AIDS or from other causes. It typically occurs as a late complication of HIV, with a subacute or chronic progression of focal neurologic signs. Cognitive impairment becomes evident over time, and MRI of the brain shows patchy nonenhancing foci of T2 hyperintensity within the subcortical white matter. Treatment involves HAART and supportive therapy when appropriate.

Opportunistic infections such as toxoplasmosis and cryptococcal meningitis are described earlier in this chapter. **Primary CNS lymphoma**, which is thought to be mediated by Epstein-Barr virus (EBV), is discussed in Chapter 19.

22 Disorders of the Spinal Cord

The central nervous system (CNS) comprises the brain and spinal cord. The spinal cord extends from the medulla, through the foramen magnum, down the spinal canal, about 45 cm (in adults) to the filum terminale, a connective tissue band anchoring the cord to the end of the canal. The brain and spinal cord are protected from external forces by the surrounding bones (the skull and vertebrae), and by the meninges, particularly the tough, resilient connective tissue of the dura mater. They are also protected chemically by the blood-brain (or blood-CNS) barrier. The spinal cord is the classic example of the applicability of neuroanatomy to clinical localization in Neurology and thus to determining diagnosis and treatment plans. So it is crucial to review the basic anatomy.

ANATOMY

In cross section, the center of the spinal cord contains the gray matter and neuron cell bodies (Fig. 22-1). The anterior horn of the grey matter contains primarily the alpha motor neurons and motor fibers innervating skeletal muscles. Surrounding the gray matter are white matter tracts. The most important descending motor tract is the corticospinal tract (CST) in the lateral portion of the cord. The CST descends from the cortex and crosses the midline in the medulla to become contralateral to its cortical origins and thus ipsilateral to the limbs it controls once below the brainstem (Fig. 22-2). The CST synapses on alpha motor neurons in the anterior horn.

Among several ascending sensory tracts are the heavily myelinated posterior (dorsal) columns, medi-

ating joint position sense. They remain ipsilateral to their origin for the length of the spinal cord, crossing in the brainstem. Fibers of the anterolateral spinothalamic tracts begin in the peripheral nerves subtending pain and temperature sensation, enter the cord and synapse within two levels, and then cross the cord and ascend contralateral to the limbs from which they convey sensation.

The spinal cord gives off motor nerve roots anteriorly and sensory roots posteriorly at each level. Seven cervical nerves exit the canal just above the corresponding vertebrae, but there is no C8 vertebra; the C8 nerve root exits just above the first thoracic vertebra. C1 has no sensory fibers. Below this, nerves exit below the corresponding vertebral bodies, from T (thoracic) 1 to T12, L (lumbar) 1 to L5, and S (sacral) 1 to S5. The corresponding level of the cord itself is typically a few bony levels above the roots—e.g., the T10 level of the cord itself may lie adjacent to the T8 vertebra. The spinal cord ends at about the L1 vertebral level. (Thus, it makes no sense to scan the lumbar spine to visualize a spinal cord lesion!)

KEY POINTS

- The corticospinal tract is the primary descending motor tract. It crosses in the medulla.
- Ascending dorsal column fibers carry position sense; they cross in the brainstem.
- The spinothalamic tract carries information on pain and temperature; it crosses the cord near the level of entry.

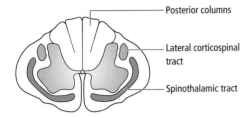

Figure 22-1 • Transverse section of the spinal cord showing the sensory pathways. The posterior columns relay information concerning proprioception and two-point discrimination. The spinothalamic tracts relay pain and temperature information. (Reproduced with permission from Ginsberg L. *Lecture Notes: Neurology*. 8th ed, Oxford: Blackwell Publishing, 2005:122.)

LOCALIZATION OF SPINAL CORD DYSFUNCTION

Spinal cord compression or dysfunction is often suspected on the basis of the neurologic examination. Localization in the cord is usually obtained by the combination of "long tract" signs and local segmental or root signs. In order to guide testing such as imaging, and to expedite treatment, it is often important to ascertain the rostral-caudal level of the lesion. Long tract motor findings include weakness and loss of motor control below the level of a lesion, plus hyperactive deep tendon reflexes and spasticity, as well as sexual and bowel and bladder dysfunction, particularly urinary retention. An indication of the spinal level can be obtained by determining the highest spinal level at which there is motor dysfunction—e.g., quadriceps weakness at L3 or L4 or finger and hand weakness at a C7 or C8 level—with preservation of motor function above that level. Nevertheless, it is difficult to ascertain motor deficits between the C8 or T1 level (the lowest levels involving upper limb function) and the L1 or L2 level (with motor deficits in the legs). There is also a sensory level, with impairment or elimination of perception of pain, temperature, position, and touch from below that level. Gait abnormalities result commonly from both motor and sensory deficits. Often a more reliable localizing sign of the level of cord dysfunction is that of a clinical abnormality at the level of lesion. This can take the form of a lost reflex (with preservation of others) or focal motor or sensory deficit at a particular level. Loss of alpha motor neurons at a given level leads to flaccid weakness in the innervated muscles.

It is important to remember that long tracts are "laminated" (with fibers to and from lower limbs

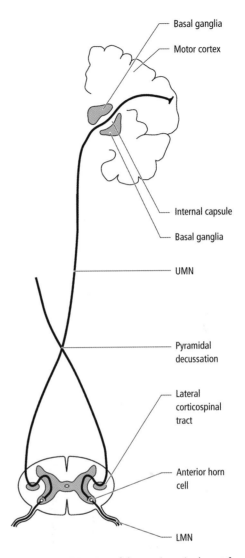

Figure 22-2 • Diagram of the corticospinal tract from the cortex to the ventral horn. (Reproduced with permission from Ginsberg L. *Lecture Notes: Neurology*. 8th ed, Oxford: Blackwell Publishing, 2005:37.)

running parallel to those from higher regions), and compression or other lesions of the cord can produce deficits *at* the level of the lesion or appearing anywhere *below* this. Extrinsic cord compression can produce misleading clinical signs because of the lamination of fibers. An evident sensory level may not indicate the true level of lesion clearly (especially with progressive compression) and the apparent level may rise over days (i.e., a lesion may produce a sensory level significantly below the lesion itself). Thus, loss of pinprick sensation seen clearly at T8 indicates that there is a lesion at this level *or above*. Without local (e.g., root) signs, the level of the lesion cannot be determined exactly, and the examination must focus carefully on *all higher* levels.

SPINAL CORD SYNDROMES

TRANSECTION

Severe trauma may cause complete transection of the spinal cord. Localization proceeds according to the principles above. If transection occurs above the level of the C3–C5 nerve roots (which control the diaphragm), respiratory insufficiency may result. Though apparently above the level of the lesion, a Horner's syndrome may result from cervical cord disease due to the transit of sympathetic fibers through the upper cervical spinal cord. Abdominal reflexes are lost with lesions above T6. Bowel and bladder dysfunction may follow lesions above the sacral cord level. A transverse myelitis may produce a similar clinical picture and may mimic a transection, but it usually develops over a longer period and eventually with evidence of inflammation, such as a spinal fluid pleocytosis.

SPINAL CORD COMPRESSION

Spinal cord compression is a neurologic emergency although it may evolve over hours to days.

Lesions causing spinal cord compression can be extradural, intradural but extramedullary, or intramedullary. Extradural (outside of the dural lining) lesions are relatively common causes of cord compression. The lesions are often in the bones or are in the intervertebral disks. Bony lesions from metastatic cancer (especially from breast and prostate cancer) are relatively common causes of cord compression. Usually, they are associated with significant pain due to the bony disease; compression of the cord itself does not hurt. Pressing or percussing on all levels of the vertebral column is important in looking for bony lesions. Other masses such as epidural abscesses and hematomas can produce acute and threatening cord compression.

Epidural abscesses can follow skin infections or tuberculosis or many other infections and may spread from a local osteomyelitis. They are often associated with radicular and other local pain. They can produce cord compression with loss of motor and sensory function below the lesion. They can extend over several spinal levels and be missed easily on radiologic studies, appearing very similar to a sheath or other lining of the spinal canal. Clinical suspicion must remain high for epidural abscesses because they are so dangerous, difficult to detect (even with good radiologic technology), and generally quite treatable with surgical drainage and antibiotics. (See also Chapter 21 on infections.)

Compressive lesions within the dura but outside of the spinal cord itself ("intradural, extramedullary"), include meningiomas and neurofibroma masses. Other lesions such as multiple sclerosis plaques and CNS gliomas can occur within the cord itself ("intramedullary"). Primary spinal cord tumors are rare.

HEMICORD SYNDROMES

When one side of the spinal cord is affected by an injury or other lesion, this can be manifested as a "hemicord" or Brown-Sequard syndrome. Classic localization in Neurology diagnoses these lesions readily. There is weakness (and usually hyperreflexia) ipsilateral to and below the lesion due to dysfunction of the corticospinal tract, as well as impaired position sense below the lesion from involvement of posterior column fibers ascending on the same side. Loss of pain and temperature perception below the level of the lesion, however, is contralateral to the lesion because nerve fibers subtending pain and temperature sensation begin contralaterally and cross below the level of the lesion. A Brown-Sequard syndrome can be caused by trauma or by cord compression, and occasionally by multiple sclerosis or other illnesses.

CENTRAL CORD LESIONS

A structural abnormality in the center of the spinal cord particularly affects spinothalamic tract fibers crossing at the level of the lesion. Deficits in pain and temperature sensation are usually bilateral and over several segments. Thus, there can be a "cape-like" loss of these sensations over the shoulders and arms, with preservation of the same sensations above and below the lesion (Fig. 22-3). The sensory loss is described as "dissociated" because pain and temperature sensation is affected, but touch and position sense is not. In addition, a variety of motor and sensory functions can be impaired below the lesion.

The classic central cord lesion is syringomyelia, an expansion of the (potential) fluid space in the center

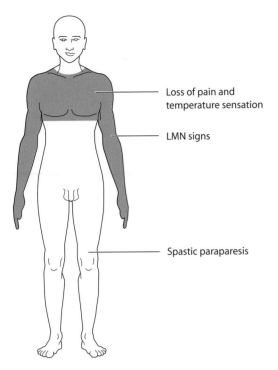

Loss of pain and
temperature sensation

LMN signs

Spastic paraparesis

Figure 22-3 • Clinical features of syringomyelia.
(Reproduced with permission from Ginsberg L. *Lecture Notes: Neurology.*
8th ed, Oxford: Blackwell Publishing, 2005:124.)

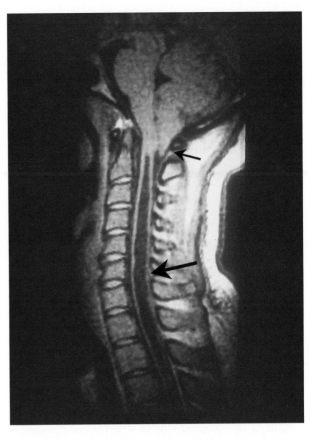

Figure 22-4 • Sagittal MRI scan of the spinal cord showing a
hypointense region in the middle of the cord that represents a
fluid-filled syrinx cavity (*large black arrow*). This syrinx is associated with a type I Chiari malformation characterized by the
downward displacement of the cerebellar tonsils through the
foramen magnum (*small black arrow*).
(Reproduced with permission from Ginsberg L. *Lecture Notes: Neurology.*
8th ed, Oxford: Blackwell Publishing, 2005:123.)

of the spinal cord, usually over several levels. Sensory
deficits are most common, as the crossing spinothalamic tracts are affected with enlargement of the cavity. Numbness may begin in the hands; loss of alpha
motor neurons in the same area may lead to wasting
and weakness, often developing over months or years.
Spasticity is usually a later sign. Loss of pain and temperature sensation entails a risk of tissue injury (such
as burns) without the patient noticing. Dorsal column
function is often preserved. About half of syrinxes are
associated with posterior skull and brain malformations such as Chiari malformations. Occasionally, the
syrinx may extend into the brainstem (syringobulbia),
causing brainstem neurologic signs.

Diagnosis is tremendously facilitated by MRI (Fig.
22-4). Treatment of syringomyelia is very controversial. Expansile central fluid cavities can be drained
and left with a shunt, draining fluid out of the cavity.
This might interrupt neurologic worsening without
necessarily reversing an earlier deficit.

Central cord lesions also include hematomyelia
(bleeding into the center of the cord), and small focal
tumors. Sometimes an external compressive lesion
can produce dysfunction in the center of the cord
even when there is no discrete lesion there.

 KEY POINTS

- Spinal cord compression causes weakness, incoordination, and sphincter dysfunction below the level
  of the lesion and often causes a sensory level at (or
  below) the lesion.

- A Brown-Sequard syndrome affects one side of the
  cord and causes motor control and position sense
  loss ipsilaterally and below the lesion, as well as loss
  of pain and temperature sensation contralaterally.

- A central cord syndrome includes motor and
  sensory dysfunction below the lesion and often a
  "cape-like" loss of pain and temperature sensation
  at levels near the lesion.

MULTIFOCAL AND DIFFUSE CORD DYSFUNCTION

Some illnesses affect the cord more diffusely. Radiation therapy and paraneoplastic syndromes affect the cord broadly. Radiation myelopathy develops 6 months to years after radiotherapy. Syphilis can affect posterior columns preferentially (tabes dorsalis), although this is rare now. Vitamin B_{12} deficiency can cause posterior column dysfunction. Demyelinating and vascular lesions may be multifocal.

CAUDA EQUINA AND CONUS LESIONS

Cauda equina lesions are those affecting the spinal nerve roots within the spinal canal in the lumbar and sacral regions, without affecting the spinal cord itself. Cauda equina lesions produce wasting, weakness, and fasciculations in the appropriately innervated muscles, often with substantial pain. Sacral root dysfunction can cause bowel, bladder, and sexual dysfunction. Cauda equina syndromes can be produced by narrowing or obstruction of the spinal canal in the lumbosacral region, by infections, and by central disks below the level of the spinal cord.

At the tip of the spinal cord, there are lesions of the conus medullaris, which includes centers controlling bowel, bladder, and sexual function. Causes include compressive lesions and intramedullary abnormalities such as tumors. Lesions here can produce a mixture of upper motor neuron findings such as hyperreflexia, Babinski signs, and particularly prominent sphincter dysfunction, as well as radicular pain. If they remain below the lumbar cord, conus lesions may leave leg strength and reflexes intact while severely affecting bowel, bladder, and sexual function.

VASCULAR DISEASE OF THE SPINAL CORD AND THE ANTERIOR SPINAL ARTERY SYNDROME

The blood supply for the anterior two-thirds of the spinal cord comes primarily from the large solitary longitudinal anterior spinal artery (ASA) running along most of the ventral surface of the cord. The cephalad portion of the ASA arises from branches of the two vertebral arteries, joining at the top of the cord. Caudally, the largest single artery supplying the ASA is the artery of Adamkiewicz, originating from perforating arteries from the aorta (of which there are several), entering the spinal canal at about the L2 level. This large artery supplies blood superiorly through much of the thoracic cord. The anterior horns and corticospinal tracts are perfused primarily from the ASA. Supplying the dorsal columns posteriorly is a plexus of many arteries rather than one large vessel, in turn fed by segmental arteries that arise from the aorta and course along the ribs, giving off radicular arteries next to the nerve roots near the cord.

The spinal cord, like the brain, can incur a stroke when the blood supply is compromised, usually by atherosclerotic disease and occasionally by vasculitis. Strokes can occur following systemic or local hypotension, or by occlusion of a vessel, sometimes when injured during aortic surgery or by dissection. The most common form of cord stroke is the anterior spinal artery syndrome. This causes weakness below the lesion, and there may be intense radicular pain or back pain and sphincter dysfunction. Sensory loss is prominent, but usually not involving position sense because posterior column function is unaffected in this syndrome—a major neurologic examination clue to the diagnosis. The thoracic cord is the least well perfused and most vulnerable area. The border between the vascular supply from the vertebral arteries above and the inferior blood supply may reach up to about T4, and that can be the clinical level of cord dysfunction. Systemic hypotension can lead to a watershed infarct affecting this area.

Strokes are diagnosed clinically; MRI can show the lesion in many cases. Angiography of the spinal cord vessels is very difficult and may lead to complications. With the sudden deficit, investigations are usually too late to help. There are no good treatments for spinal cord infarction. The prognosis is uncertain but often poor.

Strokes also include hemorrhages, and hematomas can cause serious cord deficits. Venous infarctions occur very rarely; some result from coagulopathies. Emboli to the cord are rare. Spinal AVMs are often very difficult to diagnose and may present in a stuttering fashion over months or years. Dural arteriovenous malformations may cause slowly progressive spinal cord deficits.

KEY POINTS

- The anterior spinal artery syndrome (ASAS) is a stroke in the cord affecting motor and sensory function below the lesion, usually sparing posterior column function.
- Aortic surgery and atherosclerosis are common causes of the ASAS.

TRAUMA

Spinal cord injury is a serious concern with any neck or back trauma. Motor vehicle accidents and athletic activity are relatively common causes of such injury. In the first aid of patients with neck or back trauma, the neck should be immobilized immediately until it is clear that the spinal cord is functioning properly. Airway maintenance is more difficult when the neck is immobilized, but this is crucial in severe trauma. The patient is then examined with attention to principles described earlier.

While spinal cord lesions often produce hyperreflexia and extensor plantar responses (Babinski signs), there may be flaccid weakness and complete absence of DTRs immediately after trauma, a condition called "spinal shock." Spasticity typically develops over the next few days and weeks. Flaccidity and loss of reflexes should not divert attention from the spinal cord.

High dosages of steroids (at least 100 mg of dexamethasone) are usually used for traumatic cord compression, and for compression due to tumors (with subsequent radiation therapy for some tumors). Surgical decompression is of uncertain benefit, but probably very little when paraparesis is complete or after several days of compression.

AMYOTROPHIC LATERAL SCLEROSIS

Amyotrophic lateral sclerosis (ALS; Lou Gehrig's disease) causes progressive neurologic dysfunction primarily within the spinal cord, but some evidence indicates that neuronal loss is more extensive, and some patients have an associated frontotemporal dementia. The cause of ALS is unknown in most cases. About 10% are familial (genetic) and many of these involve a mutation in the superoxide dismutase enzyme, thought to lead to excitotoxin damage.

The pathologic abnormalities of ALS involve the alpha motor neurons (lower motor neurons) of the anterior horn of the spinal cord, leading to weakness in the muscles they supply and evidence of denervation, such as fasciculations and wasting. There is also involvement of the lateral corticospinal tracts, leading to weakness, spasticity, hyperreflexia, and Babinski signs. The term "amyotrophic" refers to a loss of muscle mass from denervation and "lateral" to the corticospinal tract dysfunction. ALS causes no sensory deficits, and eye movements remain unaffected.

ALS is a relentlessly progressive illness, typically fatal within 3 to 5 years of diagnosis. Some patients lose all motor function (including respiration, but usually not sphincter control) while maintaining cognitive function and sensation. Some go on to years of mechanical ventilation assistance. Riluzole retards the speed of deterioration in ALS somewhat but does not reverse it. Causes and treatment of ALS are under intensive investigation.

In the evaluation of a patient with suspected ALS, it is crucial to look for potentially treatable illnesses that can mimic ALS. Stenosis of the spinal canal can cause denervation at several levels. Cervical spine disease can also produce hyperreflexia and Babinski signs by compression of the cord in the neck, along with lower motor neuron weakness, wasting, and fasciculations in the arms due to concomitant cervical root compression. EMG testing can show denervation above this region (e.g., in facial or tongue muscles) that cannot be caused by spine disease, corroborating a diagnosis of ALS.

Far fewer patients have primarily lateral CST dysfunction, producing spasticity and loss of motor control, without prominent alpha motor neuron loss—referred to as primary lateral sclerosis, but some of these patients will be diagnosed with ALS eventually. Cord dysfunction with progressive spasticity and weakness and severe gait disorders also occurs in hereditary spastic paraparesis, where there is the possibility of genetic diagnosis, and tropical spastic paraparesis, in which HTLV-1 testing can help make the diagnosis. Severe nutritional deficiency can also cause widespread spinal cord dysfunction.

Other illnesses involving primarily the alpha motor neurons (with wasting, fasciculations, and weakness, but without spasticity or sensory deficits) occur in the spinal muscular atrophies (SMA)—somewhat different in presentation at different ages, and often clearly genetic in origin. SMAs present (usually in childhood) with weakness and atrophy from anterior horn cell degeneration. Werdnig-Hoffmann disease is an SMA presenting in infancy. Evaluation is most appropriately done by pediatric neuromuscular specialists with command of the neurophysiology and genetic testing.

KEY POINTS

- ALS is a relentlessly progressive degenerative disease leading to loss of anterior horn cell and peripheral nerve function, with weakness and signs of denervation.
- It also affects the corticospinal tracts, causing spasticity and additional loss of motor control.
- Patients with ALS often die within a few years of diagnosis, often from respiratory failure.
- When considering a diagnosis of ALS, it is important to look for other (treatable) diagnoses such as extensive spine disease.

CONGENITAL AND DEGENERATIVE ILLNESSES OF THE SPINE

Many congenital abnormalities affect the spinal cord. A syrinx in the cervical cord, or even extending rostrally into the brainstem, can be associated with a Chiari malformation (a downward protrusion of the medulla, with or without the cerebellum, through the foramen magnum). At the caudal end of the canal, failure of proper closure of the neural tube can result in midline structural deficits referred to as "dysraphisms," some as mild as pilonidal cysts in the lumbar midline. Spina bifida is an incomplete closure of the posterior parts of the vertebrae; it may be asymptomatic. More severe deficits include larger openings of the spinal canal such as a meningocele (protrusion of the meninges into the tissues of the back beyond the spinal canal) or even myelomeningocele—with protrusion of spinal cord tissue itself. The more severe lesions are associated with paraplegia and maldevelopment of the legs. There are many related congenital abnormalities. Hypertrophy of the filum terminale can produce a "tethered cord syndrome," with pain and dysfunction of the spinal cord, especially at lower levels. This is often associated with other structural

abnormalities. Some are evident on inspection of the lower back; most can be diagnosed with MRI as prompted by clinical suspicion, and many produce severe neurologic deficits.

Herniated disks may compress the spinal cord in the cervical (or rarely thoracic) region. Herniated lumbar disks may compress lumbar nerve roots, often causing significant pain and eventually, wasting and weakness of innervated muscles. Bowel and bladder dysfunction may occur with compression of sacral roots. With severe pain and with motor deficits, surgical removal of the herniated disc can be curative, but some extruded disks are reversible on their own with time.

SPINAL CORD DIAGNOSTIC TESTS

Many different radiologic techniques can help in evaluating spinal cord problems. Plain x-rays can show bony abnormalities, such as dislocation of the vertebral bodies. Lateral views can show one vertebra displaced significantly enough on another (spondylolisthesis) to produce spinal cord or root dysfunction. Plain x-rays may show lytic lesions of the vertebrae from metastases, leading to spinal cord compression. CT scanning is also very helpful with bony abnormalities, especially when the clinical examination indicates the axial level to be scanned. MRI can produce excellent longitudinal (sagittal) views of the entire length of the spinal cord. T2 and FLAIR sequences can help to show intrinsic lesions of the spinal cord, such as tumors (sometimes with expansion of the cord itself), multiple sclerosis, and other inflammatory tissue changes, including those of a transverse myelitis. Vascular lesions such as strokes and hemorrhages are often demonstrated well. CT and MRI axial images can show root compression from disks or other structural abnormalities. The sagittal MRI is often particularly helpful in the diagnosis of a central cord lesion such as a syrinx and may help to show an epidural abscess or other lesions. Myelograms (with contrast material in the spinal fluid) are performed infrequently now, but occasionally they can demonstrate vascular abnormalities around the spinal cord or other structural problems, especially in cauda equina roots, that are not seen well on other tests. Evoked potentials can demonstrate poor conduction in the sensory tracts of the spinal cord, but they are used seldom since the development of MRI. Cerebrospinal fluid from a lumbar puncture can provide evidence of infection, inflammation, or malignancy.

The Peripheral Nervous System

The peripheral nervous system (PNS) consists of cranial nerves, spinal roots, peripheral nerves, neuromuscular junction, muscles, and autonomic ganglia. Afferent fibers connect the sensory receptors to the CNS, and efferent fibers connect the CNS to the effector (motor) apparatus. Three classically described pathologic changes affect peripheral nerve axons:

- **Wallerian degeneration:** After injury to axons and myelin, a distal disintegration of axon and myelin occurs.
- **Neuronal (or axonal) degeneration:** This develops after damage to the cell body of the neuron, resulting in the distal dying of the axon and subsequent loss of myelin.
- **Demyelination:** The myelin sheath is lost as a result of this process.

APPROACH TO PERIPHERAL NEUROPATHY

The goals in the evaluation of peripheral neuropathy (PN) are to localize the site of disease to the axon, myelin sheath, cell body, or vascular structures; identify the cause; and prescribe treatment when available.

Start by determining the types of symptoms (motor, sensory, autonomic, or mixed); the distribution of weakness (proximal or distal, symmetric or asymmetric); the nature and distribution of sensory involvement (small fiber, large fiber, or mixed); and the evolution of the condition (acute, subacute, or chronic) (Box 23-1).

The next step is to recognize a pattern of PN that will help to determine the etiology of the disease (Table 23-1). Finally, characterize the primary pathologic process by using electrodiagnostic studies, including nerve conduction studies and EMG.

KEY POINTS

- The symptoms associated with involvement of small nerve fibers are neuropathic pain (described as aching, shooting, throbbing, or burning); temperature sensations; and autonomic dysfunction (cardiac arrhythmias, orthostatic hypotension, impotence, incontinence, and constipation).
- The symptoms and signs associated with involvement of large fibers are loss of vibration and joint position sense, weakness, fasciculations, and loss of deep tendon reflexes.

INVESTIGATION OF THE PERIPHERAL NERVOUS SYSTEM

A logical and rational approach to the diagnosis of peripheral nervous system (PNS) disorders is fundamental. Tests are ordered sequentially, guided by the history, and clinical and electrodiagnostic findings. In general, first-line tests include CBC, ESR, and rheumatoid profiles (for collagen disease, leukemia, vasculitis); renal and liver function tests (for uremic and hepatic disease); glucose and Hb-

■ BOX 23-1 Approach to the Classification of Peripheral Neuropathy

Functional involvement
Motor
Sensory
Small fiber
Large fiber
Small and large fiber
Autonomic
Anatomic distribution
Asymmetric
Symmetric
Upper extremity
Lower extremity
Temporal course
Acute: GBS, porphyria, diphtheria, polio, toxins (thallium, lead, arsenic, Adriamycin), paraneoplastic, uremia, vasculitis
Subacute: deficiency states (vitamins B_1 and B_{12}), toxins, uremia, diabetes, sarcoidosis, paraneoplastic, vasculitis, toxins, drugs
Chronic: CIDP, diabetes, uremia
Relapsing: CIDP
Pathologic mechanism
Axonal
Demyelination
Combined neuropathy

CIDP, chronic inflammatory demyelinating polyneuropathy; GBS, Guillain-Barré syndrome.

A1C levels (diabetes); vitamin B_{12} and folate levels (neuropathy with macrocytosis); thyroid function tests (hypothyroid neuropathy); and serum protein electrophoresis and urine protein electrophoresis (dysproteinemias, monoclonal gammopathy, lymphoma, amyloidosis).

Second-line tests include urine porphobilinogen (acute intermittent porphyria); urine heavy metals such as lead, arsenic, and mercury; arsenic in hair and nails (arsenic neuropathy); hepatitis B antigen (Ag), antineutrophil cytoplasmic antibodies (Abs) (Wegener's granulomatosis); CT scan of the chest (cancer survey, carcinomatous neuropathy); CSF protein (Guillain-Barré syndrome, chronic inflammatory demyelinating polyneuropathy); CSF pleocytosis (Lyme disease, AIDS, paraneoplastic); serum HIV test (AIDS neuropathy); Lyme titers; anti-Hu Ab (paraneoplastic); anti-GM_1, MAG Ab (autoimmune neuropathy); and genetic testing for hereditary neuropathy.

Electrodiagnostic studies include nerve conduction studies and EMG. A nerve biopsy should be performed when indicated.

EPIDEMIOLOGY

The prevalence of PN among patients with no recognized exposure to diseases or neurotoxic agents is 2%. Diabetes mellitus is the most common risk factor, followed by alcoholism, nonalcoholic liver disease, and malignancy. Among patients with one or two risk factors, the prevalence is 12% and 17%, respectively.

The most common causes of PN in the United States are hereditary (30%), followed by cryptogenic (23%), diabetes mellitus (15%), multifocal motor neuropathy (MMN), vitamin B_{12} deficiency, and drugs (Box 23-2).

KEY POINTS

- A mnemonic for the most common causes of peripheral neuropathies is DANG THE RAPIST: diabetes, alcohol, nutritional, Guillain-Barré, trauma, hereditary, environmental (toxins and drugs), rheumatic (vascular), amyloid, paraneoplastic, infections, systemic disease, and tumors.

- **Polyneuropathy** refers to symmetric involvement of the peripheral nerves, usually of the legs more than the arms and distal more than proximal segments—the "stocking-glove" pattern.

- **Mononeuropathy** refers to involvement of a single nerve—for example, median neuropathy at the wrist, also known as carpal tunnel syndrome.

- **Mononeuropathy multiplex** refers to involvement of individual nerves in a multifocal distribution.

- **Radiculopathy** refers to involvement of nerve roots (Table 23-4).

■ **TABLE 23-1** Pattern-Recognition Approach to Peripheral Neuropathy

Pattern	Possible Causes
Symmetric proximal and distal weakness with sensory loss	GBS, CIDP
Symmetric distal weakness with sensory loss	Drug-induced, toxic, and metabolic neuropathies; hereditary neuropathies; amyloidosis
Asymmetric distal weakness with sensory loss Multiple nerves	Vasculitis; HNPP; infections such as leprosy, Lyme disease, sarcoidosis, and HIV
Single nerve	Compressive mononeuropathy and radiculopathy
Asymmetric distal weakness without sensory loss	Motor neuron disease, multifocal motor neuropathy
Asymmetric proximal and distal weakness with sensory loss	Polyradiculopathy or plexopathy, meningeal carcinomatosis or lymphomatosis, HNPP, hereditary neuropathies
Symmetric sensory loss without weakness	Cryptogenic sensory polyneuropathy; metabolic, drug-induced, or toxic neuropathies; leprosy
Asymmetric proprioceptive sensory loss without weakness	Sensory neuronopathies (ganglionopathies); consider paraneoplastic, Sjögren syndrome, vitamin B_6 toxicity, HIV-related sensory neuronopathies, *cis*-platinum toxicity
Autonomic symptoms and signs	Diabetes mellitus, amyloidosis, GBS, vincristine, porphyria, HIV-related autonomic neuropathy, idiopathic pandysautonomia

CIDP, chronic inflammatory demyelinating polyradiculoneuropathy; GBS, Guillain-Barré syndrome; HIV, human immunodeficiency virus; HNPP, hereditary neuropathy with liability to pressure palsies.

IMMUNE-MEDIATED NEUROPATHIES

GUILLAIN-BARRÉ SYNDROME (ACUTE INFLAMMATORY DEMYELINATING POLYNEUROPATHY)

Epidemiology

There are one to two cases of Guillain-Barré syndrome (GBS) per 100,000 population per year. Males and females are at equal risk. Adults are more frequently affected than children. Of those affected, 5% will die of the illness, but more than 85% make an excellent recovery.

Pathogenesis

In 60% to 70% of patients, neurologic symptoms are preceded by an acute infection (usually respiratory or gastrointestinal). Some 25% of cases in the United States are preceded by infection with *Campylobacter jejuni* and others by a herpesvirus infection, most frequently cytomegalovirus or Epstein-Barr virus. Acute inflammatory demyelinating polyneuropathy (AIDP) is considered an autoimmune disease, with neural targets represented by gangliosides. Many antiganglioside antibodies are found in GBS, the most frequent being anti-GM_1, but anti-GD_{1a}, anti-GQ_{1b}, anti-GD_{1b}, and others are found as well.

Clinical Manifestations

GBS typically presents as a rapidly evolving, ascending areflexic motor paralysis with or without sensory disturbances. Initial symptoms often consist of tingling and pins-and-needles sensations in the feet, sometimes with lower back pain. Weakness evolves over hours to days, reaching its worst within 30 days (usually by 14 days). Bulbar weakness and respiratory muscle paralysis may occur. Tendon reflexes usually

■ BOX 23-2 Classification of Peripheral Neuropathy by Etiology

Immune-mediated neuropathies	**Hereditary sensory and autonomic neuropathies**
Guillain-Barré syndrome	Neuropathy with leukodystrophy (metachromatic leukodystrophy, Krabbe disease, adrenoleukoneuropathy)
CIDP	
Multifocal motor neuropathy	
Neuropathy associated with monoclonal antibodies	**Toxic neuropathies**
	Metals: Arsenic, lead, mercury, thallium
Immune-mediated ataxic neuropathies, including carcinomatous sensory neuropathy, sensory ganglionitis associated with Sjögren syndrome, and idiopathic sensory ganglionitis	Drugs: Vincristine, cisplatin, antiretrovirals
	Substance abuse: Alcohol, glue inhalation, nitrous oxide inhalation
Vasculitic neuropathies: Rheumatoid arthritis, Sjögren syndrome, hepatitis B, Lyme disease, HIV, etc.	Industrial poisons: Acrylamide, carbon disulfide, cyanide, ethylene, hexacarbon, organophosphorous, trichloroethylene (trigeminal neuropathy)
Metabolic neuropathies	
Diabetic neuropathy	**Neuropathies associated with infections**
Thyroid disease	HIV
Hepatic neuropathy	Lyme neuropathy
Uremic neuropathy	Leprosy (the most frequent infectious cause of neuropathy in the world)
Porphyric neuropathy (acute intermittent porphyria)	
Vitamin deficiency (B_1, B_6, B_{12})	CMV and herpes
Critical illness neuropathy	**Entrapment and compressive neuropathies**
Hereditary neuropathies	Upper extremity: Carpal tunnel syndrome or median neuropathy, ulnar neuropathy, radial neuropathy
Charcot-Marie-Tooth disease	
Amyloid neuropathies	Lower extremity: Femoral and peroneal neuropathies, among others
Hereditary neuropathy with liability to pressure palsies	

CIDP, chronic inflammatory demyelinating polyradiculoneuropathy; CMV, cytomegalovirus; HIV, human immunodeficiency virus.

disappear after 3 days. Over 50% of patients develop facial weakness, and 10% have extraocular muscle paralysis. Pain is common. Autonomic dysfunction may be present, with orthostatic hypotension, transient hypertension, and cardiac arrhythmias.

The Miller-Fisher variant is characterized by gait ataxia, areflexia, and external ophthalmoplegia, usually without limb weakness. Nerve conduction studies are normal, and anti-GQ_{1b} Abs are positive in 90% of cases.

Diagnostic Evaluation

Albuminocytologic dissociation in the CSF (elevated protein but few or no cells) is characteristic. Usually the CSF protein rises after the first few days. Early electrodiagnostic findings may include prolonged distal latencies, variably prolonged or absent F waves, and possible conduction block. Early EMG changes include decreased motor unit recruitment. Routine laboratory evaluation should include CBC, ESR, liver function tests, and HIV test. The differential diagnosis includes spinal cord disease such as transverse myelitis and acute neuromuscular junction problems (myasthenia) or myopathy.

Treatment

Patients should be hospitalized. Monitoring should include frequent measurement of the forced vital capacity (FVC) and negative inspiratory pressure. An FVC below 15 mL/kg warrants transfer to the intensive care unit and likely intubation. Medical treatment includes intravenous immunoglobulin (IVIg) or plasmapheresis (equally effective). Intravenous steroids are not proven to be beneficial.

CHRONIC INFLAMMATORY DEMYELINATING POLYNEUROPATHY

Chronic inflammatory demyelinating polyradiculoneuropathy (CIDP) is sometimes called chronic GBS. Although there are many similarities, the two conditions differ in time course and in response to steroids.

Epidemiology

CIDP may occur at any age, typically in adults between the ages of 40 and 60 years.

Clinical Manifestations

Patients experience a slowly evolving weakness beginning in the legs, with widespread areflexia and loss of vibratory sense (larger fiber). Weakness of neck flexors is often present. Painful paresthesias and other sensory symptoms can occur.

Diagnostic Evaluation

Diagnosis of chronic inflammatory demyelinating polyneuropathy is supported by clinical features, time course, relapses, prominent demyelinating features in nerve conduction studies, and CSF protein elevation. About 10% have associated systemic illness such as HIV infection, monoclonal gammopathy, or Hodgkin lymphoma.

Treatment

About 90% of CIDP improves with steroids, but 50% will relapse afterward. Patients who do not respond to steroids may require plasmapheresis or intravenous immunoglobulin. Treatment is often required for years.

MULTIFOCAL MOTOR NEUROPATHY

MMN is an uncommon disorder characterized by a pure motor multiple mononeuropathy. It can occur at any age. There is a slight male predominance. Evidence supports an immune-mediated mechanism.

Clinical Manifestations

Patients present with a slowly progressive, asymmetric, predominantly distal limb weakness that usually begins in the arms. Weakness develops in the distribution of individual nerves rather than following a spinal myotome; it can be severe in muscles with relatively normal bulk. Reflexes are spared in less affected muscles. Minor sensory symptoms are common. Objective sensory deficits, upper motor neuron findings, and cranial nerve findings are usually absent.

Diagnostic Evaluation

Diagnosis is made by clinical features plus electrodiagnostic studies demonstrating conduction block in motor nerves in areas not prone to compression. CSF protein is usually normal. Nerve biopsy is nonspecific. A very high IgM anti-GM_1 is found in 60% to 80% of patients with MMN. It is important to recognize and distinguish MMN from typical motor neuron disease because MMN responds to IVIg or immunosuppressive drug therapy such as cyclophosphamide.

NEUROPATHIES ASSOCIATED WITH MYELOMA AND OTHER MONOCLONAL GAMMOPATHIES

Approximately 10% of peripheral neuropathies are associated with serum monoclonal gammopathy (M protein) that reacts with myelin-associated glycoprotein (MAG). One-third of those patients have multiple myeloma, amyloidosis, macroglobulinemia, cryoglobulinemia, lymphoma, or leukemia.

Clinical Manifestations

These neuropathies develop as symmetric sensorimotor neuropathies that usually affect the legs more than the arms. This neuropathy causes prominent large-fiber sensory loss and sensory ataxia as well as weakness.

Diagnostic Evaluation

Electrodiagnostic studies show demyelination.

Treatment

Treatment depends on the cause. If the neuropathy is due to a plasmacytoma, excision and radiation of the tumor can be curative. In other cases, plasmapheresis may have some benefit.

KEY POINTS

- Neuropathy associated with monoclonal gammopathy is primarily demyelinating.

METABOLIC NEUROPATHIES

DIABETIC POLYNEUROPATHY

Diabetic polyneuropathy is the most frequent form of diabetic neuropathy (Table 23-2) and is a common complication of diabetes mellitus; up to 60% of diabetic patients will develop neuropathy.

Epidemiology

The prevalence of diabetic neuropathy increases with the duration of diabetes; it usually develops after 5 to 10 years of the disease. Neuropathy can be present prior to overt diabetes and may be associated with impaired glucose tolerance. The pathogenesis of diabetic neuropathy is directly related to the prolonged effects of hyperglycemia.

Clinical Manifestations

Patients may report neuropathic pain and dysesthesias. More characteristic is a distal, symmetric, slowly

■ TABLE 23-2 Diabetic Neuropathies	
Type	**Comments**
Chronic progressive distal symmetric diabetic polyneuropathy	Mixed sensory-autonomic-motor polyneuropathy; variants include small-fiber (painful, usually spontaneous burning pain), large-fiber (ataxic), and autonomic
Diabetic proximal motor neuropathy (diabetic amyotrophy)	Severe thigh and back pain, followed within weeks by mild to severe hip and thigh muscle weakness with muscle atrophy; usually affects older type 2 diabetic patients
Acute axonal diabetic polyneuropathy (intensely painful acute or subacute progressive symmetric sensory axonal peripheral neuropathy)	Diabetic neuropathic cachexia (with worsening hyperglycemia); insulin neuritis (with improved hyperglycemia)
Diabetic mononeuropathy, radiculopathy, and polyradiculopathy	Can present with cranial neuropathy (third, fourth, and sixth nerves), multisegmental truncal radiculopathy, or limb mononeuropathy
Focal compression neuropathies associated with diabetes	Diabetic patients are more susceptible to compression neuropathies, such as median nerve at the wrist, ulnar nerve at the elbow, and peroneal nerve at the knee

progressive sensory loss in the lower extremities (stocking distribution, beginning with toes and feet before hands). Autonomic insufficiency can be an important feature. Weakness is a late feature.

Diagnostic Evaluation

Diagnosis is straightforward in established diabetes with typical clinical findings. It is an axonal polyneuropathy, usually involving small and large fibers.

Treatment

Glucose control is the best treatment. Symptomatic management of neuropathic pain includes the use of NSAIDs, tricyclic antidepressants, duloxetine, or anticonvulsants such as gabapentin, pregabalin, lamotrigine, and others.

KEY POINTS

- Diabetic polyneuropathy is the most common and important of the diabetic neuropathies.
- It usually involves small and large fibers.
- The neuropathy is distal and symmetric, with a stocking-glove distribution.
- Neuropathic pain may respond to anticonvulsants such as gabapentin.

OTHER METABOLIC NEUROPATHIES

Uremic Neuropathy

Uremic neuropathy is a symmetric, distally predominant sensorimotor axonal polyneuropathy. Footdrop and leg weakness are major manifestations.

Porphyric Neuropathy

Porphyric neuropathy is usually associated with acute intermittent porphyria. It is an acute or subacute sensorimotor axonal PN manifested by paresthesias and dysesthesias of the extremities sometimes with rapidly evolving weakness or paralysis (mimicking GBS), with areflexia and abdominal pain.

Critical Illness Neuropathies

Critical illness neuropathies develop in 50% of patients with severe medical illness who have been in the intensive care unit for more than 2 weeks. The etiology is unclear; often it may be related to an infection. Electrodiagnostic studies show an axonal neuropathy.

HEREDITARY NEUROPATHIES

Hereditary neuropathies are the most prevalent inherited neurologic disease and also the most common cause of polyneuropathy in patients referred to neurologic clinics in Western countries.

Charcot-Marie-Tooth disease (CMT) is the most common inherited PN, with an estimated prevalence of 40 per 100,000 adults and 19 per 100,000 children. CMT typically presents in adolescence with symmetric, slowly progressive distal muscular atrophy of the legs and feet; in most cases, it eventually involves the hands. Hammer toes and pes cavus are common. The age of onset, severity, and rate of progression can vary, even within the same family.

KEY POINTS

- CMT-2 is the only axonal motor neuropathy of the CMT family; the others are primarily demyelinating.
- Hereditary sensory and autonomic neuropathy (HSAN) is a hereditary neuropathy that affects autonomic sensory or motor nerves.
- There is no specific drug or gene therapy for hereditary neuropathies.

INFECTIOUS NEUROPATHIES

PN occurs in a number of infections, including viral, bacterial, parasitic, and prion disease. Most such peripheral neuropathies are beyond the scope of this chapter.

HIV NEUROPATHIES

HIV neuropathies include the following:

- **Distal sensory polyneuropathy:** occurs in more than 30% of patients with AIDS. It may be HIV-related, nucleoside treatment–related, or due to other neurotoxic medications.
- **Mononeuropathy and multiple mononeuropathies:** usually occur late in the illness, sometimes associated with superimposed infection (herpes,

cytomegalovirus, hepatitis C, and syphilis), lymphomatous infiltration, or necrotizing vasculitis.

- **Acute inflammatory demyelinating polyneuropathy:** is similar to GBS and responsive to plasmapheresis and IVIg.
- **Lumbosacral polyradiculoneuropathy:** is uncommon but usually associated with cytomegalovirus infection. It is a devastating complication and presents as a rapidly progressive flaccid paraparesis, with sphincter dysfunction, perineal sensory loss, and lower limb areflexia.

NEUROPATHY OF LEPROSY

Leprosy is among the most common of all neuropathies in the world. It is caused by *Mycobacterium leprae* and characterized by sensory and motor involvement. It usually presents as a mononeuropathy multiplex or mononeuropathies with predilection for cooler areas such as distal limbs, nose, and ears. Deep tendon reflexes (DTRs) are usually preserved. There is often nerve hypertrophy, which can be palpated. Axonal damage, myelin changes, and nerve fiber loss are cardinal features of lepromatous leprosy.

ENTRAPMENT NEUROPATHIES

Entrapment neuropathies are a common group of mononeuropathies produced by nerve entrapment (pressure, stretch, friction, and so forth). They are reviewed in Table 23-3.

KEY POINTS

- Leprosy is among the most common causes of neuropathy in the world.
- HIV neuropathies are common.
- Tips to remember about peripheral neuropathies are found in Table 23-5.

AUTONOMIC NEUROPATHIES

Autonomic neuropathies are a group of disorders that affect the sympathetic and parasympathetic nervous systems. Autonomic dysfunction may result from a lesion affecting one or more areas of the CNS or PNS and can be acquired or inherited. They can be primary or secondary—i.e., associated with another neuropathy or a systemic disorder.

CLINICAL MANIFESTATIONS

Symptoms include orthostatic hypotension, diarrhea, constipation, early satiety, tachycardia or palpitation, blurred vision, urinary retention, and erectile dysfunction. **Pandysautonomia** refers to an acquired disorder, usually immune in nature, often following a viral infection, in which both the sympathetic and parasympathetic nervous systems are affected. Postural orthostatic tachycardia syndrome (POTS) occurs most commonly in women, with orthostatic light-headedness and near-syncopal episodes.

Autonomic neuropathy can be a prominent presentation in patients with diabetic neuropathy or a part of the more generalized polyneuropathy syndrome of diabetes. Autonomic neuropathy can also be seen in GBS, amyloid neuropathy, Chagas disease, paraneoplastic disorders, toxic and drug-induced neuropathies (from vincristine, cisplatin, acrylamide, amiodarone, etc.), and in systemic disorders like multiple system atrophy (MSA) and Lambert-Eaton myasthenic syndrome, and others.

DIAGNOSTIC EVALUATION

Investigations include recording cardiovascular, sudomotor, gastrointestinal, genitourinary, respiratory, and pupillary autonomic functions. These include heart rate (R to R) variability with different maneuvers (deep breath, Valsalva, etc.), tilt-table testing, sudomotor responses (quantitative sudomotor axon reflex test [QSART]), and plasma and urinary catecholamines. The evaluation aims to assess the degree of autonomic system dysfunction with emphasis on localizing the site of the lesion. Additional testing will help to determine the cause of the dysfunction (primary or secondary).

TREATMENT

The prognosis and management of autonomic neuropathy depend on the diagnostic category and primary cause if identified. Avoidance of exacerbating factors is recommended. Symptomatic therapy includes stockings (to avoid orthostatic hypotension); fludrocortisone (0.1 mg daily up to four times a day) to reduce salt loss; midodrine (10 mg two or three times daily) or phenylephrine for vasoconstriction; and prevention of postprandial hypotension and vasodilation.

■ TABLE 23-3 Entrapment Neuropathies

Nerve	Clinical Features	Exam	Etiology
Upper extremity			
Median nerve: at the wrist is called carpal tunnel syndrome	Numbness or tingling involving one or more of the first four digits. Symptoms may awaken patient from sleep.	Weakness and atrophy of the thenar muscles, particularly APB. Decreased sensation in the volar aspect of the first three and a half digits. Tinel's and Phalen's signs may be present.	Compression of the median nerve at the wrist within the space known as the carpal tunnel.
Ulnar nerve: at the elbow	Paresthesias and pain in the fifth digit and the medial half of the fourth. Difficulty spreading the fingers.	Weakness and atrophy in the FDI and ADM.	Compression of the ulnar nerve in the cubital tunnel at the elbow.
Radial nerve	Wristdrop and sensory loss on the dorsal aspects of the hand.	Weakness includes triceps, brachioradialis, supinator, and wrist and finger extensors. The triceps is affected by axillary compression but spared by spiral groove compression. Weakness of wrist extensors causes wristdrop.	Compression of the radial nerve at the level of the axilla ("Saturday night palsy"); the spiral groove, or in the forearm (posterior interosseous neuropathy).
Lower extremity			
Meralgia paresthetica	Burning sensation and variable loss of sensation over the anterolateral thigh.	Area of sensory change over the lateral aspect of the thigh. Tender palpation of the inguinal ligament. No motor involvement.	Entrapment of the lateral femoral cutaneous nerve near the inguinal ligament.
Femoral neuropathy	Leg weakness on attempting to stand or walk. Pain in the anterior thigh is common.	Weakness of the quadriceps muscles, absent or diminished patellar reflex, and sensory loss over the anterior thigh— and, with saphenous nerve involvement, the medial leg/foot. Adductors intact (differentiates from an L2–3 radiculopathy).	Usually trauma from surgery, stretch injury (prolonged lithotomy position in childbirth), diabetes mellitus, and other inflammatory processes.
Peroneal neuropathy	Usually presents with footdrop with minimal sensory complaints.	Weakness of extensor hallucis longus, tibialis anterior, and the peroneal muscles (eversion of the foot); sensory loss over the dorsal part of the foot is mild.	Entrapment of the peroneal nerve between the neck of the fibula and the insertion of the peroneus longus muscle.

ADM, abductor digiti minimi; APB, abductor pollicis brevis; FDI, first dorsal interosseus.

■ **TABLE 23-4** Root Syndromes

Segment	Sensation	Motor Deficit	Reflexes
Cervical			
C5	Pain in lateral shoulder; sensory loss over deltoid	Paresis of deltoid, supraspinatus, and biceps	Impairment of biceps reflex
C6	Radial side of the arm to thumb	Paresis of biceps and brachioradialis	Impairment or loss of biceps reflex
C7	Between second and fourth finger	Triceps, wrist extensors and flexors, pectoralis major muscles	Impairment or loss of triceps reflex
Lumbosacral			
L3	Often none; sometimes medial thigh and knee	Quadriceps; adductor may be affected (differentiates from femoral neuropathy)	Loss of knee jerk; loss or impaired adductor reflex
L4	Medial leg below knee to medial malleolus	Quadriceps and anterior tibial muscles	Decreased knee jerk
L5	Dorsum of foot to great toe	Extensor hallucis longus, extensor digitorum longus, inversion, and eversion of foot	None
S1	Lateral border of the foot	Plantar flexion, toe flexion	Decreased or absent ankle jerk

■ **TABLE 23-5** Tips to Remember in Peripheral Neuropathies

Type of Neuropathy	Tips
Neuropathies that may begin proximally	Sensory: porphyria, occasionally Charcot-Marie-Tooth and Tangier disease Motor: GBS, CIDP, diabetes
Neuropathies that may begin in the arms rather than the legs	Lead toxicity, leprosy, sarcoidosis, porphyria, entrapments, diabetes, vasculitic neuropathy, Tangier disease
Predominantly sensory neuropathies	Autoimmune: Miller-Fisher syndrome, IgM paraproteinemia, paraneoplastic, Sjögren syndrome Toxic: pyridoxine and doxorubicin Infectious: diphtheria, HIV Nutritional: vitamin E deficiency
Painful neuropathies	Diabetic neuropathy, Fabry disease, leprosy, alcoholic neuropathy, HSAN I, isoniazid, pellagra, paraneoplastic, infectious, vasculitic, HIV, inflammatory
Neuropathies that are predominantly motor	GBS, porphyria, and multifocal motor neuropathy
Neuropathy associated with cranial nerve involvement	Diphtheria, sarcoidosis, diabetes, GBS, Sjögren syndrome, polyarteritis nodosa, Lyme disease, porphyria, Refsum disease, syphilis, arsenic
Causes of mononeuritis multiplex	Trauma, diabetes, vasculitis, leprosy, HIV, Lyme, sarcoidosis, tumor infiltration, lymphoid granulomatosis, HNPP
Neuropathies associated with palpable peripheral nerves	CMT and Dejerine-Sottas, amyloidosis, Refsum disease, leprosy, acromegaly, neurofibromatosis

CIDP, chronic inflammatory demyelinating polyradiculoneuropathy; CMT, Charcot Marie Tooth; GBS, Guillain Barré syndrome; HIV, human immunodeficiency virus; HNPP, hereditary neuropathy with liability pressure palsies; HSAN, hereditary sensory and autonomic neuropathy.

Disorders of the Neuromuscular Junction and Skeletal Muscle

Myasthenia gravis (MG) and the Lambert-Eaton myasthenic syndrome (LEMS) are the two most common diseases of the neuromuscular junction (NMJ) (Table 24-1). Fatigable muscle weakness is the defining clinical feature of these disorders. In order to understand the clinical manifestations, pathophysiology, and approach to the treatment of these diseases, it is necessary to have some understanding of the anatomy and physiology of the NMJ. Nerve and muscle have both undergone structural and functional specialization at the NMJ, their point of contact. At the presynaptic bouton, secretory vesicles containing acetylcholine are concentrated at active zones formed by clusters of P/Q-type voltage-gated calcium channels. Across the synaptic cleft, the muscle membrane is thrown into folds at what is known as the **muscle endplate**. Acetylcholine receptors are clustered at the peaks of these folds. Depolarization of the nerve terminal, mediated by a sodium-dependent action potential, leads to activation of the voltage-gated calcium channels, which in turns leads to calcium influx into the presynaptic bouton. The rise in intracellular calcium triggers the release of acetylcholine via a process known as **exocytosis**, whereby the synaptic vesicles dock at the active zones and then fuse with the presynaptic membrane to release their contents into the synaptic cleft. The acetylcholine molecules diffuse across the cleft to bind to the acetylcholine receptors. This generates an inward sodium current through the acetylcholine-receptor ion pore, which leads to depolarization of the muscle endplate. This, in turn, triggers activation of the voltage-dependent

sodium channels that line the troughs of the endplate membrane folds, resulting in muscle contraction. The action of acetylcholine is terminated when it is metabolized by acetylcholinesterase in the synaptic cleft.

MYASTHENIA GRAVIS

Acquired MG is an immunologic disorder in which antibodies are directed against the postsynaptic (muscle) nicotinic acetylcholine receptor (nAChR). Blockade and downregulation of these nAChRs reduce the probability that a nerve impulse will generate a muscle action potential.

EPIDEMIOLOGY

Acquired MG is the most common disorder of NMJ transmission. Its incidence is bimodal, with a peak in the second and third decades of life (during which women are more commonly affected) and a peak in the seventh and eighth decades (when it is more common in men). Earlier-onset MG is often associated with thymic hyperplasia, whereas thymoma is seen more commonly in the patients with later-onset disease.

PATHOGENESIS

In acquired MG, antibodies are directed against the postsynaptic nAChR. These antibodies directly

■ **TABLE 24-1** Disorders of the Neuromuscular Junction and Skeletal Muscle

Disease	Clinical Phenotype	Dysfunctional Protein
Myasthenia gravis	Fatigable proximal muscle weakness; prominent ocular and bulbar involvement	Muscle nicotinic acetylcholine receptor
Lambert-Eaton myasthenic syndrome	Fatigable proximal muscle weakness; ocular and bulbar involvement rare; prominent autonomic symptoms	P/Q-type voltage-gated calcium channel
Duchenne and Becker muscular dystrophy	Childhood onset of proximal muscle weakness, including neck flexors; no ocular or bulbar involvement	Dystrophin
Limb-girdle muscular dystrophy	Proximal muscle weakness; no ocular or bulbar involvement	Sarcoglycan and several others, including calpain, caveolin, dysferlin, etc.
Myotonic dystrophy	Distal muscle weakness and stiffness; myotonia; systemic features (ptosis, balding, etc.)	Dystrophica myotonica protein kinase (DMPK)
Emery-Dreifuss muscular dystrophy	Early onset of joint contractures; humeroperoneal pattern of muscle weakness	Emerin and lamin A/C
Hypokalemic periodic paralysis	Episodes of generalized weakness lasting hours to days	Skeletal muscle L-type voltage-gated calcium channel
Hyperkalemic periodic paralysis	Episodes of generalized weakness lasting minutes to hours	Voltage-gated sodium channel

block the binding of acetylcholine and lead to a complement-mediated attack and internalization of receptors. The result is distortion of the endplate with loss of the normal postjunctional folds and a reduction in the concentration of the receptors. Thus, even though acetylcholine is released normally from the presynaptic bouton, its effect at the endplate is reduced, with the result that the nerve impulse is less likely to generate a muscle action potential. This failure of neuromuscular transmission is what accounts for the weakness in patients with MG. Fatigability occurs because of depletion of presynaptic vesicles with sustained activity.

CLINICAL MANIFESTATIONS

Fatigable muscle weakness is characteristic. The specific symptoms depend on the distribution of this weakness. Ocular involvement is most common, manifesting as ptosis and diplopia. The pupils are never involved. Bulbar muscle weakness is next most frequent and manifests as dysarthria or dysphagia. Limb weakness is usually proximal and symmetric. Symptoms are typically worse with sustained activity or toward the end of the day. Examination is directed toward demonstrating weakness and fatigability. The patient should be asked to sustain a gaze or limb posture for a few minutes as well as following a brief period of exercise or repetitive muscle activity. DTRs are usually preserved or, if reduced, are in proportion to the degree of muscle weakness.

Most patients with MG have generalized disease, but as many as 15% may have involvement restricted to the ocular muscles. The sensitivity of the ancillary diagnostic tests depends on whether the disease is generalized or restricted.

Presentation with respiratory muscle weakness, termed **myasthenic crisis**, constitutes a medical emergency. Respiratory muscle weakness may be present even in patients who do not appear short of breath, underscoring the importance of obtaining formal measures of pulmonary function—forced expiratory volume in 1 second (FEV_1) and negative inspiratory force (NIF)—in every patient with active disease. Myasthenic crisis should be distinguished from cholinergic crisis (a state of increased cholinergic drive due to overmedication with cholinesterase inhibitors). Apart from respiratory muscle weakness, cholinergic crisis is also characterized by the presence of increased bronchial secretions, salivation, diarrhea, nausea, vomiting, and diaphoresis.

DIAGNOSTIC EVALUATION

The diagnosis of MG is primarily clinical, but support for the diagnosis may be obtained from various tests. Edrophonium chloride (Tensilon) is an antiacetyl-cholinesterase agent. It is administered intravenously and the patient observed for improvement in muscle strength. Antibodies against the nAChR may be detected in about 80% of patients with generalized MG and 55% of patients with ocular MG. Elevated titers confirm the diagnosis but negative titers do not exclude it. Seronegative MG is clinically indistinguishable from seropositive disease. Antibodies directed against MuSK (muscle-specific kinase) may be present in some patients with generalized seronegative disease. Repetitive nerve stimulation reveals a decremental response that is seen more commonly in proximal muscles. Single-fiber electromyography is the most sensitive clinical test of neuromuscular transmission. The characteristic finding in MG is increased jitter.

TREATMENT

Antiacetylcholinesterase drugs such as pyridostigmine inhibit the synaptic degradation of acetylcholine and thus prolong its effect. Although pyridostigmine provides adequate symptomatic therapy for many patients with MG, it does not affect the underlying immunopathology. Immune-modulating therapy thus serves as the mainstay for most patients with MG. There are few controlled trials of immunosuppressive therapy, but steroids, steroid-sparing agents such as azathioprine and cyclosporine, plasmapheresis, and intravenous immunoglobulin (IVIg) have all been used with some success. Plasmapheresis and IVIg provide rapid (but relatively short-lived) immunosuppression for patients with severe disease. Steroids and steroid-sparing agents are the mainstay for long-term immune therapy. The place and timing of thymectomy are not clear, but most would agree that it facilitates easier immunosuppression in young patients.

Patients who present with respiratory muscle weakness (myasthenic crisis) warrant admission to an intensive care unit, careful monitoring of respiratory function with intubation, and mechanical ventilation if necessary. Plasmapheresis or IVIg as well as high-dose steroids are appropriate under such circumstances, given their relatively rapid onset of action. Cholinesterase inhibitors are typically ineffective in patients with myasthenic crisis and should be discontinued (a practical measure that obviates the need to distinguish myasthenic from cholinergic crisis).

KEY POINTS

- MG is mediated by antibodies directed against the muscle nAChR.
- It presents with fatigable muscle weakness.
- MG is treated with acetylcholinesterase inhibitors, steroids, and immunosuppressive therapy.

LAMBERT-EATON MYASTHENIC SYNDROME

EPIDEMIOLOGY

LEMS is an uncommon condition that is usually associated with an underlying small cell lung carcinoma. It is caused by antibodies directed against the presynaptic P/Q-type voltage-gated calcium channel. By reducing presynaptic calcium entry, these antibodies reduce the release of acetylcholine, leading to weakness.

CLINICAL MANIFESTATIONS

Patients present with fatigable proximal weakness. DTRs are reduced or absent. In contrast to MG, bulbar and ocular symptoms are rare, but autonomic complaints (dry eyes, dry mouth, and impotence) are common. The characteristic finding is that of muscle facilitation: with brief intense exercise, muscle strength increases, and reflexes may appear transiently. Fatigue develops with sustained activity.

DIAGNOSTIC EVALUATION

The presence of elevated anti–voltage-gated calcium channel antibody titers together with an incremental response on repetitive nerve conduction studies helps to establish the diagnosis.

TREATMENT

The diagnosis of LEMS should prompt a thorough search for an underlying malignancy, even though a tumor is not always found. Initial therapy is directed at the underlying malignancy; in many patients, no further therapy is required. Steroids, azathioprine, IVIg, and plasmapheresis have all been used, but with less success than in MG. 3,4-diaminopyridine is the most effective medication for improving muscle strength in patients with LEMS, but it is not FDA-approved in the United States.

KEY POINTS

- LEMS is mediated by anti–voltage-gated calcium channel antibodies.
- It has a strong association with underlying small cell lung cancer.

SKELETAL MUSCLE DISORDERS

Disorders of skeletal muscle are a diverse group of conditions that do not lend themselves to easy classification. Discussion of these diseases is further complicated by the array of terminology used commonly. A few words of clarification may help. **Myopathy** is a nonspecific term used to refer to disorders of skeletal muscle. Muscular **dystrophy** refers to a group of hereditary conditions in which muscle biopsy demonstrates **dystrophic** changes (fiber splitting, increased connective tissues). **Myotonia** is a state of increased, sustained muscle contraction or impaired relaxation. The term **congenital** indicates onset of clinical disease in the early infantile period. **Myositis** implies an inflammatory process.

Broadly speaking, it is still useful to think of these disorders as inherited or acquired. The inherited disorders encompass the muscular dystrophies, the congenital myopathies, and the channelopathies as well as the metabolic and mitochondrial myopathies. The acquired disorders include the inflammatory myopathies, endocrine and drug- or toxin-induced myopathies, and a group of myopathies associated with other systemic illnesses. With recent advances in molecular genetics, there has been a shift toward thinking about and classifying at least the hereditary disorders on the basis of the underlying molecular defect. The approach adopted here is an attempt to synthesize clinical classification with newly acquired knowledge of the genetic basis of many of the inherited skeletal muscle disorders.

There is no single defining clinical feature of disorders of skeletal muscle. However, the selective involvement of particular groups of muscles (i.e., focal patterned weakness) is highly suggestive of a myopathic process. A detailed history and examination with particular attention to the age of onset, the presence of a family history, the nature of the symptoms and pattern of weakness as well as the tempo of the disease should allow a reasonable preliminary diagnosis to be made. Investigations like serum CK, EMG, and muscle biopsy should then lead to a definitive diagnosis in most cases.

The symptoms of muscle disease may be negative (weakness and fatigue) or positive (muscle pain, cramps, or stiffness). Weakness is the most common and important symptom; a detailed history of the sorts of activities with which the patient has difficulty provides a good indication of the pattern of weakness. Generalized fatigue or tiredness does not indicate a muscle disease, particularly when this is an isolated symptom. Muscle pain (myalgia) is a common symptom and also does not usually imply primary disease of muscle, particularly when it is an isolated symptom. Myalgias may be a feature of the inflammatory and metabolic myopathies. Patients with myotonia may complain of difficulty releasing a handgrip or of opening their eyes after squeezing them shut tightly.

The tempo of the symptoms is of major diagnostic importance. For example, acute or subacute onset of progressive weakness is a feature of some of the inflammatory myopathies, whereas chronic, slowly progressive (over years) weakness is most often encountered in the muscular dystrophies. Episodic weakness suggests one of the channelopathies or metabolic myopathies. The age of onset may also help point to a particular disease process. For example, among the dystrophies, the onset of Duchenne muscular dystrophy (DMD) is usually around the age of 3, while many of the limb-girdle dystrophies begin only during adolescence. Of the inflammatory myopathies, dermatomyositis (DM) may occur at any age, but polymyositis is rare in children, and inclusion body myositis (IBM) usually affects the elderly. Finally, the family history may be very helpful, and the specific pattern of inheritance should be determined.

DYSTROPHINOPATHIES

DMD and Becker muscular dystrophy (BMD) result from different mutations of the same gene, dystrophin, and are thus said to be **allelic**.

CLINICAL MANIFESTATIONS

DMD and BMD should be thought of as a single disorder representing a spectrum of severity, with DMD more severe than BMD. Inheritance is X-linked, and onset is usually in childhood. The child may use an arm to push down on his or her thighs when arising from the floor (Gowers sign), and there may be pseudohypertrophy of the calf muscles. Proximal muscle weakness, including neck flexors, predominates; there is usually sparing of ocular and bulbar muscles. DMD is relentlessly progressive, with the child becoming wheelchair-bound by the age of 10 or 12. Although primarily a disorder of skeletal muscle, cardiac and gastrointestinal smooth muscle involvement as well as CNS involvement are common. In DMD, death usually occurs around age 20 because of respiratory insufficiency and aspiration. Life expectancy is also reduced in BMD, but usually not so severely.

DIAGNOSTIC EVALUATION

The CK level is typically markedly elevated in DMD and moderately so in BMD. A normal CK level provides strong presumptive evidence against the diagnosis. Muscle biopsy shows dystrophic features, with absent or reduced staining for dystrophin.

KEY POINTS

- DMD and BMD are X-linked disorders that result from mutations in the dystrophin gene.
- They present clinically as proximal muscle weakness in young boys.

LIMB-GIRDLE MUSCULAR DYSTROPHIES

The limb-girdle muscular dystrophies are a group of hereditary conditions in which the proximal muscles of the arms and legs are affected predominantly.

CLINICAL MANIFESTATIONS

Most of these disorders are characterized by weakness of the limb-girdle muscles, with relative sparing of facial, extraocular, and pharyngeal musculature. Cardiomyopathy is less frequent than in the dystrophinopathies.

CLASSIFICATION

There are both autosomal dominant and recessive varieties. Recessive inheritance is more common. The most frequent causes are mutations in calpain-3, dysferlin, one of the sarcoglycans, or FKRP (Fukudin related protein). Some are due to mutations in proteins known as the sarcoglycans, which form part of the multimolecular dystrophin-associated glycoprotein complex.

DIAGNOSTIC EVALUATION

CK level is usually elevated. The EMG is myopathic, and biopsy demonstrates nonspecific dystrophic changes. Immunohistochemistry and Western blot analysis on muscle biopsy, as well as DNA analysis on whole blood may help to distinguish the diffferent limb-girdle muscular dystrophies.

KEY POINTS

- Limb-girdle muscular dystrophies are characterized clinically by shoulder and hip girdle weakness with relative sparing of extraocular, pharyngeal, and facial muscles.
- They affect both boys and girls and may resemble the dystrophinopathies, requiring muscle biopsy for differentiation.

MYOTONIC DYSTROPHY

The classic form of myotonic dystrophy is the most common inherited skeletal muscle disorder affecting adults. Inheritance is autosomal dominant and the genetic defect is either an unstable CTG expansion in the DMPK (dystrophia myotonica protein kinase) gene or a CCTG expansion in the ZNF9 gene.

CLINICAL MANIFESTATIONS

Myotonic dystrophy is a multisystem disease. Weakness and stiffness of distal muscles are usually the presenting symptoms in young adults. Action and percussion myotonia are often present. Proximal weakness develops later in the course of the disease. Systemic findings include cataracts, ptosis, arrhythmias, dysphagia (from esophageal myotonia), insulin resistance, testicular atrophy, and frontal balding. Neurobehavioral features (changes in affect, personality, and motivation) as well as cognitive dysfunction are also observed commonly.

DIAGNOSTIC EVALUATION AND TREATMENT

CK level is usually normal or only mildly elevated. EMG demonstrates myotonia. DNA testing for the CTG expansion is now available. Cardiac evaluation is important to screen for and prevent arrhythmias. There is no specific treatment for the muscle weakness, but drugs such as phenytoin and carbamazepine may reduce the myotonia. Management is otherwise supportive.

KEY POINTS

- Myotonic dystrophy is the most common adult-onset muscular dystrophy.
- It is a trinucleotide (CTG) repeat disorder.
- Myotonic dystrophy presents with distal muscle weakness and myotonia.

EMERY-DREIFUSS MUSCULAR DYSTROPHY

Emery-Dreifuss muscular dystrophy is primarily caused by mutations in the **emerin** gene on the X chromosome. A rare autosomal dominant form of the disease results from mutations in the **lamin A** and **lamin C** genes on chromosome 1. **Emerin** is a trans (nuclear) membrane protein, and the lamin A and C genes also localize to the nuclear membrane.

CLINICAL MANIFESTATIONS

This disorder is characterized by the early onset of joint contractures (predominantly affecting the elbows, ankles, and cervical spine), a slowly progressive humeroperoneal pattern of weakness and atrophy, and a cardiomyopathy that manifests as conduction abnormalities. The appearance of contractures prior to the onset of weakness and atrophy helps to distinguish this disorder from the other muscular dystrophies. The pattern of weakness is described as humeroperoneal because of early involvement of biceps, triceps, peroneal, and tibial muscles. Both tachy- and bradyarrhythmias may occur. Although female carriers do not develop weakness or atrophy, they are at risk for the cardiac complications.

DIAGNOSTIC EVALUATION AND TREATMENT

CK levels are typically mildly to moderately elevated. EMG is myopathic, and muscle biopsy usually demonstrates nonspecific dystrophic changes. The diagnosis may be confirmed by reduced or absent immunostaining for **emerin.** No specific treatment is available. Range-of-motion and stretching exercises may reduce the severity of contractures. Pacemaker placement may be lifesaving for patients with severe cardiac conduction abnormalities.

KEY POINTS

- Mutations in the emerin and lamin A/C genes are responsible for Emery-Dreifuss muscular dystrophy.
- Early contractures affecting the elbows, ankles, and cervical spine are characteristic.
- Weakness occurs in a humeroperoneal distribution.
- Cardiac conduction defects are an important cause of morbidity.

CHANNELOPATHIES

The channelopathies are a group of disorders characterized by ion channel dysfunction. The clinical manifestations are determined by the specific ion channel involved.

The periodic paralyses (PP) are autosomal dominant conditions that derive their designation from their cardinal manifestation, episodic muscle weakness. Attacks of weakness are usually associated with a change in serum potassium concentration; they are therefore classified accordingly into hypokalemic and hyperkalemic varieties. Hypokalemic PP is the result of a mutation in the pore-forming α 1S-subunit of the skeletal muscle calcium channel that results in secondary dysfunction of the Na^+,K^+-ATPase. Hyperkalemic PP results from mutations in the skeletal muscle voltage-gated sodium channel.

KEY POINTS

- The periodic paralyses are characterized by episodic muscle weakness.
- They are caused by mutations in skeletal muscle membrane ion channels.

MITOCHONDRIAL MYOPATHIES

The mitochondrial myopathies are a heterogeneous group of disorders with systemic manifestations.

INHERITANCE

Mitochondrial DNA is entirely maternally inherited; this is therefore the usual mode of inheritance for mitochondrial disorders. Given that over 90% of mitochondrial proteins are encoded by nuclear genes, however, virtually all other patterns of inheritance may occur as well.

CLINICAL MANIFESTATIONS

A number of characteristic syndromes have been identified. These include myoclonic epilepsy with ragged red fibers (MERRF); mitochondrial myopathy, encephalopathy, lactoacidosis, and stroke (MELAS); progressive external ophthalmoplegia (PEO); and the Kearns-Sayre syndrome.

DIAGNOSTIC EVALUATION

There are no characteristic clinical or electrophysiologic findings in the mitochondrial myopathies, but a common finding is the co-occurrence of a myopathy and a peripheral neuropathy. Serum or CSF lactate and pyruvate are often increased. The histopathologic changes are also nonspecific and include the presence of ragged red fibers and variability of cytochrome oxidase staining.

 KEY POINTS

- The mitochondrial myopathies are clinically and genetically heterogeneous.
- The myopathy is frequently accompanied by other systemic manifestations (e.g., seizure, stroke, migraine, diabetes).
- Serum lactate and pyruvate are often increased.
- Muscle biopsy may show ragged red fibers.

DISTAL MYOPATHIES

The distal myopathies are a group of largely hereditary conditions in which muscle weakness at onset is predominantly distal. Distal muscle weakness, however, may occur atypically in acquired disorders such as polymyositis and inclusion body myositis, in which weakness is usually more proximal. Distal weakness may also occur in some of the other muscular dystrophies (e.g., fascioscapulohumeral, scapuloperoneal, and Emery-Dreifuss humeroperoneal).

INFLAMMATORY MYOPATHIES

The noninfectious immune-mediated inflammatory myopathies include polymyositis (PM), dermatomyositis (DM), and inclusion body myositis (IBM).

CLINICAL MANIFESTATIONS

PM and DM are characterized by proximal (usually symmetric) muscle weakness. Weakness in IBM is often asymmetric and may affect both proximal and distal muscles. Early selective involvement of forearm and finger flexors, as well as of knee extensors (quadriceps) and ankle extensors, should arouse suspicion of this diagnosis. Pharyngeal and neck flexor muscles may be affected, but facial and respiratory muscles are usually spared. IBM is often diagnosed only when patients thought to have PM fail to respond to steroids. DM is distinguishable by the associated purplish discoloration of the eyelids (heliotrope) and papular erythematous scaly lesions over the knuckles (Gottron patches).

Extramuscular manifestations are frequent in DM. Cardiac manifestations include conduction defects, tachyarrhythmias, myocarditis, and congestive cardiac failure. Interstitial lung disease associated with the presence of anti-Jo-1 antibodies occurs in approximately 10% of patients. DM may occur in the context of systemic sclerosis or other mixed connective tissue disease, and there is an increased incidence of malignancy in patients with DM. In contrast to DM and IBM, PM is more often associated with other autoimmune diseases, including Crohn's disease, vasculitis, sarcoidosis, MG, and others.

PATHOGENESIS

DM is a microangiopathic disorder in which antibodies and complement are directed primarily against intramuscular blood vessels. Inflammation is due to muscle ischemia. PM is mediated by CD8+ T lymphocytes, while IBM is likely both an inflammatory and neurodegenerative disorder.

DIAGNOSTIC EVALUATION

CK is elevated in more than 90% of patients with an inflammatory myopathy. While this is the most sensitive and specific marker for muscle breakdown, levels do not correlate with the degree of weakness. EMG demonstrates myopathic changes (often with accompanying denervation changes due to muscle fiber necrosis) and is useful in selecting a muscle for biopsy. The characteristic muscle biopsy findings in PM are endomysial inflammation with invasion of nonnecrotic muscle fibers with CD8+ T-cells. The diagnosis of IBM is made by demonstrating endomysial inflammation and basophilic rimmed vacuoles.

TREATMENT

Corticosteroids are the mainstay of treatment in PM and DM, but they are of no benefit in IBM. IVIg has been shown to be beneficial in DM, but its role in PM is less clear. Plasmapheresis is probably not beneficial. Steroid-sparing agents such as azathioprine and methotrexate should be reserved for patients with refractory disease.

KEY POINTS

- The inflammatory myopathies are characterized by muscle pain, weakness, and elevated CK level.
- Proximal muscle involvement is found in PM and DM, but distal muscle weakness is more common in IBM.
- PM and DM are steroid-responsive; IBM is resistant.

ENDOCRINE AND DRUG- OR TOXIN-INDUCED MYOPATHIES

THYROTOXIC MYOPATHY

Although weakness is rarely the presenting complaint of patients with thyrotoxicosis, it is found on examination in many. Proximal muscle weakness and atrophy with normal or brisk reflexes are the most common clinical features, but rarely distal weakness may be the earliest manifestation. Bulbar and respiratory muscle involvement is uncommon. If Graves disease is the cause of thyrotoxicosis, then the differential diagnosis of muscle weakness should include myasthenia gravis. The pathogenesis of thyrotoxic myopathy is unknown but may reflect enhanced muscle catabolism. CK level is typically normal, and EMG demonstrates myopathic units. Treatment of the underlying thyrotoxic state with β-blockers should improve muscle strength.

HYPOTHYROID MYOPATHY

Myopathic symptoms develop in about one-third of patients with hypothyroidism. The typical presentation is that of proximal muscle weakness, fatigue, myalgias, and cramps. Reflexes may demonstrate delayed relaxation. There may be an associated distal polyneuropathy. CK level is typically elevated (and can be 10 times normal). EMG shows nonspecific myopathic changes. Weakness usually improves following thyroid replacement, but recovery may lag behind a return to the euthyroid state.

STEROID MYOPATHY

Myopathy may result from increased glucocorticoids from either endogenous production or exogenous administration. The latter is more common, and although any synthetic glucocorticoid can cause myopathy, it is more common with fluorinated compounds (e.g., triamcinolone and dexamethasone). Doses in excess of the equivalent of 30 mg of prednisone per day are associated with an increased risk of myopathy. The risk is reduced with alternate-day regimens. Typically, weakness begins after chronic administration of steroids, but it may occur within a few weeks. Weakness is predominantly proximal, with sparing of the ocular, bulbar, and facial muscles. CK level is usually normal. EMG is usually normal. Muscle biopsy typically demonstrates type II fiber atrophy, but this finding is nonspecific. Treatment requires a reduction in the steroid dose, switching to an alternate-day regimen or using a non-fluorinated compound.

DRUG- OR TOXIN-INDUCED MYOPATHY

Many drugs and toxins have been implicated as causes of myopathy. Typically they produce a syndrome

■ TABLE 24-2 Drug- or Toxin-Induced Myopathies

Disorder	Drug or Toxin	Clinical Syndrome
Necrotizing myopathy	HMG-CoA reductase inhibitors; cyclosporin; propofol; alcohol	Acute or insidious onset of proximal muscle weakness; CK level typically elevated
Steroid myopathy	Fluorinated glucocorticoids	Proximal muscle weakness; CK level usually normal
Mitochondrial myopathy	Zidovudine	Acute or insidious onset of proximal muscle weakness; CK level normal or only mildly increased
Inflammatory myopathy	Cimetidine; procainamide; L-dopa; phenytoin; lamotrigine; D-penicillamine	Acute onset of proximal muscle weakness; CK level typically increased
Critical illness myopathy	Corticosteroids plus neuromuscular blocking agents in patients with sepsis	Acute or subacute onset of generalized weakness; CK level may be normal or elevated

CK, serum creatinine kinase; HMG-CoA, hydroxymethylglutaryl coenzyme A.

characterized by proximal myopathy and increased serum CK level. Some of the more commonly encountered drugs that induce myopathies are listed in Table 24-2.

KEY POINTS

- Proximal muscle weakness is frequent in patients with either hypothyroidism or hyperthyroidism.
- Proximal myopathy may result from excessive circulating steroids, either from increased endogenous production or exogenous administration.
- CK level is usually normal in the metabolic myopathies except for hypothyroidism, in which it is typically elevated.

NEUROLEPTIC MALIGNANT SYNDROME

NMS is a disorder characterized by fever, depressed level of arousal, muscle rigidity, autonomic dysfunction and fever. It is most commonly encountered in the context of treatment with antipsychotics (haloperidol > chlorpromazine, fluphenazine > risperidone, olanzapine, clozapine, quetiapine) but may also occur with L-dopa withdrawal in patients with Parkinson's disease and in association with the use of tricyclic antidepressants, phenelzine, and metoclopramide. Although the etiology of this disorder is unclear, it has been suggested to result from central dopaminergic blockade. Management requires discontinuation of the offending drug, aggressive fluid resuscitation, and other supportive measures, usually in the context of an intensive care unit. Intravenous benzodiazepines, bromocriptine, amantadine, or dantrolene may be helpful.

25 Pediatric Neurology

Neurologic disorders in children are encountered commonly by pediatricians and general physicians. Many neurologic diseases that affect infants and children also affect adults, such as infection, epilepsy, inflammatory and demyelinating diseases, peripheral neuropathies, and myopathies; but some are characteristic of early ages, including developmental disorders, malformations, and genetically determined conditions. Seizures are among the most common neurologic problems in childhood (see Chapter 15).

The history is the most important component of the evaluation of a child with a neurologic problem. It shares the same principles as described for the adult history but also requires a complete review of the pregnancy, labor, and delivery, especially if a perinatal injury or congenital infection is suspected.

DEVELOPMENT AND MATURATION

One of the most important elements of the neurologic history is a developmental assessment of the child. The Denver Developmental Screening Test is an efficient and reliable method to assess achievement of developmental milestones. It evaluates four components of development: gross motor skills, fine motor adaptive skills, language, and personal-social interaction. Table 25-1 summarizes developmental milestones by age. This is based on averages and therefore can be used only with an understanding of the variability among children. Table 25-2 gives a brief description of primitive reflexes and their significance.

CEREBRAL PALSY

Cerebral palsy (CP) is a static disorder due to pre- or perinatal damage to cerebromotor pathways. It can be acquired or genetic. CP occurs in about 2.7 per 1,000 births. Risk factors for CP include hypoxic-ischemic insult to the brain in the perinatal period, prematurity, low birth weight, chorioamnionitis, prenatal viral infections, and prenatal strokes.

CLASSIFICATION

The most commonly used classification of CP is based on the distribution of the affected limbs:

- **Hemiparetic:** Weakness and spasticity are seen on one side of the body. Signs include fisting on the affected side, early hand preference, and increased reflexes with upgoing toes on the affected side.
- **Diparetic:** There is spasticity of all four limbs, affecting the legs more than the arms. The children are usually of normal intelligence and are less likely to have seizures than children with other forms of CP.
- **Spastic quadriplegic:** All four limbs are affected. Seizures usually occur within the first 48 hours of life. The infant may show signs of cerebral hypotonia (see later discussion).

CLINICAL MANIFESTATIONS

CP may be diagnosed as early as the first week of life: infants may have flaccid weakness, asymmetric limb

	TABLE 25-1 Developmental Milestones			
Age	Adaptive/Fine Motor Skills	Gross Motor Skills	Language	Personal/Social
1 month	Grasp reflex; hand fisted	Raises head slightly when prone	Facial response to sounds	Stares at face
2 months	Follows objects with eyes past midline	Lifts head from prone to 45 degrees	Coos	Smiles in response to others
4 months	Hands open; brings objects to mouth	Sits, head steady; rolls to supine	Laughs and squeals; toward voice	Smiles spontaneously
6 months	Palmar grasp of objects; starts transfer of objects	Sits independently; stands with hands held	Babbles (consonant sounds); mimics sounds	Reaches for toys; recognizes strangers
9 months	Pincer grasp; claps hands	Pulls to stand	Says "mama," "dada," nonspecifically; comprehends "no"; associates word and action ("bye-bye," "no," etc.)	Finger-feeds self; waves bye-bye
1 year	Helps to turn pages of book; tower of two blocks	Stands independently; walks with one hand held	2 to 4 words; follows command with gesture	Points to indicate wants
18 months	Turns pages of book; imitates vertical lines	Walks up steps	10 to 20 words; points to four body parts; obeys simple commands	Feeds self with spoon; uses cup
2 years	Solves single-piece puzzles	Jumps; kicks ball	Combines 2 to 3 words; uses "I" and "you"; 50 to 300 words	Removes coat; verbalizes wants
3 years	Copies circle; draws person with three body parts; imitates horizontal lines; towers of six cubes; draws circles	Throws ball overhand; walks up stairs, alternating feet	Gives full name, age, and sex; names two colors	Toilet trained; puts on shirt and knows front from back
4 years	Counts four objects; identifies some numbers and letters; uses scissors	Hops on one foot	Understands prepositions (under, on, behind, in front of); asks "how" and "why"	Dresses with little assistance; shoes on correct feet
5 years	Prints first name; counts 10 objects; draws triangle; draws person with several parts	Skips, alternating feet	Asks meaning of words; understands conjunctions and past tenses; knows colors	Ties shoes

movements, or seizures. In older children, spasticity, dystonia, developmental delay, and drooling are common presentations.

DIAGNOSTIC EVALUATION

The diagnosis of CP is based on the clinical symptoms and signs. The cause may not be determined, but the presence of a static (not worsening) disorder is suggestive. One must rule out other entities that may present with dystonia, ataxia, or spasticity but which progress with time (e.g., metabolic disorders, metachromatic leukodystrophy, and movement disorders such as levodopa-responsive dystonia). MRI is indicated only to exclude other structural causes such as tumor, stroke, or AVMs.

■ **TABLE 25-2** Primitive Reflexes			
Reflex	**Significance**	**Appears**	**Disappears**
Moro	Elicited by head extension. Two phases: extension and abduction of arms and leg extension, followed by slower abductions of arms.	Term newborns	3 months
	Asymmetry indicates central nervous system disease such as hemiparesis, spinal cord lesion or brachial plexus injury.		
Tonic neck	Turning head: arm and leg extended on the side of the turn, with flexion on the other side (fencing posture). If infant is unable to move out of posture, implies possible brain pathology.	1 month	5 months
Traction response	Lift baby by traction in both hands. Head lag after 6 months is pathologic and indicates hypotonia.	Birth	6 months
Parachute	Elicited by plunging suspended infant downward. Arms should thrust forward symmetrically as if breaking the fall. Also elicited with baby in sitting position and pushed forward. Arms should try to break the fall. Asymmetry suggests hemiparesis, spinal cord lesion, or brachial plexus pathology.	6 months	Persists throughout life

TREATMENT

In general, a multidisciplinary approach is necessary, with early infant stimulation, physical and occupational therapy, orthopedic and psychological evaluation, and speech therapy.

KEY POINTS

- Cerebral palsy (CP) is a static disease; if the disease is progressing, it is not CP.
- It occurs in almost 3 per 1,000 births.
- The most common abnormality is spasticity.

MENTAL RETARDATION AND DEVELOPMENTAL DELAY

Mental retardation is the failure to develop normal mental capacities. It can be classified by the results of standard intelligence tests such as the Stanford-Binet IQ and the Wechsler Preschool and Primary Scale of Intelligence–Revised. Normal IQ is 100 with a standard deviation of 15. Mental retardation is classified as follows:

- Mild: IQ between 55 and 70
- Moderate: IQ between 40 and 55
- Severe: 25 to 40
- Profound: less than 25

There are many causes of mental retardation. Among them are prenatal and postnatal trauma (e.g., intracerebral hemorrhage and hypoxic-anoxic encephalopathy); congenital and postnatal infection (e.g., congenital rubella, syphilis, cytomegalovirus, toxoplasmosis, and HIV infection); chromosomal abnormalities (e.g., Down syndrome, fragile X syndrome, Angelman syndrome, Prader-Willi syndrome); chromosomal translocations (e.g., cri du chat syndrome); inherited metabolic disorders (e.g., hypothyroidism, galactosemia, Tay-Sachs disease); and toxic, nutritional, and environmental causes. Table 25-3 summarizes some chromosomal abnormalities associated with mental retardation.

Developmental delay is the failure to acquire age-appropriate cognitive, language, fine or gross motor skills, or social skills. The Denver Developmental Assessment is a standard test that can help establish the diagnosis. Many of the etiologies of developmental delay are similar to those responsible for mental retardation and include intrauterine toxins and infections, genetic abnormalities, migrational disorders, hypoxic-ischemic encephalopathy, and inborn errors of metabolism. Most often, though, no cause for developmental delay is found, in which case it is labeled idiopathic.

■ TABLE 25-3 Mental Retardation Syndromes Associated with Chromosomal Abnormalities

Condition	Epidemiology	Genetic Defect	Clinical Characteristics
Down's syndrome	Most common inherited MR	Trisomy 21	MR; upslanting palpebral fissures; protuding tongue; simian crease; Brishfield spots
Fragile X syndrome	Relatively common males form of MR; affects males more than females	Defect in the X chromosome; mutation in the 5′ end of the gene with amplification of a CGG repeat (200 or more copies)	20% males are normal; 30% of carrier females are mildly affected; moderate mental retardation; behavioral problems; somatic abnormalities: long face, enlarged ears, and macro-orchidism
Prader-Willi syndrome	Uncommon inherited disorder	Absence of segment 11 to 13 on the long arm of the paternally derived chromosome 15	Mental retardation; decreased muscle tone; short stature; emotional lability and insatiable appetite (obesity)
Angelman's syndrome	Uncommon neurogenetic disorder	Deletion of segment 11 to 13 on the maternally derived chromosome 15	Mental retardation; abnormal gait; speech impairment; seizures; inappropriate happy behavior that includes laughing, smiling, and excitability ("happy puppet" syndrome)
Rett's syndrome	Progressive neuro-developmental disorder; generally affects only females; incidence of 1 in 10,000 births	Causal gene is MeCP2, found on the long arm of chromosome X (X 28).	Normal development until 6 to 18 months; a first sign is hypotonia; autistic-like behavior; stereotyped hand movements (wringing and waving); lag in brain and head growth; gait abnormalities; seizures

MR, mental retardation.

Treatment for both mental retardation and developmental delay includes referral to early intervention programs for special education and training.

KEY POINTS

- Mental retardation implies a substantially below-average cognitive ability and adaptive behavior.
- Developmental delay implies inability to achieve developmental milestones at the usual age. It is not synonymous with mental retardation.

AUTISTIC SPECTRUM DISORDERS

Autism is a developmental disorder of brain function. Usually, the etiology is unknown. Autism is the most common of the disorders that fall under the banner of **pervasive developmental disorder**.

CLINICAL MANIFESTATIONS

Autism is characterized by a combination of social, behavioral, and language abnormalities with onset before age 3. Marked deficiencies in social and communication skills manifest as a lack of attachment to other members of the family and poor social interactions. A restricted range of behaviors, interests, and activities is demonstrated and may include repetitive and stereotyped behaviors such as toe walking, rocking, flapping, banging, and licking. Abnormal language features include echolalia and stereotyped speech.

DIAGNOSTIC EVALUATION

The diagnosis is clinical. Differential diagnosis includes other causes of speech and language problems, such as deafness, mental retardation, and seizures (Landau-Kleffner syndrome). **Asperger syndrome** can be considered a variant of autism characterized by social isolation and eccentric behavior with normal intelligence and language development.

KEY POINTS

- Autism is characterized by a combination of social, behavioral, and language abnormalities.

TREATMENT

The treatment of autism includes support and behavior modification. No cures are available at present.

DEVELOPMENTAL REGRESSION AND INHERITED NEURODEGENERATIVE DISORDERS

Developmental regression is defined as a loss of previously attained developmental milestones. It is often related to an inherited neurodegenerative disorder. It is one of the most distressing complaints confronted by pediatricians and neurologists. An extensive battery of diagnostic tests is the wrong approach. A complete history, physical and neurologic examination, and additional tests based on those findings are fundamental in reaching an accurate diagnosis. Always differentiate regression from developmental delay (see previous). Table 25-4 shows common causes of

---

■ TABLE 25-4 Causes of Progressive Encephalopathy

Onset before Age 2	Onset after Age 2
Mitochondrial disorders	AIDS
Hypothyroidism	Congenital syphilis
Neurocutaneous syndromes	Subacute sclerosing panencephalitis
Tuberous sclerosis complex	Enzymatic lysosomal disorders
Neurofibromatosis	Gaucher disease
Gray matter disorders	Gangliosidosis
Infantile ceroid lipofuscinosis	Late-onset Krabbe disease
Rett syndrome	Metachromatic leukodystrophy
White matter disorders	Other gray matter disorders
Alexander disease	Ceroid lipofuscinosis
Canavan disease	Huntington disease
Neonatal adrenoleukodystrophy	Mitochondrial disorders (MERRF)
Pelizaeus-Merzbacher disease (peroxisomal disorders)	Other white matter disorders
Disorders of amino acid metabolism	Adrenoleukodystrophy
Homocystinuria	Alexander disease
Maple syrup urine disease	
Phenylketonuria	
Enzymatic disorders	
Gangliosidosis	
Gaucher disease	
Krabbe disease	
Mucopolysaccharidoses	
Metachromatic leukodystrophy	

AIDS, acquired immunodeficiency syndrome; MERRF, myoclonic epilepsy with ragged red fibers.

progressive encephalopathy at different ages that can produce developmental delay or regression.

The inherited neurodegenerative diseases are classified according to the involved cellular element: the lysosome, peroxisome, mitochondria, Golgi apparatus, and cell membrane. Whatever the cellular and molecular mechanism responsible, it is possible to recognize common patterns of disease expression according to the age of onset, symptoms, and systems involved. The most common clinical features of neurometabolic diseases presenting in infancy and childhood are developmental delay or regression.

Lysosomal disorders are caused by genetic defects of lysosomal enzymes and cofactors that result in the accumulation of undegraded substrates in lysosomes. They are classified according to the accumulated material: sphingolipidoses, mucopolysaccharidoses, mucolipidoses, glycogen storage disease type II, sialidoses, and neuronal ceroid lipofuscinosis. Some of the most important characteristics of these clinical entities are reviewed in Table 25-5.

Peroxisomal disorders are a heterogeneous group of syndromes characterized by abnormalities in lipid metabolism. Multiple enzyme deficiencies have been characterized. They are rare. The most important are X-linked adrenoleukodystrophy and Zellweger syndrome (see Table 25-5). Most of the degenerative diseases of infancy and childhood are not treatable. However, attempts to reach a final diagnosis are important in order to provide parents with genetic counseling, prognosis, and further management advice.

KEY POINTS

- Neurodegenerative diseases involving the white matter include metachromatic leukodystrophy, Krabbe disease, adrenoleukodystrophy, Pelizaeus-Merzbacher disease, Canavan disease, and Alexander disease.
- Peripheral nerve involvement is found in metachromatic leukodystrophy, Krabbe disease, Canavan disease, and adrenoleukodystrophy.
- Congenital macular cherry-red spots (red color of the macula compared with a pale retina) are found in Tay-Sachs disease, Sandhoff disease, Niemann-Pick disease, Gaucher disease, metachromatic leukodystrophy, and sialidoses.

NEUROCUTANEOUS DISORDERS

Neurocutaneous disorders (phakomatoses) are characterized by lesions in the CNS and PNS, skin, eyes, and other organs. A summary of neurocutaneous disorders and their clinical features is given in Table 25-6.

THE HYPOTONIC INFANT

Hypotonia is a reduction in postural tone. It may be the manifestation of a CNS or PNS disorder or of both.

The most common cause of hypotonia is **cerebral hypotonia**, a static encephalopathy from pre- or perinatal brain injury. The most useful diagnostic finding in this group of disorders is not the hypotonia but the other signs of CNS dysfunction. Seizures, microcephaly, dysmorphic facies, and mental retardation point to the brain as the source of hypotonia. Usually, DTRs are increased and plantar reflexes are extensor.

Other causes of hypotonia include spinal cord disease (e.g., transection during breech presentation), anterior horn cell lesions (spinal muscular atrophy), neuromuscular junction abnormalities, and myopathies (congenital, metabolic, etc.). The physical exam and presence or absence of "central" signs may help to localize the site of disease.

KEY POINTS

- Hypotonia can be central, peripheral, or both.
- Cerebral hypotonia is usually associated with other signs of CNS dysfunction (seizures, developmental delay, etc.).
- Infants with severe hypotonia but only marginal weakness usually do not have a disorder of the lower motor unit.

ATTENTION DEFICIT–HYPERACTIVITY DISORDER

CLINICAL MANIFESTATIONS

The essential features of attention deficit–hyperactivity disorder (ADHD) are inappropriate inattention, impulsivity, and hyperactivity for age. Children with

■ TABLE 25-5 Inherited Neurodegenerative Disorders

Disorder	Metabolic Defect	Chromosome and Inheritance	Notes
Tay-Sachs disease	Hexosaminidase A	15, autosomal recessive	Cherry-red spot. More common in Ashkenazi Jews.
Niemann-Pick disease	Sphingomyelinase	11, autosomal recessive	Cherry-red spot. More common in Ashkenazi Jews.
Gaucher disease	Glucocerebrosidase	1, autosomal recessive	Cherry-red spot. Gaucher cells in bone marrow.
Krabbe disease	Galactosylceramide β-galactosidase	14, autosomal recessive	Globoid cells with periodic–acid Schiff (PAS)-positive granules.
Hurler syndrome	α-L-iduronidase	4, autosomal recessive	Clouding of the cornea. Characteristic facies and dwarfism.
Hunter syndrome	Iduronate sulfatase	X-linked	Hurler phenotype without corneal clouding.
Metachromatic leukodystrophy	Arylsulfatase A	22, autosomal recessive	Cherry-red spot. Demyelinating disorder. Can present as schizophrenia in adults. Positive urine sulfatides.
Adrenoleukodystrophy	Very long chain fatty acid oxidation	X-linked	White matter hyperintensity on MRI. May present as a neuropathy or myelopathy in adults.
Alexander disease	Glial fibrillary acidic protein	11 or 17, autosomal recessive	Rosenthal fibers on biopsy. Macrocephaly. Dysmyelination of the CNS.
Canavan disease	Aspartoacylase	17, autosomal recessive	Macrocephaly. Dysmyelination of the CNS.
Pelizaeus-Merzbacher disease	Proteolipid protein	X-linked	Pendular nystagmus. Dysmyelination of the CNS.
Leigh disease	Mitochondrial	Autosomal recessive or X-linked	Bilateral putaminal hyperintensity on MRI.
Rett syndrome	Methyl-CpG-binding protein-2	X-linked	Occurs exclusively in girls. Microcephaly, autism, and hand-wringing.
Neuronal ceroid lipofuscinosis	Excess lipofuscin storage	Variety of mutations, autosomal recessive	Dementia, myoclonus, ataxia, retinitis pigmentosa. Variety of forms with different ages of onsets and severities.

■ TABLE 25-6 Neurocutaneous Syndromes

	Inheritance	Neurologic Findings	Cutaneous Findings	Other Findings
Neurofibromatosis 1	Autosomal dominant; chromosome 17	Optic nerve gliomas	Café-au-lait spots, neurofibromas, axillary or inguinal freckles	Lisch nodules in the iris
Neurofibromatosis 2	Autosomal dominant; chromosome 22	Bilateral acoustic neuromas	Café-au-lait spots are less common than in NF-1	
Tuberous sclerosis	Autosomal dominant; TSC 1—chr 9, TSC 2—chr 16	Cortical tubers, subependymal nodules and astrocytomas, mental retardation, seizures	Adenoma sebaceum, ash-leaf spots, shagreen patches	Angiomyolipomas of kidneys, cardiac rhabdomyoma
Ataxia telangiectasia	Autosomal recessive; chromosome 11	Truncal ataxia, progressive dementia	Telangiectasias	Immunodeficiency and susceptibility to infections, leukemia, lymphoma
von Hippel-Lindau	Autosomal dominant; chromosome 3	Cerebellar hemangioblastomas, ataxia		Renal lesions including hemangiomas and carcinomas, pheochromocytoma
Sturge Weber	Sporadic	Venous angioma of the pia mater, seizures, hemiparesis, mental retardation	Port-wine stain in the distribution of the ophthalmic nerve	

NF, neurofibromatosis; TSC, tuberous sclerosis complex.

the hyperactive-impulsive subtype are fidgety, leave their seats in the classroom, and have difficulty playing quietly. Children with the inattentive-distractible subtype do not pay close attention to details, have difficulty organizing tasks, and are forgetful in daily activities. There are many causes of ADHD, but most often there is a family history, implying a genetic etiology.

DIAGNOSTIC EVALUATION

A diagnosis is made by clinical history and neuropsychological screening tests. Children usually have normal IQs but low scores on tests of sustained attention. Imaging and laboratory tests are generally not helpful.

TREATMENT

The standard medical treatment of ADHD is with stimulant drugs like methylphenidate and dextroamphetamine. It is important to emphasize parent participation in the treatment program and behavioral modifications like goal setting, incentives, and punishments.

KEY POINTS

- Children with ADHD usually have a positive family history for the disorder.
- Stimulants like methylphenidate and dextroamphetamine are often effective treatments for ADHD.

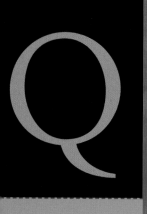

Questions

1. A 78-year-old woman with dementia and rigidity is hospitalized with dehydration. During her hospitalization, she becomes agitated and has prominent visual hallucinations. After a dose of haloperidol, she becomes very rigid and mute. The most likely type of dementia in this patient is:
   a. Alzheimer disease (AD)
   b. Parkinson disease (PD)
   c. Dementia with Lewy bodies
   d. Pick disease
   e. Vascular dementia

2. A 32-year-old woman presents to the ER complaining of blurred vision and pain in the right eye. Your evaluation shows decreased visual acuity in the right eye that does not correct with pinhole testing. There is a relative afferent pupillary defect (RAPD) on the right, and testing of the right visual field shows a small central scotoma. The most likely localization of the lesion is the:
   a. Optic chiasm
   b. Optic nerve
   c. Optic tract
   d. Occipital cortex
   e. Optic radiations

3. In the course of evaluating an infant with developmental regression, a pediatric neurologist notes a cherry-red spot on funduscopic examination. Which of the following diagnoses is consistent with that finding?
   a. Alexander disease
   b. Hurler syndrome
   b. Krabbe disease
   d. Niemann-Pick disease
   e. Canavan disease

4. A 62-year-old woman presents with progressive distal symmetric paresthesias and dysesthesias, with preserved muscle strength. She smokes cigarettes. Your electrodi-

agnostic study indicates that this is likely a sensory neuronopathy. Which one of the following tests will help to find the possible etiology?
   a. Anti-GM$_1$ antibodies
   b. Anti-DNA antibodies
   c. Anti-Hu antibodies
   d. MRI of the spine
   e. CT myelogram

5. A 40-year-old woman is evaluated in the ER after a motor vehicle accident resulting in left facial injuries. Examination after she recovers acutely demonstrates that her left seventh and eighth cranial nerves remain dysfunctional. Which of the following skull structures may have been affected by her injury?
   a. Cribriform plate
   b. Optic canal
   c. Superior orbital fissure
   d. Internal auditory meatus
   e. Jugular foramen

6. A 54-year-old woman was seen in the ER complaining of a severe headache. Head CT was normal, and an LP was performed. The opening pressure was 14 cm H$_2$O, and CSF analysis showed the following: 150 red blood cells, xanthochromic fluid, protein 55 (slightly increased), 15 white blood cells (90% lymphocytes), and normal glucose. Which of the following statements is true?
   a. The xanthochromia may have been caused by a traumatic tap.
   b. The lymphocytic pleocytosis indicates an active infectious process.
   c. Viral meningitis is unlikely because of the normal CSF glucose.
   d. The lymphocytic pleocytosis is likely reactive to the presence of blood within the CSF.
   e. The opening pressure is elevated and reflects pseudotumor cerebri.

7. A 29-year-old woman is brought into the ER in an unresponsive state. Her temperature is 37°C, heart rate 84 per minute, respirations 10, and blood pressure 152/84. On examination, she withdraws to noxious stimulation only. Her right pupil is 10 mm and does not constrict to light. Her left pupil is 5 mm and reacts normally. Which of the following is clinically contraindicated?
   a. Raising the head of the bed
   b. Intravenous administration of mannitol
   c. Hyperventilation
   d. LP
   e. Neurosurgical consultation

8. A patient presents with gradually worsening weakness of the proximal arm and leg muscles symmetrically over several months. On examination, neck flexors and extensors are found to be weak also. There is no muscle pain or tenderness. What is the most likely site of dysfunction in the nervous system?
   a. Peripheral nerve
   b. Brachial plexus
   c. Spinal nerve root
   d. Internal capsule
   e. Muscle

9. An 8-year-old boy is brought to a child psychiatrist for evaluation of potential attention deficit–hyperactivity disorder. His mother states that his teachers have been concerned about his attention because they frequently have to repeat instructions to him. At home his brother has noticed that he will stare for several seconds at a time, during which he does not respond to questions. An EEG demonstrates a 3-Hz spike-and-wave pattern. Which of the following is the most appropriate treatment?
   a. Methylphenidate (Ritalin)
   b. Ethosuximide (Zarontin)
   c. Clonidine (Catapres)
   d. Fluoxetine (Prozac)
   e. Carbamazepine (Tegretol)

10. A 28-year-old woman comes to the ER with a severe unilateral throbbing headache accompanied by photophobia and phonophobia. These headaches started in her teens and she has one every month. Which of the following medications is effective as abortive treatment?
    a. Propranolol
    b. Sumatriptan
    c. Verapamil
    d. Amitriptyline
    e. Valproic acid

11. A 42-year-old man is brought to the neurologist for evaluation of a few months' history of personality changes. His family indicates that, over the previous year, he has made unusual movements with his hands, and he seems to have some memory difficulties. His father died in his 50s with a similar clinical syndrome, including prominent chorea and dementia. The most likely genetic abnormality will be localized on chromosome:
    a. 19
    b. 6
    c. 4
    d. 11
    e. 21

12. A 55-year-old woman with a history of ovarian cancer and moderate alcohol consumption is seen in the Neurology ambulatory clinic with a 1-month history of progressive unsteadiness of gait and dysarthria. Examination confirms the presence of both gait and limb ataxia as well as nystagmus. These symptoms were fairly abrupt in onset, progressed over a period of a few weeks, and now appear to have stabilized, but there has been no sign of spontaneous improvement. Which of the following statements is correct?
    a. The findings of gait ataxia, dysarthria, and nystagmus indicate diffuse involvement of the cerebellum and suggest that alcohol consumption is the likely cause.
    b. The constellation of symptoms and their temporal evolution are most consistent with paraneoplastic cerebellar degeneration, a disorder associated with underlying gynecologic malignancy.
    c. The constellation of symptoms and their temporal evolution are most consistent with paraneoplastic cerebellar degeneration (PCD), but ovarian cancer is an unusual cause of this syndrome.
    d. The symptoms and signs indicate cerebellar hemispheric dysfunction and are most suggestive of a metastasis from the underlying ovarian cancer.
    e. The sudden onset of symptoms and diffuse cerebellar involvement suggest midline cerebellar hemorrhage as the cause.

13. A 45-year-old man with multiple sclerosis (MS) comes to the Neurology clinic complaining of urinary incontinence. He indicates that he experiences increased urgency and frequency of urination. The most likely urodynamic finding in this patient is:
    a. An atonic bladder
    b. A spastic bladder
    c. Stress incontinence
    d. Absence of abnormalities
    e. Overflow incontinence

14. A 65-year-old man complains of a 3-month history of intermittent urinary incontinence. Urodynamic studies

show an atonic bladder. Which of the following is most likely responsible for his problem?

a. Diabetes
b. Old stroke
c. Multiple sclerosis
d. Right parietal tumor
e. Pineal tumor

15. A 35-year-old man is seen in the Neurology outpatient clinic with the complaint that his fingers occasionally "get stuck" when he tries to open jars. On examination you find subtle weakness of the fingers and toes as well as percussion myotonia. You suspect the diagnosis of myotonic dystrophy. Which of the following statements is true?

a. Myotonic dystrophy is a systemic disorder that may also cause cataracts, diabetes, mental retardation, and cardiac arrhythmias.
b. Myotonic dystrophy is primarily a disorder of skeletal muscle.
c. Myotonic dystrophy should not be considered in the differential diagnosis because it is an inherited disorder that typically manifests itself either at birth or early in life.
d. Myotonic dystrophy is an autosomal recessive disorder caused by a triplet expansion in the DMPK gene.
e. Electromyography is usually normal in myotonic dystrophy and genetic testing is essential to confirm the diagnosis.

16. An 18-year-old woman is brought to the Neurology clinic by her mother, who explains that her daughter has been behaving strangely recently and appears to have paranoid delusions. She has a slight tremor of both hands and the examiner notes that there is a brownish discoloration of the cornea in the vicinity of the limbus. Laboratory studies show a mild transaminitis. Which of the following test results are most likely?

a. Increased serum copper and ceruloplasmin with decreased 24-hour urinary copper
b. Increased serum copper with decreased serum ceruloplasmin and increased 24-hour urinary copper
c. Decreased serum copper and ceruloplasmin and increased 24-hour urinary copper
d. Increased 24-hour urinary copper but decreased copper staining on liver biopsy
e. Increased serum copper and 24-hour urinary copper with decreased serum ceruloplasmin

17. A 40-year-old woman with SLE develops weakness of her right finger and wrist extensors and pain on the right dorsum of her hand several months after being diagnosed

with left carpal tunnel syndrome and right sciatic neuropathy. What is the most likely diagnosis?

a. Mononeuropathy multiplex
b. Axonal polyneuropathy
c. Demyelinating polyneuropathy
d. Neuromuscular junction disease
e. Polyradiculopathy

18. A 70-year-old man develops the acute onset of an inability to speak. Examination reveals that he struggles to pronounce a complete word and cannot string words together. He is unable to repeat a sentence but can follow simple and multistep commands. What is the most likely diagnosis?

a. Global aphasia
b. Conduction aphasia
c. Broca aphasia
d. Wernicke aphasia
e. Transcortical motor aphasia

19. A 28-year-old woman is brought to the ER by her husband. In addition to having neck stiffness, she has had a fever for several days, has been somewhat confused, and has not been "acting like herself." LP shows 9 white blood cells with a lymphocytic predominance, 32 red blood cells, protein = 63, and glucose = 65. Gram stain is negative. What is the most likely diagnosis?

a. Bacterial meningitis
b. Viral meningitis
c. Fungal meningitis
d. Meningitis from tuberculosis
e. Subarachnoid hemorrhage

20. A healthy 32-year-old man is brought to the ER after he stopped speaking suddenly, fell to the ground, lost consciousness, and shook for 2 minutes. After the event, he was noted to have a tongue laceration and urinary incontinence. He has no history of similar events. His physical exam shows a mild right hemiparesis. Routine labs and a head CT are normal. An EEG performed the next day is normal. The normal EEG suggests that this man:

a. Had a pseudoseizure and does not require anticonvulsants.
b. Needs admission for long-term video-EEG monitoring.
c. Probably had a seizure, and the normal EEG result is not surprising.
d. Requires hyperventilation to elicit an absence seizure on EEG.
e. Has actually had an ischemic stroke rather than a seizure.

21. Two days after coronary artery bypass surgery, a 62-year-old man with hypertension complains that "there is another man's arm in bed" with him. When asked to hold up his arms, the patient raises his right arm only. When asked about his left arm, he claims it is the examiner's or another patient's. What is the most likely diagnosis?

a. Right hemispheric stroke with neglect
b. Left hemispheric stroke with neglect
c. Conversion disorder
d. Adjustment disorder
e. Alien-limb phenomenon

22. A 35-year-old man with no known history of seizures is brought in by paramedics in status epilepticus. Which of the following medications is used as initial therapy for this condition?

a. Benzodiazepines
b. Barbiturates
c. Propofol
d. Carbamazepine
e. Lamotrigine

23. Subfalcine herniation most often results in which of the following?

a. Ipsilateral third nerve palsy
b. Contralateral third nerve palsy
c. Ipsilateral hemiparesis
d. Contralateral hemiparesis
e. Bilateral leg weakness

24. A 23-year-old woman presents with loss of vision in the right eye accompanied by slight pain in that eye over a period of 3 days. She has 20/200 acuity, red desaturation, and an afferent pupillary defect in the right eye. The remainder of her examination and MRI are normal. A diagnosis of optic neuritis is made. Which of the following is true about treatment?

a. Interferon beta-1b will hasten recovery from this episode.
b. Mitoxantrone is the most effective treatment.
c. Medical treatment is not likely to help optic neuritis.
d. Oral corticosteroids are preferred for the treatment of optic neuritis.
e. Corticosteroids may delay the development of multiple sclerosis.

25. A 22-year-old right-handed woman develops horizontal diplopia acutely. Your evaluation shows normal right lateral gaze but difficulty with adduction of the right eye while looking to the left and nystagmus in the abducting left eye. What is the most likely anatomic localization?

a. Left paramedian pontine reticular formation (PPRF) producing a right internuclear ophthalmoplegia (INO)
b. Right PPRF producing a right one-and-a-half syndrome
c. Right medial longitudinal fascicle (MLF) producing a right INO
d. Left medial longitudinal fascicle producing a right INO
e. Lateral geniculate nuclei

26. A 55-year-old man with a history of tick bite and erythema chronicum migrans is diagnosed with Lyme disease. He asks his primary care physician about neurologic symptoms he should watch for. Which of the following is an early neurologic manifestation of Lyme disease?

a. Facial nerve palsy
b. Painful polyradiculopathy
c. Spinal cord compression
d. Leukoencephalopathy
e. Generalized epilepsy

27. A 34-year-old man is seen in the Neurology outpatient clinic with symptoms of headache and bilateral lower motor neuron (LMN) facial weakness. There is no history of a skin rash. Neurologic examination discloses a relative afferent papillary defect in the right eye as well as the bilateral facial weakness.

a. Guillain-Barré syndrome (GBS) is the most likely diagnosis, and he should have an LP to help confirm the diagnosis.
b. Lyme disease is the most likely diagnosis, and *Borrelia* serology should be sent to confirm the diagnosis.
c. Sarcoidosis is likely the correct diagnosis, and appropriate investigations include MRI of the brain, LP, and chest x-ray.
d. Multiple sclerosis (MS) is most likely the correct diagnosis, as bilateral facial weakness and optic neuropathy are both common manifestations of this disease.
e. Vasculitis, causing mononeuritis multiplex, is the most likely diagnosis, and so the patient should be referred for rheumatologic evaluation.

28. A 64-year-old man with a history of hypertension presents to the ER with the sudden onset of numbness of his left leg, arm, and face. His motor examination is normal. What is the most likely site of his lesion?

a. Right thalamus
b. Left thalamus
c. Left postcentral gyrus
d. Right precentral gyrus
e. Right corona radiata

29. While playing baseball with some friends, a 15-year-old boy, who was not wearing a helmet, was hit accidentally on the side of the head with a ball. He was knocked unconscious briefly but recovered fully. Two hours later he became increasingly lethargic, so his parents brought him to the ER. When you evaluate the patient, he is barely arousable to your voice. He has mild weakness on the left side of his body, and his right pupil is slightly larger than the left pupil; the right pupil does not appear to react to light. What is the most likely cause of the patient's symptoms and signs?

a. Concussion
b. Epidural hematoma

c. Diffuse axonal injury

d. Ischemic infarct

e. Drug intoxication

30. Which of the following syndromes or diseases could cause bilateral weakness and loss of pain and temperature sensation with preservation of joint position sense in both legs?
a. Amyotrophic lateral sclerosis (ALS)
b. Vitamin B_{12} deficiency
c. Brown-Séquard syndrome
d. Anterior spinal artery syndrome
e. Tabes dorsalis

31. A 2-year-old child presents with new seizures. Her mother tells you that the child is not walking yet. He has a 5-year-old brother with a seizure disorder and mental retardation. On examination, using the Wood's lamp, you find hypomelanotic lesions. The most appropriate next test is:
a. Skeletal surveillance
b. Skin biopsy
c. Head CT or MRI
d. No need for further tests
e. LP

32. A 3-year-old boy is brought to his pediatrician for evaluation of repetitive behaviors, delay of language development, and social isolation. He otherwise has normal motor development. Which of the following is a required feature of autism but not of Asperger syndrome?
a. Abnormal language development
b. Social isolation
c. Onset after age 3
d. Failure to meet milestones for gross motor development
e. Failure to meet milestones for fine motor development

33. A 62-year-old woman with a history of small cell lung carcinoma presents to the Neurology clinic complaining of bilateral paresthesias of the lower extremities. She has no history of diabetes or family history of polyneuropathy. She describes severe pain in the soles of her feet when standing and has difficulty walking. On examination, there is severe pain to light touch over both soles. On your sensory examination description, you will state that this patient has:
a. Hyperesthesia
b. Paresthesia
c. Allodynia
d. Sensory loss
e. Hypesthesia

34. A 38-year-old man presents to the ER complaining of mild headache. He had neck trauma a week earlier. The exam shows anisocoria, with the right pupil being 3 mm and the left 5 mm, both reactive to light. What other findings will help to localize the lesion?
a. Look at the pupils in the dark and check tongue deviation.
b. Look for evidence of ptosis in the left eye and anhidrosis on the left face.
c. Look for evidence of ptosis in the right eye and anhidrosis in the right face.
d. Look for evidence of horizontal diplopia and a cut in the right visual field.
e. Look for evidence of dysarthria and hemiparesis.

35. A 35-year-old woman presents to the ER reporting a few days of progressive ascending muscle weakness. She had a viral infection a few weeks earlier. On examination, you find diffuse weakness and areflexia. The most likely finding in the CSF is:
a. High protein–high cell count
b. High protein–low cell count
c. Low protein–high cell count
d. Low protein–low cell count
e. Normal CSF

36. A 33-year-old man is seen in the ER for difficulty walking. He has paresthesias in his feet and a left footdrop. Initial physical exam shows mild distal weakness in both legs, with absent ankle jerks and reduced reflexes throughout. While the patient is waiting in the ER, his weakness worsens, involving the arms, but he has no difficulty breathing. You want to admit the patient to the intensive care unit. What will be your best argument to convince your ER attending to do so?
a. Absence of upper extremity reflexes
b. Decreased gag reflex
c. A forced vital capacity FVC below 25 mL/kg
d. The patient's weakness is worsening very quickly, and you fear that he may need mechanical ventilation
e. You don't have an argument in this case

37. A 35-year-old man who is HIV-positive presents with radicular pain in the legs and associated bladder distention. The most likely agent responsible for these symptoms is:
a. Cytomegalovirus
b. *Clostridium*
c. *Toxoplasma*
d. *Cryptococcus*
e. *Pneumocystis carinii*

38. A 45-year-old woman presents to the ER with "dizziness," by which she means that she feels a spinning sensation. The sensation is intermittent and seems to be exacerbated by head movement. She has some nausea with the episodes but otherwise has no other symptoms, such as double vision, weakness, hearing loss, tinnitus, or difficulty swallowing. What diagnosis is most likely?
a. Vestibular neuronitis
b. Ménière disease

c. Brainstem infarction

d. Benign positional paroxysmal vertigo (BPPV)

e. Cerebellar infarction

39. A 32-year-old woman is seen in the Neurology outpatient clinic with symptoms of diplopia and ptosis that fluctuate during the course of the day. Examination shows fatigable proximal weakness. You suspect that she has myasthenia gravis (MG). Which of the following statements concerning MG is true?

a. It is an autoimmune disorder caused by antibodies that are directed against presynaptic nicotinic acetylcholine receptors.

b. It is an autoimmune disorder caused by antibodies directed against postsynaptic muscarininc acetylcholine receptors.

c. It is an autoimmune disorder caused by antibodies directed against presynaptic voltage-gated calcium channels.

d. It is an autoimmune disorder caused by antibodies directed against postsynaptic nicotinic acetylcholine receptors.

e. It is an autoimmune disorder caused by antibodies directed against the synaptic enzyme acetyl-cholinesterase.

40. A patient complains of difficulty chewing. On examination he is found to have decreased strength of his muscles of mastication. Which of the following cranial nerves is responsible for this motor function?

a. Trigeminal

b. Facial

c. Oculomotor

d. Glossopharyngeal

e. Hypoglossal

41. The following patients are being evaluated in a neurologic intensive care unit. For which one would the Glasgow Coma Scale (GCS) be used most commonly to follow his or her clinical status?

a. A 75-year-old man in coma after cardiac arrest

b. A 29-year-old woman with delirium after medication overdose

c. A 69-year-old woman with a thromboembolic stroke and Broca aphasia

d. A 20-year-old man who is unresponsive after head trauma

e. A 59-year-old man with subarachnoid hemorrhage after aneurysm rupture

42. A 68-year-old man taking warfarin falls while in the hospital, is found on the floor, and is difficult to rouse. He has a new right hemiparesis and an intracranial hemorrhage is

suspected. What is the most appropriate initial radiologic study?

a. Head CT with contrast

b. Head CT without contrast

c. Skull x-ray

d. Cerebral angiography

e. Brain perfusion scan

43. A 75-year-old man presents to your office with a 1-month history of progressive pain in the left temporal area and pain in his jaw while eating. On laboratory testing, the patient is found to have an elevated ESR of 94. What is the treatment of choice?

a. Sumatriptan

b. Carbamazepine

c. Verapamil

d. Surgical resection of brain tumor

e. Prednisone

44. A 35-year-old man presents with his spouse to your office for difficulty concentrating. Further history also reveals that he has fallen asleep while driving as well as in the middle of important business meetings, despite sleeping at least 8 hours each night. He denies hallucinations or a history of his knees buckling while laughing. His wife reports that he snores loudly while sleeping. His examination is normal with the exception of moderate obesity. Which of the following tests would be most helpful in diagnosing this patient's disorder?

a. Multiple sleep latency test (MSLT)

b. EEG

c. MRI of the brain

d. LP

e. Polysomnography

45. A previously healthy 21-year-old presents to the ER after being involved in a high-speed motor vehicle accident. You note that the patient is unresponsive, makes no spontaneous movement, and has a dilated pupil on the right that is nonreactive to light. What is the best explanation for these signs?

a. Infarction of the left occipital lobe

b. Concussion from the motor vehicle accident

c. Uncal herniation

d. Cervical neck fracture

e. Diffuse axonal injury

46. An 84-year-old man is transferred from another hospital with a reported hypertensive hemorrhage. The films from that hospital are not available, and there are no further details. Which of the following is the most likely location of his hemorrhage?

a. Pons

b. Midbrain

c. Internal capsule

d. Frontal lobe

e. Corpus callosum

47. A 28-year-old man was recently diagnosed with obstructive sleep apnea. Of the following choices, which is the most appropriate treatment?

a. Pemoline

b. Methylphenidate

c. CPAP

d. Benzodiazepine

e. Clomipramine

48. A 45-year-old man with a prior history of migraine headaches with aura presents to the ER complaining of a progressive headache for the last month that is different from his usual migraine. There is no associated nausea or vomiting. His neurologic examination is completely normal. Your next step in management should be:

a. Brain imaging study

b. Abortive migraine treatment

c. Preventive migraine treatment

d. Reassurance and discharge home

e. Administration of pure oxygen

49. Which of the following features is most commonly associated with a pituitary adenoma?

a. Homonymous hemianopia

b. Bitemporal hemianopia

c. Ring enhancement on brain imaging with contrast

d. Seizures

e. Hemiparesis

50. A 24-year-old construction worker falls from a ladder and fractures his cervical spine with resulting signs of upper motor neuron (UMN) dysfunction. Which of the following signs is characteristic of a UMN lesion?

a. Hypotonia

b. Decreased reflexes

c. Flexor plantar response

d. Spasticity

e. Absent reflexes

51. A 67-year-old woman presents to the ER with a new onset of headache, nausea, vomiting, and unsteadiness of gait. Her history is significant for atrial fibrillation, for which she is chronically anticoagulated with warfarin. She also has a pacemaker in place. You are concerned about the possibility of a cerebellar hemorrhage. The imaging modality of choice is:

a. A CT scan, because this is the imaging modality most sensitive to the presence of acute intracranial blood.

b. An MRI, because blood in the posterior fossa will not be visualized on CT.

c. An MRI, because CT is contraindicated by the presence of a pacemaker.

d. A CT scan, because it provides the best images of the contents of the posterior fossa.

e. A SPECT scan to show metabolic activity in the cerebellum.

52. A 22-year-old woman presents with acute bilateral facial nerve palsy and intermittent peripheral nerve symptoms for over 3 weeks. You find elevated Lyme titers in serum and CSF. What treatment would you choose first?

a. Oral doxycycline

b. Intravenous ceftriaxone

c. Oral amoxicillin

d. Oral amoxicillin and doxycycline

e. Fluconazole

53. A 58-year-old man is seen in the Neurology ambulatory clinic with a 3-month history of right-sided resting tremor. On examination, he is noted to have mild masking of facial expression and there is diminished swing of the right arm when he walks. You suspect that he may have early idiopathic Parkinson disease. Which of the following statements concerning this disorder is true?

a. Most cases are familial with mutations in the α-synuclein or parkin genes.

b. It is characterized by the death of dopaminergic neurons in the substantia nigra pars reticulata.

c. The four cardinal features of this disorder are tremor, rigidity, bradykinesia, and postural instability.

d. Impairment of vertical gaze is a common manifestation of this disorder.

e. Early falls are a common problem in this disorder.

54. A 5-year-old boy is seen in the Pediatric Neurology clinic. His motor milestones have been delayed, and examination discloses proximal muscle weakness with difficulty arising from the floor. There is pseudohypertrophy of his calf muscles. He has an older brother with Duchenne muscular dystrophy (DMD) who is confined to a wheelchair. Which of the following statements concerning DMD is true?

a. It is an autosomal recessive disorder caused by mutation in the dystrophin gene.

b. It is an autosomal dominant disorder caused by mutation in the dystrophin gene.

c. DMD and limb-girdle muscular dystrophy are allelic disorders, both being due to mutations in the dystrophin gene.

d. It is a disorder caused by mutation in the dystrophin gene, which is located on the X chromosome.

e. DMD and Becker muscular dystrophy are allelic disorders, due to mutations in the dystrophin gene on chromosome 4.

55. A 9-year-old boy presents with difficulty walking. Neurologic examination demonstrates, among other things, that he performs rapid alternating movements poorly, with a lack of proper rhythm and coordination. This finding, called dysdiadochokinesis, is most typically associated with dysfunction of which of the following brain structures?
   a. Basal ganglia
   b. Medulla
   c. Cerebellum
   d. Parietal lobe
   e. Thalamus

56. An ischemic stroke involving the right side of the pons could lead to which of the following patterns of weakness?
   a. Left facial weakness and right body weakness
   b. Right facial weakness and left body weakness
   c. Right facial weakness and right body weakness
   d. Left arm weakness and right leg weakness
   e. Right arm weakness and left leg weakness

57. A 27-year-old woman with complex partial seizures is well controlled on carbamazepine. Which of the following is a characteristic side effect of this medication?
   a. Thrombocytopenia
   b. Agitation
   c. Diabetes insipidus
   d. Nephrolithiasis
   e. Hyponatremia

58. A 53-year-old construction worker is brought to the ER with a severe, sudden-onset headache accompanied by vomiting. A CT scan of his head demonstrates a subarachnoid hemorrhage. Which of the following is a common cause of subarachnoid hemorrhage?
   a. Tearing of bridging veins
   b. Laceration of the middle meningeal artery
   c. Aneurysmal rupture
   d. Amyloid angiopathy
   e. Arteriovenous malformation rupture

59. A 45-year-old woman has an MRI scan of the brain for evaluation of progressive headaches. The MRI scan shows a lesion that enhances in a homogeneous manner with contrast administration. Which of the following lesions is most likely to account for the appearance of the MRI scan?
   a. Glioblastoma multiforme
   b. Meningioma
   c. Brain abscess
   d. Toxoplasmosis
   e. Granuloma

60. A 75-year-old man is brought to the ER after having lost consciousness briefly in his bathroom. By the time he arrives he is feeling fine and is able to give a clear account of what happened. He recalls walking to the bathroom to urinate. Shortly thereafter he became light-headed and felt as if his vision were graying out. These symptoms lasted for about 30 seconds. The next thing he recalls is awakening on his bathroom floor. His wife notes that he was unconscious only briefly. Which of the following descriptions pertinent to this clinical scenario is correct?
   a. The symptoms of light-headedness and graying out of vision are atypical symptoms described by patients with syncope.
   b. He has micturition syncope.
   c. Orthostatic hypotension is the likely explanation for his syncopal episode.
   d. Vasovagal syncope is the likely explanation for his syncopal episode.
   e. Vestibular neuronitis is the likely explanation for his symptoms.

61. A 36-year-old man comes to the ER with a 4-day history of fever and a generalized unwitnessed seizure 2 hours earlier. MRI of the brain with gadolinium shows contrast enhancement of both temporal lobes and, in a nontraumatic tap, 10,000 RBCs and 15 white blood cells. What is the most likely organism responsible for this clinical picture?
   a. Enterovirus
   b. *Streptococcus* species
   c. *Cryptococcus neoformans*
   d. Herpes simplex virus (HSV-1)
   e. *Meningococcus*

62. A 55-year-old woman comes to the Neurology clinic complaining of numbness in the last two fingers of her right hand; it tends to worsen at night. On examination, you find a positive Tinel sign at the right elbow (percussion of the ulnar nerve at the right elbow produces a tingling sensation in the last two fingers of the right hand). You are convinced that this is an ulnar neuropathy at the right elbow and perform electrodiagnostic studies. Why do you think that this is a peripheral nerve problem?
   a. The acuteness of presentation
   b. The physical examination findings
   c. The symptoms described by the patient
   d. You don't think this is a peripheral nerve problem.
   e. There is no CNS complaint.

63. A 25-year-old man is now comatose after suffering blunt-force trauma to the head. On the basis of the clinical history, neurologic exam, and head CT scan, he is diagnosed with an epidural hematoma. Of the following choices, which is the best treatment option?
   a. Neurosurgical decompression
   b. Hyperventilation
   c. Administration of mannitol

d. Conservative management with close monitoring of vital signs and neurologic status
e. Administration of tissue plasminogen activator

64. A 19-year-old man is admitted to a Neurology service with an episode of transverse myelitis. Workup includes an MRI of his head and LP. Which of the following distinguishes acute disseminated encephalomyelitis (ADEM) from multiple sclerosis (MS)?
a. Presence of oligoclonal bands in the CSF
b. Pleocytosis with neutrophilic predominance
c. Monophasic course
d. Multiple lesions on MRI
e. A positive family history of ADEM

65. A 55-year-old man with type 2 diabetes presents with a 5-week history of pain in his right knee, followed by weakness and atrophy of his right quadriceps. Exam shows weakness of the right quadriceps and iliopsoas muscles and an absent right knee jerk. This presentation is most characteristic of what?
a. Diabetic distal symmetric polyneuropathy
b. Proximal diabetic neuropathy or diabetic amyotrophy
c. Mononeuropathy multiplex
d. Stroke
e. These conditions are not seen in diabetics.

66. A 19-year-old man is accidentally hit on the left side of the head with a baseball bat while playing a game with some friends. He loses consciousness and is taken to an emergency room. A head CT scan showed a lenticular shaped hyperdensity in the epidural space over the left temporal region that is exerting some mild mass effect on the brain. Which of the following mechanisms best explains the patient's head CT scan results?
a. Tearing of bridging veins
b. Laceration of the middle meningeal artery
c. Impact of the brain over bony prominences of the skull
d. Rotational acceleration and deceleration of the head
e. Rupture of a cerebral aneurysm

67. A 56-year-old woman is referred to the Neurology clinic by her optometrist, who noted that she had limited movement of her eyes. The patient herself notes only that she has fallen a few times in recent months. Examination confirms that there is marked limitation of vertical eye movements (both up and down gaze). There is mild rigidity in both arms and legs but no tremor. Her postural reflexes are poor. Which of the following is the most likely diagnosis?
a. Parkinson disease (PD)
b. Progressive supranuclear palsy (PSP)
c. Corticobasal ganglionic degeneration
d. Miller-Fisher syndrome (MFS)
e. Chronic progressive external ophthalmoplegia (PEO)

68. A 65-year-old obese woman is referred to the Neurology clinic with complaints of burning pain in both feet, which has been present for several months. You suspect that she may have a small fiber peripheral neuropathy. The most likely findings on examination are:
a. Symmetric weakness and atrophy of intrinsic muscles of the feet with loss of ankle reflexes
b. Symmetric stocking pattern diminution of pinprick and temperature sensation
c. Symmetric stocking pattern diminution of vibration and joint position sense with absent ankle reflexes
d. Symmetric stocking pattern diminution of all sensory modalities with absent DTRs in the arms and legs
e. Symmetric stocking pattern diminution of vibration and joint position sense with retained ankle reflexes

69. A 45-year-old man presents with a several-month history of weakness in his lower and upper extremities. On examination, in addition to weakness in multiple muscle groups, he demonstrates atrophy, hyperreflexia, spasticity of the legs, and bilateral Babinski signs. Fasciculations in multiple muscles are also noted. His sensation to pain, temperature, and joint position sense appear intact. What is his most likely diagnosis?
a. Amyotrophic lateral sclerosis (ALS)
b. Vitamin B_{12} deficiency
c. Anterior spinal artery syndrome
d. Central cord syndrome
e. Brown-Séquard syndrome

70. A 25-year-old man presents to your office with excessive daytime sleepiness, visual hallucinations while falling asleep, and a history of transiently losing tone in his extremities and falling to the ground when he is angry or laughing. Of the following choices, what would be his single best treatment option?
a. Pemoline
b. Venlafaxine
c. Clomipramine
d. CPAP
e. Methylphenidate

71. A 54-year-old man is seen in the Neurology clinic with complaints of resting tremor of the left hand and a general feeling of slowing down. As an example, he explains that it takes him at least 20 minutes to get dressed in the morning. You suspect that he has idiopathic Parkinson disease (PD). If you are correct, examination would be most likely to show which of the following combinations of physical signs?
a. Asymmetric rest tremor, asymmetric rigidity, and poor postural reflexes
b. Symmetric rest tremor, asymmetric rigidity, and poor postural reflexes
c. Asymmetric rest tremor, symmetric rigidity, and poor postural reflexes

d. Symmetric rest tremor and rigidity and poor postural reflexes

e. Asymmetric rest tremor, symmetric rigidity, and impairment of vertical gaze

72. A 55-year-old man with a history of hypertension is seen in the ER with complaints of clumsiness and incoordination; these began 2 days earlier and have increased in severity. He also reports double vision on lateral gaze, which resolves when one eye is covered. He is awake, alert, and oriented. Examination shows restricted eye movements in all directions, with eye abduction in both directions most limited. DTRs are absent, and there is impaired joint position sense. The most likely diagnosis is:

a. Brainstem stroke

b. Cerebellar infarction with compression of the brainstem

c. Miller-Fisher syndrome (MFS)

d. Myasthenia gravis (MG)

e. Alcoholic cerebellar degeneration

73. A 44-year-old woman presents to the ER complaining of urinary incontinence and lower back pain. What will be the most useful next diagnostic procedure to try in the effort to find the etiology of her problem?

a. Urodynamic studies

b. Blood testing including glucose level

c. MRI of the spine

d. Post-void residual

e. LP

74. A 48-year-old woman reports recurrent episodes of stabbing unilateral pain associated with tearing and conjunctival injection. Which of the following is characteristic of chronic paroxysmal hemicrania as opposed to cluster headache?

a. Unilateral pain

b. Conjunctival injection

c. Male predominance

d. Indomethacin responsivity

e. Headache duration of hours

75. A 75-year-old right-handed man with hypertension, diabetes, and hypercholesterolemia is seen in the ER. His family explains that he has had difficulty doing things around the house for the last few days. The patient himself admits that he has found it difficult to get dressed and to prepare his breakfast, but he feels healthy otherwise. On examination his speech is fluent, and he is able to name objects and repeat short phrases without difficulty. He is, however, unable to mimic certain activities described by the examiner, although he seems to have no difficulty understanding what it is that he is supposed to do.

a. He likely has a form of Wernicke aphasia due to a lesion in the left superior temporal lobe.

b. He likely has a form of apraxia due to a lesion in the right frontal lobe.

c. He likely has a form of Wernicke aphasia due to a lesion in the left inferior frontal lobe.

d. He likely has a form of apraxia due to a lesion in the right parietal lobe.

e. He likely has a form of apraxia due to a lesion in the left parietal lobe.

76. The most reliable method for distinguishing between a "traumatic" spinal tap (lumbar puncture) and a subarachnoid hemorrhage is the presence of:

a. Increased opening pressure

b. Increased red cell count

c. Increased white cell count

d. Xanthochromia

e. Pain upon needle insertion

77. The magnetic resonance imaging sequence that is most sensitive for the presence of blood breakdown products (e.g., after a hemorrhage) is:

a. T1

b. T2

c. Contrast-enhanced T1

d. FLAIR

e. Susceptibility

78. Which of the following disorders is most closely associated with REM sleep behavior disorder?

a. Alzheimer disease

b. Multiple sclerosis

c. Multiple system atrophy

d. Myasthenia gravis

e. Primary lateral sclerosis

79. Which of the following vascular malformations is the most likely to result in an intracranial hemorrhage?

a. Arteriovenous malformation

b. Capillary telangiectasia

c. Cavernous hemangioma

d. Developmental venous anomaly

e. Vein of Galen

80. An 81-year-old right-handed man with hypertension and hypercholesterolemia presents with the sudden onset of a dense right hemiplegia. His language is normal, and he has normal eye movements and pupillary reactions. He has no sensory deficits. What is the most likely localization of his stroke?

a. Left motor cortex

b. Left internal capsule

c. Left thalamus

d. Left midbrain

e. Left lateral medulla

81. In which of the following disorders would the highest elevation of creatine kinase (CK) be expected?
a. Becker muscular dystrophy
b. Duchenne muscular dystrophy
c. Lambert-Eaton myasthenic syndrome
d. Limb-girdle muscular dystrophy
e. Myotonic dystrophy

82. A 68-year-old man with no major medical problems attends his annual visit with his primary care physician. The doctor wishes to perform a brief screening neurologic examination. Which of the following parts of the neurologic exam would be the most sensitive for the detection of potential abnormalities in multiple different parts of the nervous system?
a. Deep tendon (muscle stretch) reflexes
b. Gait evaluation
c. Visual field examination
d. Joint position sense testing
e. Total weight-lifting capacity

83. A 78-year-old woman with a history of coronary artery disease and hypercholesterolemia develops the sudden onset of paralysis of all four extremities. On examination her eyes are open, she appears alert, and she can consistently respond to complex questions and commands by blinking her eyes but otherwise has minimal facial movement and no movement of the extremities. This condition is best described as:
a. Locked-in syndrome
b. Persistent vegetative state
c. Brain death
d. Coma
e. Stupor

84. A 30-year-old man is found to have increased intracranial pressure after a head injury. Which of the following treatments can serve to lower intracranial pressure?
a. Lowering the head of the bed
b. Intravenous fluid load
c. Depression of respiratory rate
d. Mannitol
e. Basilar artery stent

85. An 80-year-old man has developed gradually worsening memory over the past several years. His wife also reports that he appears to have vivid visual hallucinations at times, and his alertness has been fluctuating on a day-to-day basis. Examination demonstrates bradykinesia and rigidity in the extremities, without any dyskinesias. What is the most likely diagnosis?
a. Alzheimer disease
b. Dementia with Lewy bodies
c. Vascular dementia
d. Huntington disease
e. Progressive supranuclear palsy

86. A 71-year-old with a clinical diagnosis of Alzheimer disease comes to autopsy after a fatal motor vehicle accident. Which of the following is a neuropathological hallmark of Alzheimer disease?
a. Lewy bodies in the substantia nigra
b. Lewy bodies in cortical neurons
c. Prominent atrophy of caudate
d. Spongiform changes in cortex
e. Neurofibrillary tangles

87. A 34-year-old man comes for neurologic consultation because of paroxysmal episodes of speech difficulty that have occurred recently. The best way to distinguish whether these are seizures or other types of events is:
a. History
b. Neurologic examination
c. Brain MRI
d. Routine EEG
e. Empiric anticonvulsant trial

88. A 16-year-old college student is seen in the emergency room for fever, confusion, and headache. Lumbar puncture is performed. Which of the following cerebrospinal fluid profiles is most consistent with acute bacterial meningitis?
a. Normal white blood cell count, high protein, low glucose
b. Normal white blood cell count, high protein, high glucose
c. Elevated white blood cell count, high protein, low glucose
d. Elevated white blood cell count, high protein, high glucose
e. Decreased white blood cell count, high protein, high glucose

89. A 55-year-old man presents with headache and right hand weakness. On examination you find bilateral papilledema and upper motor neuron weakness in the right arm and leg. MRI with contrast shows an enhancing mass in the left frontal region, crossing the corpus callosum in a "butterfly" pattern with surrounding edema. Prior to requesting a biopsy, you discuss with your resident that this is most likely a:
a. Meningioma
b. Astrocytoma
c. Glioblastoma
d. Ependymoma
e. Schwannoma

90. You evaluate a 22-year-old woman complaining of visual problems. Your examination shows bitemporal visual field defects. Where is the lesion?
a. Right optic nerve
b. Right occipital lobe
c. Left optic radiation
d. Optic chiasm

e. This visual field defect is nonphysiologic, suggesting a psychiatric explanation.

91. You are asked to evaluate a 33-year-old construction worker who is complaining of paresthesias in the first and second digits of his right hand. Your physical examination shows no weakness but a mild decrease in light touch over the thumb. You request a nerve conduction study to rule out carpal tunnel syndrome, and it turns out to be normal. On repeated history, the patient indicates that on occasion, he gets a sharp, "electric" pain travelling from his neck to the right hand. What are you missing?
a. A median neuropathy at the wrist
b. A neuromuscular junction disorder affecting distal hand muscles
c. A C8–T1 radiculopathy
d. A lower trunk brachial plexopathy
e. A C6-7 radiculopathy

92. A 75-year-old man underwent surgery to correct a large abdominal aortic aneurysm. The procedure appeared to go well, but you are called a few hours later to evaluate the patient who states that he cannot move or feel his legs. On the way to the ICU, you consider the possible causes of his symptoms and plan your physical examination. What is the most important test to help localize the lesion?
a. MRI of the spine
b. Sensory level
c. Reflexes in lower extremities
d. Plantar flexion reflex
e. Toe position sense

93. A 19-year-old man presents to the emergency department with 2 days of ascending weakness. He had diarrhea 3 weeks earlier. He looks comfortable. On examination, you find moderate weakness in all limbs, with normal strength in facial muscles. You suspect Guillain-Barré syndrome and recommend admission to Neurology. What should be done first?
a. Spinal tap to look for albuminocytologic dissociation
b. Call for an emergency EMG to verify diagnosis
c. Send the patient for a whole spine MRI to rule out cord compression
d. Obtain pulmonary function tests, including FVC
e. Start high-dose steroids and then move to the floor

94. A 55-year-old woman is seen in the emergency room with the complaint that when she rolled over in bed in the morning she felt acutely vertiginous for about 30 seconds, with associated nausea and vomiting. Over the course of the day, the vertigo has recurred, each time precipitated by turning her head. She has no other symptoms and feels well in between the episodes of vertigo. She is known to have poorly controlled diabetes and hypertension. When examined in the emergency room, she is found to have rotatory and downbeating nystagmus during the Dix-Hallpike maneuver with the head tilted one way but not the other. The neurologic examination is otherwise entirely normal. Which of the following is the most likely diagnosis?
a. Meniere disease
b. Cerebellar stroke
c. Benign positional paroxysmal vertigo (BPPV)
d. Perilymph fistula
e. Vestibular neuronitis

95. A 77-year-old woman with a history of migraine in her 20s and 30s is seen by her primary care physician with the complaint that she has experienced headaches again for the first time in many years. Upon further enquiry she reports a sense of generalized fatigue and notes that there is discomfort over her right temple when she brushes her hair. The neurologic examination is normal. Which of the following would be the most appropriate clinical course?
a. Reassurance that her headaches likely represent recurrence of her old migraines. No further investigations are needed
b. MRI of the brain to rule out an intracranial mass lesion, as new-onset headaches in the elderly are commonly caused by raised intracranial pressure
c. Lumbar puncture to rule out high or low pressure headaches
d. ESR, CRP, and temporal artery biopsy, as giant cell arteritis is the most likely diagnosis
e. Explanation that she likely has trigeminal neuralgia, given the distribution of her symptoms over the right temporal region

96. A 63-year-old man with poorly controlled hypertension is brought to the emergency room after being found by his wife in a confused state. He had been fine when she left to go shopping, but when she returned several hours later, she found that he wasn't making any sense when talking. When you examine him you find that his naming is impaired and his verbal fluency is reduced, but other language functions are intact. You note that his speech is soft. Which of the following conclusions is most accurate?
a. The reduced verbal fluency, together with an anomia, is most suggestive of a posterior (Broca) aphasia.
b. The hypophonia, together with the evidence for a language impairment, is most suggestive of a subcortical aphasia.
c. He does not have an aphasia given that his language functions other than verbal fluency and naming are intact.
d. The impaired ability to name objects (anomia) is most suggestive of a conduction aphasia.
e. The soft speech, together with the anomia and reduced verbal fluency, suggests that he has a transcortical motor aphasia.

97. A 27-year-old African-American woman with diabetes presents to the outpatient Neurology clinic with subacute onset of bilateral facial weakness. She explains that the symptoms have developed over the course of the last few days. She also reports having a slightly raised and tender rash over the anterior aspects of both shins. On examination you find bilateral lower motor neuron facial palsy as well as tender erythematous nodules over both shins. Which of the following is the most likely diagnosis?

a. Guillain-Barré syndrome
b. Lyme disease
c. Neurosarcoidosis
d. Diabetes
e. Tuberculosis

98. Ataxia may be a manifestation of which vitamin deficiency?

a. Vitamin A
b. Vitamin B
c. Vitamin C
d. Vitamin D
e. Vitamin E

99. Which of the following are the cardinal features of idiopathic Parkinson disease?

a. Tremor, bradykinesia, rigidity, and postural instability
b. Bradykinesia, dementia, tremor, and rigidity
c. Rigidity, hallucinations, tremor, and postural instability
d. Tremor, rigidity, bradykinesia, and gaze palsy
e. Tremor, autonomic dysfunction, bradykinesia, and rigidity

100. Which of the following statements regarding higher cortical function is true?

a. Aphasia is characterized by a problem with articulation of words.
b. Apraxia is defined by the inability to carry out an automatic or unlearned motor task.
c. Agnosia is an inability to recognize objects through a sensory modality even when the primary sensory modality is unimpaired.
d. Neglect is a form of apraxia in which there is insufficient attention paid to one hemispace.
e. Agraphia is a disorder in which affected individuals are unable to draw pictures.

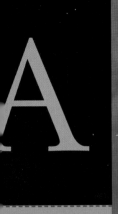

Answers

1. c (Chapter 12)

The presence of visual hallucinations is an early symptom of dementia with Lewy bodies (DLB). Other characteristics include cognitive decline, fluctuations of alertness, extrapyramidal symptoms, and an extraordinary sensitivity to neuroleptics. Visual hallucinations and sensitivity to neuroleptics are not early signs of AD, PD, Pick disease, or vascular dementia.

2. b (Chapter 4)

Decreased visual acuity that does not correct with pinhole testing, an RAPD, and a central scotoma is characteristic of optic nerve disease. A lesion affecting the optic chiasm will produce a bitemporal heteronymous hemianopia. If a lesion affects the optic tract, the optic radiations (in both temporal and parietal areas) or the occipital cortex (unilaterally), it will produce a homonymous hemianopia; that in the occipital cortex may be "macular sparing."

3. d (Chapter 25)

Niemann-Pick disease, Gaucher disease, and Tay-Sachs disease are all associated with cherry-red spots in the macula. Niemann-Pick disease is an autosomal recessive disorder caused by sphingomyelinase deficiency. Alexander disease and Canavan disease are dysmyelinating disorders with prominent macrocephaly but not cherry-red spots. The classic ophthalmologic finding of Hurler syndrome is clouding of the cornea rather than a cherry-red spot in the macula. Krabbe disease is an autosomal recessive disorder caused by galactosylceramide §-galactosidase deficiency. It does not produce a cherry-red spot in the macula.

4. c (Chapter 23)

One possible etiology of sensory neuronopathies is a paraneoplastic disorder, in particular small cell lung cancer. This is generally associated with positive anti-Hu antibodies (anti-neuronal antibodies) and can also be associated with paraneoplastic encephalomyelitis, ataxia, and autonomic neuropathy. Anti-GM$_1$ has been associated with multifocal motor neuropathy with conduction block. MRI of the spine would not help at this stage. Other causes of sensory neuronopathy include Sjögren syndrome, pyridoxine intoxication, and chemotherapy (cisplatin). Chest CT to search for occult malignancy is also recommended.

5. d (Chapter 1)

Each cranial nerve courses through a particular foramen, or opening, in the skull. Skull base fractures and other such injuries can result in damage to these structures and injury to the associated cranial nerves. The seventh (facial) and eighth (vestibulocochlear) nerves both course through the internal auditory meatus, which may have been damaged in this woman's case.

6. d (Chapter 2)

This woman has had a subarachnoid hemorrhage. Bleeding into the subarachnoid (CSF) space typically initiates an inflammatory response, one manifestation of which is a lymphocytic pleocytosis. Xanthochromia is the result of breakdown of blood within the subarachnoid space. Its presence in a bloody CSF sample helps to distinguish intrathecal hemorrhage from a traumatic tap. The CSF glucose is typically normal in both subarachnoid hemorrhage and viral meningitis. It is frequently low in bacterial, mycobacterial, and carcinomatous meningitis. An opening pressure of 14 cm H_2O is within the normal range of 6 to 15 cm H_2O.

7. d (Chapter 3)

This patient's clinical presentation suggests increased intracranial pressure (ICP) from a right hemispheric lesion.

The "blown" right pupil suggests that herniation of the right hemisphere has compressed the right oculomotor nerve. Choices A through C are all measures that acutely decrease ICP, while neurosurgery may be needed as a more definitive intervention. Performing an LP in this situation could be dangerous and could actually precipitate worsening herniation.

8. e (Chapter 5)

Symmetric proximal weakness usually suggests a primary muscle problem, as does weakness of neck flexors and extensors. The absence of muscle pain and tenderness does not argue against a primary muscle pathology. The other listed choices would not usually result in this pattern of weakness.

9. b (Chapter 15)

This child likely has absence seizures, which are frequently diagnosed after a teacher or parent notices inattention, "daydreaming," or staring episodes. Absence seizures last a few seconds each, can occur many times a day, and have a classic EEG appearance. Ethosuximide and valproic acid are typical drugs of choice.

10. b (Chapter 10)

This woman is suffering from a migraine headache. Sumatriptan is effective as abortive treatment. The other medications are effective in decreasing the severity and frequency of attacks and are used as preventive therapy.

11. c (Chapter 12)

This case represents an early onset of dementia with associated personality changes and movement disorder (chorea)—the classic triad of HD. HD is linked to chromosome 4p16.3, also known as the HD gene, encoding for a protein called huntingtin. The mutation produces an unstable CAG repeat sequence with more than 40 repeats. HD is not linked to the other chromosomes listed.

12. b (Chapter 8)

PCD is typically a pancerebellar syndrome with clinical manifestations including ataxia, dysarthria, and nystagmus. The underlying malignancy is typically a gynecologic one or breast cancer. The temporal evolution is typically that of acute or subacute onset with fairly rapid progression over weeks to months, followed by stabilization. Metastatic cerebellar disease would more likely affect a cerebellar hemisphere and produce lateralized cerebellar dysfunction. Alcoholic cerebellar degeneration typically affects the vermis, and the characteristic manifestation is that of a gait ataxia. Stroke (ischemic or hemorrhagic), although abrupt in onset, would not be expected to progress over a period of weeks to months.

13. b (Chapter 9)

MS characteristically produces an upper motor neuron bladder or spastic bladder with increased frequency and urgency. Stress incontinence is an involuntary loss of urine during coughing, sneezing, laughing, or other physical activities that increase intra-abdominal pressure. An atonic bladder is characterized by overflow incontinence and increased capacity and compliance.

14. a (Chapter 9)

Atonic bladder implies an LMN lesion at the level of the conus medullaris, cauda equina, sacral plexus, or peripheral nerves. It is characterized by overflow incontinence and increased capacity and compliance. Diabetes is the only one in the group able to produce that type of lesion.

15. a (Chapter 24)

Myotonic dystrophy is a multisystem disorder that may also cause frontal balding, diabetes, and gastrointestinal symptoms. It is the most common adult-onset muscular dystrophy. It is inherited in an autosomal dominant fashion and is caused by a triplet repeat expansion in the DMPK gene. EMG typically shows myotonic discharges.

16. b (Chapter 16)

She likely has Wilson disease, an autosomal dominant disorder of copper metabolism that presents with neuropsychiatric symptoms as well as a movement disorder. The pigment changes in the cornea are Kayser-Fleischer rings and are characteristic of Wilson disease.

17. a (Chapter 5)

The patient's current symptoms are suggestive of a right radial neuropathy. Multiple sequential mononeuropathies, each affecting a single peripheral nerve, are known as mononeuropathy multiplex. Pain is a typical feature. Patients with rheumatologic conditions are susceptible; vasculitis may be involved.

18. c (Chapter 11)

Broca aphasia is characterized by effortful nonfluent speech and an inability to repeat, with relatively preserved comprehension. Transcortical motor aphasia is similar but features preserved repetition.

19. b (Chapter 21)

Along with the clinical picture, a CSF profile of lymphocytic pleocytosis, elevated protein, normal glucose, and a negative Gram stain point to a viral or aseptic meningitis. The clinical presentations of problems A through D could appear very similar, but the CSF analysis is crucial in identifying the responsible organism. Bacterial meningitis tends to produce a granulocytic pleocytosis. Fungal meningitis is usually associated with hypo-glycorrhacia (defined as a CSF-serum glucose ratio below 0.4). Subarachnoid hemorrhage characteristically produces a large number of RBCs (thousands).

20. c (Chapter 2)

About 50% of patients with epilepsy have normal routine EEGs. A seizure is a clinical diagnosis, and this patient's convincing story supersedes the negative EEG. Long-term video-EEG monitoring is not required to prove the diagnosis of seizure. While hyperventilation can help to elicit absence seizure activity on EEG, his history and age make an absence seizure unlikely. Although an ischemic stroke can precipitate a seizure, this man's history is most suggestive of seizure. The right hemiparesis is more likely a Todd paralysis rather than an ischemic stroke.

21. a (Chapter 11)

This patient exhibits a form of neglect, in which he does not recognize his left arm as his. Right frontal or parietal lesions are the most common etiology. In the alien-limb phenomenon, patients retain awareness of the limb but feel that it is not under their control.

22. a (Chapter 15)

Benzodiazepines are the first agents used in the treatment algorithm for status epilepticus. Typically, phenytoin and then phenobarbital are used subsequently. Propofol is used if status epilepticus becomes refractory, while carbamazepine and lamotrigine are anti-epileptic drugs that are not available in parenteral form.

23. e (Chapter 17)

Subfalcine herniation may result in compression of the anterior cerebral artery with leg weakness as the result. Ipsilateral third nerve palsy is the first sign of uncal (not subfalcine) herniation. Continued uncal herniation may result in compression of the contralateral cerebral peduncle against the free edge of the tentorium, leading to ipsilateral hemiparesis (the "Kernohan's notch" phenomenon). Contralateral third nerve palsy and contralateral hemiparesis are not features of subfalcine herniation.

24. e (Chapter 20)

Intravenous corticosteroids may delay but not prevent the development of MS in a patient with optic neuritis. They are preferred to oral corticosteroids. Inteferon beta-1b and mitoxantrone are used for MS but not in the treatment of isolated optic neuritis.

25. c (Chapter 4)

Lesions of the MLF produce an INO. The clinical characteristics of a right INO include inability to adduct the right eye in left lateral gaze plus nystagmus of the abducting left eye. Adduction during convergence is maintained because this action does not depend on the MLF. "One-and-a-half syndrome" occurs as a consequence of a lesion involving the PPRF or sixth-nerve nucleus and the adjacent ipsilateral MLF. This produces an ipsilateral gaze palsy and INO on the contralateral side; the only eye movement present in the lateral plane is abduction of the contralateral eye.

26. a (Chapter 21)

Aseptic meningitis and cranial nerve palsies (such as facial nerve palsy) are among the early manifestations when the nervous system becomes involved in Lyme disease. Painful polyradiculopathy or leukoencephalopathy are two (typically later) nervous system complications of Lyme. Spinal cord compression and generalized epilepsy would not be expected to occur as a direct consequence of this disorder.

27. c (Chapter 18)

Sarcoidosis is one of the most common causes of bilateral LMN facial weakness. It is also an important cause of a lymphocytic meningitis (hence the headache) and may cause a variety of other cranial neuropathies, including optic neuropathy (hence the relative afferent papillary defect). MS is another important cause of optic neuritis, but bilateral facial weakness would be unusual. GBS may cause bilateral facial weakness but typically in the context of areflexia and generalized weakness; the relative afferent papillary defect would be unusual. Lyme disease may cause bilateral facial weakness similarly (although unilateral facial weakness would be more common); the afferent papillary defect would not be expected. Vasculitis is an extremely unusual cause of bilateral facial weakness.

28. a (Chapter 14)

Because of the sudden onset of symptoms along with the patient's stroke risk factors, he most probably has had a pure sensory stroke. The most likely lesion is in the contralateral thalamus, because the sensory pathways cross prior to synapsing in the thalamus. The left postcentral gyrus is on the wrong side to explain the patient's deficit. Also, it is unusual to have sensory loss of the face, arm, and leg equally from a stroke affecting the postcentral gyrus. This is because the middle cerebral artery provides blood to the face and arm regions of the cortex, while the anterior cerebral artery supplies blood to the leg region. The precentral gyrus is predominantly involved in motor pathways and not the sensory system. A lesion of the right corona radiata would be expected to cause a left hemiparesis rather than left hemisensory loss.

29. b (Chapter 17)

The middle meningeal artery travels between the skull and the dura. When this vessel is damaged (typically due to trauma resulting in a skull fracture that lacerates that artery),

ANSWERS

blood accumulates in the epidural space, resulting in an epidural hematoma. Patients often have a brief episode of loss of consciousness at the time of trauma, followed by a lucid interval and then clinical deterioration as the bleeding continues. Diagnosis and treatment constitute an emergency, because the blood will continue to collect and may cause brain herniation if untreated.

Diffuse axonal injury or an ischemic infarct would be expected to have a sudden onset without a progressive decline in function. Likewise, a concussion should not cause progressive neurologic decline and, like drug intoxication, would not result in the physical signs seen in this case.

30. d (Chapter 22)

ALS is a motor neuron disease with involvement of the lower motor neurons and corticospinal tracts. Weakness, muscle atrophy, and muscle fasciculations are prominent features. Sensory findings are not typical of ALS. Vitamin B_{12} deficiency classically results in degeneration of the dorsal columns and corticospinal tracts. Therefore joint position sense loss and weakness are typical features, whereas pain and temperature are spared. Brown-Séquard syndrome results from hemisection of the spinal cord. The classic features are ipsilateral weakness and loss of joint position sense with contralateral loss of pain and temperature sensation below the lesion. Tabes dorsalis is a late complication of neurosyphilis and is characterized by isolated dorsal column dysfunction resulting in loss of joint position sense. Anterior spinal artery syndrome usually results from infarction of the anterior spinal artery, causing ischemia to the anterior two-thirds of the spinal cord. Therefore dorsal columns are spared but weakness and loss of pain and temperature sensation result because of involvement of the ventral horns and spinothalamic tracts.

31. c (Chapter 25)

This patient meets the diagnostic criteria for tuberous sclerosis complex (TSC). A head CT or MRI may identify cortical tubers, subependymal giant cell astrocytomas, or other lesions. The other tests do not help in the evaluation of TSC.

32. a (Chapter 25)

A diagnosis of autism requires a combination of social, behavioral, and language abnormalities with onset before age three. Asperger syndrome shares social isolation and eccentric behavior with autism. Language is normal in Asperger syndrome. Neither gross nor fine motor delay is a required feature of either condition.

33. c (Chapter 6)

Allodynia is pain provoked by normally innocuous stimuli; hyperesthesia is increased sensitivity to sensory stimuli, and paresthesias are abnormal spontaneous sensations. "Hypesthesia" refers to decreased sensation.

34. c (Chapter 4)

This patient appears to have a Horner syndrome on the right, likely produced by a carotid dissection as a consequence of neck trauma. Horner syndrome is characterized by unilateral miosis, ptosis, and (sometimes) ipsilateral facial anhidrosis as a result of impaired sympathetic innervation. Examine the pupils in the dark (turn the lights off and look at the pupils during the first 5 to 10 seconds). A dilation lag in the small pupil and anisocoria greater in darkness means a sympathetic defect in the smaller pupil and will help with the diagnosis.

35. b (Chapter 23)

This patient appears to have a Guillain-Barré syndrome. Albuminocytologic dissociation means high protein with almost no cells in the CSF, which is characteristic of this syndrome. Immediately after the onset of weakness, however (the first 3 to 4 days), the CSF could be completely normal. Additional studies to corroborate the diagnosis include nerve conduction studies and EMG to demonstrate slowing of conduction velocities, prolongation of F-wave latency, and possible conduction block.

36. d (Chapter 23)

This patient appears to have acute ascending weakness with loss of reflexes characteristic of Guillain-Barré syndrome or acute inflammatory demyelinating polyradiculoneuropathy. His exam worsens while in the ER, and that should be an indication that he is deteriorating quickly and needs to be admitted to the ICU for close observation. An FVC below 15 mL/kg is an indication for intubation and mechanical ventilation.

37. a (Chapter 23)

Cytomegalovirus (CMV) infection is the most common cause of polyradiculitis or cauda equina syndrome in an immunocompromised individual. The other agents do not affect the nerve roots or cauda equina primarily. Cytomegalovirus polyradiculitis occurs in about 2% of AIDS cases and is characterized by the subacute onset of a flaccid paraparesis, sacral pain, paresthesias, and sphincter dysfunction. PCR evaluation of the CSF for CMV can provide a definitive diagnosis. Treatment is with ganciclovir or foscarnet or, in severe cases, both drugs.

38. d (Chapter 7)

Her symptoms consist of a feeling of movement—which is vertigo. The intermittent nature of her vertigo, the exacerbation with head movement, and the absence of brainstem signs are consistent with BPPV. In order to confirm the diagnosis, one can perform the Dix-Hallpike maneuver at the bedside. Brainstem and cerebellar infarctions rarely present with isolated vertigo, and Meniere disease is characterized by hearing loss and tinnitus along with episodic vertigo.

39. d (Chapter 24)

The primary antigenic target in autoimmune MG is the post-synaptic acetylcholine receptor. Presynaptic voltage-gated calcium channels are the target of the Lambert-Eaton myasthenic syndrome.

40. a (Chapter 1)

The trigeminal nerve is responsible for the muscles of mastication. The facial nerve innervates the muscles of facial expression, the oculomotor nerve subserves eye movements, the glossopharyngeal nerve innervates some pharyngeal muscles, and the hypoglossal nerve moves the tongue.

41. d (Chapter 3)

The GCS—which provides a composite assessment of unresponsive patients based on their eye movements, motor function, and language ability—is typically used for patients after head trauma. It has prognostic value for head-injured patients and is easy for nonphysicians to use.

42. b (Chapter 3)

A noncontrast head CT is the imaging study of choice in suspected intracranial hemorrhage. This allows for the easiest delineation of acute blood, which should appear hyperdense (bright) on this study. Head CT with contrast, skull x-ray, and brain perfusion scan do not help to identify acute blood. Cerebral angiography would be indicated only if a ruptured aneurysm or other vascular anomaly were suspected as the cause of an intracranial hemorrhage.

43. e (Chapter 10)

The patient's clinical presentation is typical for temporal arteritis: age over 50, pain over the temporal arteries, jaw claudication, and an elevated ESR. Definitive diagnosis is made by temporal artery biopsy. Treatment with prednisone for several months must be initiated early, because involvement of the ophthalmic artery can lead to blindness if diagnosis and treatment are delayed.

44. e (Chapter 13)

The patient's history and obesity are most consistent with a diagnosis of obstructive sleep apnea. While narcolepsy is also associated with excessive daytime sleepiness, patients typically have associated hypnagogic hallucinations or cataplexy, which are absent in this patient. Therefore, polysomnography is the test that would be most helpful in confirming the diagnosis. The MSLT is useful for diagnosing narcolepsy while MRI of the brain, LP, and EEG would be of no diagnostic value in this patient.

45. c (Chapter 17)

Uncal herniation results from mass lesions of the middle cranial fossa. This patient most likely has a hemorrhage in the middle cranial fossa from head trauma. If large enough, the mass lesion causes displacement of the medial portion of the temporal lobe (uncus) downward over the tentorium cerebelli. This typically results in compression of the brainstem and entrapment of the third cranial nerve. This compression can cause coma due to disruption of the ascending arousal system from the brainstem. It causes an ipsilateral dilated pupil due to compression of the parasympathetic nerve fibers (traveling with the third cranial nerve) that normally cause pupillary constriction. Diffuse axonal injury can result in coma but would not be expected to be responsible for a unilateral dilated pupil that is nonreactive to light.

46. a (Chapter 14)

Intracerebral hemorrhages caused by hypertension are most often found in the basal ganglia, thalamus, pons, and cerebellum, in order of decreasing frequency.

47. c (Chapter 13)

Pemoline and methylphenidate are stimulants used for the treatment of narcolepsy. Clomipramine is a tricyclic antidepressant used for the treatment of cataplexy. Because obstructive sleep apnea is characterized by repetitive episodes of upper airway obstruction during sleep, treatment is often with CPAP, which helps maintain airway patency during sleep. Alcohol and sedating drugs such as benzodiazepines can decrease upper airway tone, resulting in worsened symptoms. Last, obesity is a risk factor for obstructive sleep apnea, so weight loss may prove beneficial in obese patients.

48. a (Chapter 19)

A headache that is either different from the normal pattern or progressive deserves to be investigated further with a brain imaging study. Slowly progressive brain tumors can be associated with a normal neurologic exam or minor abnormalities. Nausea and vomiting need not be present, especially in the early stages of a tumor. Administration of pure oxygen is an effective treatment for cluster headaches, but the patient's description is not consistent with this diagnosis.

49. b (Chapter 19)

Seizures or hemiparesis are not usual features of pituitary adenoma. Varying degrees of bitemporal hemianopia (a visual field deficit in the temporal visual fields bilaterally) may be caused by compression of the optic chiasm. A homonymous hemianopia results from dysfunction of the optic radiations or visual cortex posterior to the chiasm. On brain imaging with contrast, pituitary adenomas usually enhance in a homogeneous manner and do not typically exhibit ring enhancement.

50. d (Chapter 22)

Signs of UMN or corticospinal tract dysfunction include hypertonia, spasticity, increased reflexes, and an extensor plantar response (Babinski sign). Signs of lower motor neuron (LMN) dysfunction include hypotonia, decreased or absent reflexes, and a flexor plantar response (downgoing toe). Weakness may be present with either UMN or LMN dysfunction.

51. a (Chapter 2)

CT is the imaging modality of choice for demonstrating acute intracranial bleeding. While it is true that MRI provides better visualization of the contents of the posterior fossa, a cerebellar hemorrhage usually will be visible on CT. Patients with pacemakers and other implanted metal objects cannot undergo MRI. Although MRI with diffusion-weighted imaging is the most sensitive modality for ischemic stroke, a susceptibility-weighted MRI sequence is preferred for detecting intracranial blood.

52. b (Chapter 21)

In the presence of severe Lyme disease with CNS involvement, as in this case, intravenous antibiotics followed by oral therapy comprise the first choice. Here, intravenous ceftriaxone is the first choice. The combination of oral amoxicillin and doxycycline is the most common treatment for uncomplicated Lyme disease. Fluconazole is an antifungal and has no value in the treatment of *Borrelia burgdorferi* infection.

53. c (Chapter 12)

Pathologically, PD is characterized by progressive death of dopaminergic neurons of the substantia nigra pars compacta. Most cases of PD are sporadic, but there are reports of familial cases in which mutations in the parkin and α-synuclein genes have been described. Impairment of vertical gaze is a common feature of progressive supranuclear palsy (PSP), a neurodegenerative disorder that is also characterized by parkinsonian features. Despite the gait manifestations of PD, early falls are actually uncommon (but are common in PSP).

54. d (Chapter 24)

DMD and BMD are allelic disorders due to mutations in the dystrophin gene, located on the X chromosome. The inheritance pattern is X-linked. The limb-girdle muscular dystrophies are a heterogeneous group of disorders, some with autosomal dominant and some with autosomal recessive inheritance. Mutations in a wide variety of genes have been reported in patients with limb-girdle muscular dystrophy, including the sarcoglycan genes.

55. c (Chapter 1)

The cerebellum is the primary brain structure involved in coordination, although other components of the motor pathways are involved as well. Testing for rapid alternating movements is part of the coordination exam. The other choices listed have less, or no, primary role in coordination.

56. b (Chapter 5)

"Crossed signs" can occur with unilateral lesions in the pons if descending motor fibers heading for the ipsilateral facial nucleus are affected, with the descending fibers heading for the contralateral spinal cord. With right pontine lesions, the right face and left body could be weak.

57. e (Chapter 15)

Characteristic side effects of carbamazepine include hyponatremia, agranulocytosis, and the risk for Stevens-Johnson syndrome. Except for the hyponatremia, these side effects are rare.

58. c (Chapters 14 and 17)

Tearing of bridging veins produces a subdural hematoma. Laceration of the middle meningeal artery causes an epidural hematoma. Amyloid angiopathy is a cause of lobar hemorrhage in the elderly. Although arteriovenous malformation (AVM) rupture is a cause of subarachnoid hemorrhage, aneurysmal rupture is a more common cause.

59. b (Chapter 19)

Meningiomas enhance in a bright and mainly homogeneous manner. Certain tumors (particularly glioblastoma multiforme and metastatic lesions), brain abscesses, toxoplasmosis, granulomas, and active demyelinating lesions typically show ring enhancement after contrast administration. While lymphomas can enhance in a homogeneous manner, they can also be ring-enhancing.

60. b (Chapter 7)

Micturition syncope is a form of reflex or neurogenic syncope that involves the triggering of cardioinhibitory and/or vasodepressor responses. The symptoms of light-headedness and graying of vision are typically reported by patients with syncope. Other symptoms might include a heavy feeling at the base of the neck, buckling at the knees, and tinnitus. Although orthostatic hypotension is a common cause of syncope, the occurrence of syncope after micturition, rather than upon standing, suggests that this is not the cause in this case. Vasovagal syncope is another common cause of syncope but typically occurs in the setting of acute pain or with a strong emotional response. Vestibular neuronitis is characterized by vertigo, and there is no associated loss of consciousness.

61. d (Chapter 21)

In HSV infection, the MRI often shows contrast enhancement and edema of the temporal lobes. An EEG can also be helpful and may show sharp-wave discharges in the temporal lobes. Treatment for viral meningitis is mainly supportive, because there are no specific treatments for most viral infections. If

HSV infection is suspected, however, treatment should begin promptly with intravenous acyclovir even while tests are pending, because mortality is close to 70% in untreated cases.

62. b (Chapter 23)

Physical examination is the most important information to define symptoms as belonging to the peripheral nervous system (PNS). Sensory symptoms can have a central or peripheral origin. The acuteness of the presentation does not help localization in this case. Paresthesias may be seen in both PNS and CNS dysfunction.

63. a (Chapter 17)

Neurosurgical decompression is the treatment of choice for an epidural hematoma that has resulted in uncal herniation. This is a neurosurgical emergency, so conservative management would only result in further neurologic decline. While hyperventilation and administration of mannitol may help to decrease intracranial pressure, these are temporizing measures; neurosurgical decompression is necessary to remove the accumulating blood. Because the patient has a hemorrhage, tissue plasminogen activator, which is used in acute ischemic strokes, would be contraindicated.

64. c (Chapter 20)

ADEM is a monophasic demyelinating illness. MS is characterized by multiple white matter lesions separated in space and time and is therefore not monophasic. Oligoclonal bands in the CSF are more common in MS than in ADEM. The pleocytosis of ADEM is lymphocytic. Both MS and ADEM can produce multiple lesions on MRI. ADEM is acquired and commonly occurs after viral infections or vaccinations. A positive family history is more likely to be relevant for a patient with MS.

65. b (Chapter 23)

This is a common presentation of proximal diabetic neuropathy, also known as diabetic amyotrophy. It represents a form of polyradiculoneuropathy that has a predilection for the lumbosacral plexus and in general tends to recover spontaneously over months to years. The etiology is likely different from the more common distal symmetric polyneuropathy seen in diabetes.

66. b (Chapter 17)

The patient's symptoms and head CT findings are consistent with an epidural hematoma, which results from laceration of the middle meningeal artery. The classic head CT finding of an epidural hematoma is a hyperdense region with a biconvex or lenticular shape. Tearing of bridging veins results in a subdural hematoma. Impact of the brain over the bony prominences of the skull results in cerebral contusions. On head CT, these areas appear as hyperdensities within the brain parenchyma and not

in the epidural or subdural spaces. Diffuse axonal injury results from rotational acceleration and deceleration of the head and can be associated with either a normal head CT scan or hemorrhages within the deep white matter of the brain. Lastly, rupture of a cerebral aneurysm results in subarachnoid hemorrhage and not an epidural hematoma.

67. b (Chapter 16)

Progressive supranuclear palsy is a disorder characterized by parkinsonism, supranuclear impairment of eye movements (vertical gaze typically affected more prominently than horizontal gaze), and impaired postural reflexes. Corticobasal ganglionic degeneration and PD may also cause rigidity and poor postural reflexes, but are not typically associated with eye movement abnormalities. The MFS and chronic PEO are both associated with eye movement abnormalities, but these disorders affect the external ocular muscles rather than the supranuclear gaze centers and are not associated with extrapyramidal features.

68. b (Chapter 18)

Small-fiber neuropathy typically produces symptoms of neuropathic pain, and examination discloses impaired temperature and pinprick sensation. Other sensory modalities are mediated by large fibers. Weakness and atrophy reflect involvement of motor fibers rather than small-fiber sensory function.

69. a (Chapter 22)

The patient exhibits both upper motor neuron signs (hyperreflexia, spasticity, and Babinski signs) and lower motor neuron signs (atrophy and fasciculations), which are the hallmark of ALS. Weakness can occur with either lower motor neuron (LMN) or upper motor neuron (UMN) dysfunction. None of the other options listed would cause widespread findings in both. Vitamin B_{12} deficiency classically results in degeneration of the dorsal columns (loss of joint position sense) and corticospinal tracts (UMN signs). Anterior spinal artery syndrome usually results from infarction of the anterior spinal artery, causing ischemia to the anterior two-thirds of the spinal cord. Therefore dorsal columns are spared, but weakness and loss of pain and temperature sensation result because of involvement of the ventral horns and spinothalamic tracts. Central cord syndrome is most common in the cervical cord and typically results in loss of pain and temperature sensation in a cape-like distribution. Brown-Séquard syndrome results from hemisection of the spinal cord. The classic features are ipsilateral weakness and loss of joint position sense with contralateral loss of pain and temperature sensation below the lesion.

70. e (Chapter 13)

The patient's history of excessive daytime sleepiness, visual hallucinations while falling asleep (hypnagogic hallucinations),

ANSWERS

and transient loss of tone triggered by emotional states (cataplexy) is characteristic of narcolepsy. Of the choices listed, methylphenidate is the best option, as it will treat the excessive daytime sleepiness and cataplexy. Clomipramine and venlafaxine are primarily effective for treating the cataplexy but will not improve the patient's daytime sleepiness. CPAP is a treatment for obstructive sleep apnea. Pemoline is an effective medication, but due to possible hepatic toxicity, it is usually reserved for use when other medications have failed.

71. a (Chapter 16)

The extrapyramidal features of idiopathic PD are typically asymmetric. Postural reflexes may be impaired in a number of extrapyramidal disorders including idiopathic PD. Impaired vertical gaze is more typical of progressive supranuclear palsy than of idiopathic PD.

72. c (Chapter 8)

MFS is a disorder characterized by ataxia, ophthalmoplegia, and areflexia. It is considered a variant of the Guillain-Barré syndrome and is associated with the finding of anti-GQ1b antibodies in the serum. Stroke (involving either the brainstem or cerebellum) should be sudden in onset and typically would not be expected to progress over a period of several days. Ophthalmoplegia may be seen in both MG and the MFS, but areflexia is not a feature of MG. Alcoholic cerebellar degeneration may be associated with a peripheral neuropathy and loss of joint position sense and deep tendon reflexes but should not produce ophthalmoplegia (unless associated with Wernicke encephalopathy, in which case confusion should also be present).

73. c (Chapter 9)

Acute urinary incontinence is an emergency. MRI of the spine will help to determine whether an acute lesion is responsible for the incontinence (cauda equina or conus medullaris syndrome, spinal cord compression, etc.). Determination of the PVR would not help in this situation, and urodynamic studies are not indicated in the acute setting. Lumbar puncture is not indicated in this situation.

74. d (Chapter 10)

Both chronic paroxysmal hemicrania and cluster headache are unilateral and can produce conjunctival injection. Chronic paroxysmal headache is more common in women, whereas cluster headache is more common in men. Response to indomethacin is seen in chronic paroxysmal hemicrania but not in cluster headache. Episodes of chronic paroxysmal hemicrania typically last for 20 minutes rather than hours.

75. e (Chapter 11)

Although the patient's symptoms are somewhat nonspecific, examination shows that he has normal language function but

with inability to perform certain actions described by the examiner. "Apraxia" refers to the inability to perform a learned motor task and it is typically caused by lesions in either the frontal or parietal lobe of the dominant hemisphere.

76. d (Chapter 2)

Xanthochromia is the yellow discoloration of the supernatant (if blood has been present for a few hours) in a spun sample of CSF that characterizes the presence of blood due to a subarachnoid hemorrhage. In a traumatic tap, the red cells precipitate, and the supernatant is colorless. Increased opening pressure, increased white cell count, and pain upon needle insertion may or may not be present in either condition. Increased red cell count is seen in both subarachnoid hemorrhage and a traumatic tap.

77. e (Chapter 2)

While T1 and T2 images may detect blood breakdown products, susceptibility imaging or gradient-echo imaging is the most sensitive technique for determining the presence of intracranial hemorrhage. Contrast-enhanced T1 is more useful for detecting the presence of a brain tumor. FLAIR imaging is the single best MRI technique for screening for most types of intracranial lesions.

78. c (Chapter 13)

Synucleinopathies are associated with REM sleep behavior disorder. Examples of synucleinopathies are Parkinson disease, Lewy body dementia, and multiple system atrophy. Alzheimer disease, multiple sclerosis, myasthenia gravis, and primary lateral sclerosis are not synucleinopathies and are not associated with REM sleep behavior disorder.

79. a (Chapter 14)

Of the vascular malformations, arteriovenous malformations are at the greatest risk to bleed, with a rate of bleeding of approximately 2% to 3% per year. Capillary telangiectasias, cavernous hemangiomas, and developmental venous anomalies are vascular malformations which rupture much less frequently, and are thus less likely to result in an intracranial hemorrhage. The vein of Galen is a normal anatomic structure.

80. b (Chapter 14)

The patient has a pure motor stroke involving the right side. Possible localization for this syndrome includes the left corona radiata, left internal capsule, and the left side of the base of the pons. Infarction of the motor cortex capable of producing a right hemiplegia would also likely cause an aphasia. Thalamic strokes produce more prominent sensory than motor deficits. Infarction of the midbrain sufficient to produce a hemiplegia would also be associated with eye movement abnormalities. The lateral medullary (Wallenberg) syndrome is associated with ipsilateral ataxia, ipsilateral Horner syndrome, and ipsilateral facial sensory loss, with contralateral impairment of pain and temperature in the arm and leg, nystagmus, and vertigo. Weakness is absent in a Wallenberg syndrome because motor fibers travel more anteriorly within the medulla.

81. b (Chapter 24)

Duchenne muscular dystrophy is associated with a marked elevation of the serum CK level. Becker muscular dystrophy and limb-girdle muscular dystrophy are also associated with increased CK levels, but the elevations are less marked than for Duchenne dystrophy. Myotonic dystrophy may be associated with a normal CK or only mild elevation. Lambert-Eaton myasthenic syndrome is a neuromuscular junction disorder which is not typically associated with elevations in CK.

82. c (Chapter 1)

The ability to walk in a steady, coordinated manner requires the concerted functioning of multiple parts of the nervous system, including motor pathways, sensory tracts, and the cerebellum, among other things. Testing for gait abnormalities is thus a sensitive way to detect abnormalities in many different nervous system functions.

83. a (Chapter 3)

Locked-in syndrome, which generally occurs with large lesions in the base of the pons, such as infarcts from cardiac embolism or basilar artery stenosis, is characterized by loss of all significant motor function except eye blinking or perhaps vertical eye movements, with preservation of awareness and cognitive function. A large pontine lesion will typically affect corticobulbar and corticospinal fibers bilaterally, but blinking and vertical eye movements are preserved because of intact midbrain function.

84. d (Chapter 3)

Mannitol is an osmotic diuretic which can be used to lower increased intracranial pressure, although the benefit may be transient. Lowering the head of the bed, loading intravenous fluids, or a decrease in respiratory rate would all have the effect of raising intracranial pressure. Basilar artery stenting is not an appropriate intervention for increased intracranial pressure.

85. b (Chapter 12)

Dementia with Lewy bodies may be the second most common type of dementing illness after Alzheimer disease. It is characterized by a parkinsonian motor syndrome, visual hallucinations, and marked fluctuations in alertness, as well as an exquisite sensitivity to neuroleptic medications.

86. e (Chapter 12)

The two neuropathological hallmarks of Alzheimer disease are amyloid plaques and neurofibrillary tangles. The presence of Lewy bodies in the substantia nigra suggests Parkinson disease, and in cortical neurons suggests dementia with Lewy bodies. Prominent atrophy of the caudate is seen in Huntington disease. Spongiform changes in cortex suggest the possibility of Creutzfeldt-Jakob disease.

87. a (Chapter 15)

The diagnosis of seizures is a clinical one. Except on the rare occasions when a paroxysmal event is directly observed by the physician, the best way to distinguish a seizure from other episodes of neurologic dysfunction such as syncope, migraine, or transient ischemic attack is by detailed characteristics obtained from the history. The other listed choices may contribute to the diagnostic workup but none is as important as the history in making the diagnosis.

88. c (Chapter 21)

A CSF leukocytosis, elevated protein, and depressed glucose level form the characteristic profile in acute bacterial meningitis. Viral meningitides typically do not depress the CSF glucose. Fungal and tuberculous meningitides can share a common profile with bacterial meningitis except that the leukocytosis predominantly involves lymphocytes rather than neutrophils (except initially).

89. c (Chapter 19)

The typical "butterfly" pattern is characteristics of glioblastoma multiforme. There are other tumors that can cross white matter tracts, like lymphoma. The other options are very unlikely to produce this radiologic pattern. Moreover, the usual location of meningiomas, ependymomas, and schwannomas is not those found on this MRI.

90. d (Chapter 4)

Bitemporal visual field defects are seen in conditions affecting the optic chiasm, such as suprasellar tumors. Lesions in the left optic radiation produce a right homonymous hemianopia, and lesions of the right occipital lobe a left homonymous hemianopia. Optic nerve lesions produce unilateral visual field defects.

91. e (Chapter 6)

Sensory symptoms in the thumb can be related to median neuropathies (as in a carpal tunnel syndrome) but also to higher lesions such as those seen in a C6 radiculopathy. Lower trunk brachial plexopathy or C8 or T1 radiculopathies could involve the 4th and 5th digits and intrinsic muscles of the hand (including those innervated by the median nerve). The fact that the EMG did not show median neuropathy at the wrist, plus the history of radicular pain, makes a C6 or C7 radiculopathy the most likely cause. Neuromuscular junction disorders do not present with pain or sensory symptoms.

ANSWERS

92. e (Chapter 22)

The patient appears to have an anterior spinal artery syndrome (ASAS), a well-recognized complication of abdominal aortic surgery. It usually includes a dissociated sensory loss as the anterior two-thirds of the spinal cord is perfused by the ASA, while the posterior third (posterior columns) is perfused by posterior spinal arteries. Therefore, the corticospinal and spinothalamic tracts are affected in ASAS, but the posterior columns remain intact, with preservation of joint position sense. A sensory level should be present but may not help to define the location of the lesion (nor will reflexes). MRI of the spine can help corroborate your clinical diagnosis but not show much quickly.

93. d (Chapter 23)

The patient has ascending weakness, and the preceding gastrointestinal syndrome makes Guillain-Barré syndrome more likely. Other tests need to be considered to confirm the diagnosis, but it is important to know the current respiratory status before any other test. If the FVC is less than 15 mL/kg, the patient should be transferred to the ICU and intubated. If the FVC is normal, the patient should have frequent FVC checks early during hospitalization, because a very rapid deterioration can occur. Steroids are not a treatment option for Guillain-Barré, which is treated with IVIg or plasmapheresis.

94. c (Chapter 8)

This is a very characteristic history of BPPV. Typically episodes of vertigo are brief, lasting 10 to 30 seconds, with no symptoms in between attacks. The absence of any other associated symptoms, the normal neurologic examination, and the characteristic nystagmus when the affected ear is closer to the ground during the Dix-Hallpike maneuver, are all highly characteristic. Meniere disease is associated with tinnitus and hearing loss. A cerebellar stroke would not produce recurrent positional symptoms and would likely be associated with other neurologic deficits.

95. d (Chapter 10)

This history is very characteristic of giant cell (temporal) arteritis. Other symptoms might include jaw claudication. Testing the ESR and CRP and proceeding to temporal artery biopsy are critical if the feared complication of blindness from an anterior ischemic optic neuropathy is to be avoided. Migraine is very unlikely; it would be a mistake to assume that a new headache in a 77-year-old woman represents recurrence of an old problem. MRI and LP are of no value in suspected GCA.

96. b (Chapter 11)

The anomia (impaired naming) and reduced verbal fluency indicate the presence of an aphasia (language disorder). The reduced verbal fluency does suggest an anterior location, but the hypophonia is most suggestive of a subcortical (usually thalamic) syndrome.

97. c (Chapter 18)

The rash on her shins likely represents erythema nodosum. Sarcoidosis is one of the most common causes of bilateral lower motor neuron facial palsy, especially in the African-American population.

98. e (Chapter 18)

Vitamin E deficiency may cause ataxia, myelopathy, and polyneuropathy. Vitamin B deficiency may cause subacute combined degeneration of the cord and dementia.

99. a (Chapter 16)

Tremor, bradykinesia, rigidity, and postural instability are the four cardinal features of idiopathic Parkinson disease. Dementia may occur but is late and is not characteristic. Hallucinations may occur as part of diffuse Lewy body disease and are frequently encountered in idiopathic PD, but are not a cardinal feature. Gaze palsy suggests the diagnosis of progressive supranuclear palsy rather than idiopathic PD. Autonomic dysfunction is common in PD, but if prominent should raise the prospect of multiple system atrophy.

100. c (Chapter 11)

Aphasia is a language (not a speech) disorder. Apraxia is the inability to carry out a learned motor task. Neglect is not a form of apraxia. Agraphia describes an inability to write.

Appendix: Evidence-Based Resources

Chapter 2

Hasbun R, Abrahams J, Jekel J, et al. Computed tomography of the head before lumbar puncture in adults with suspected meningitis. N Engl J Med 2001;345:1727–1733.

Kidwell CS, Chalela JA, Saver JL, et al. Comparison of MRI and CT for detection of acute intracerebral hemorrhage. JAMA 2004;292:1823–1830.

Warach S, Chien D, Li W, et al. Fast magnetic resonance diffusion-weighted imaging of acute human stroke. Neurology 1992;42:1717–1723.

Young GR, Humphrey PR, Shaw MD, et al. Comparison of magnetic resonance angiography, duplex ultrasound, and digital subtraction angiography in assessment of extracranial internal carotid artery stenosis. J Neurol Neurosurg Psychiatry 1994;57:1466–1478.

Chapter 3

Booth CM, Boone RH, Tomlinson G, et al. Is this patient dead, vegetative, or severely neurologically impaired? Assessing outcome for comatose survivors of cardiac arrest. JAMA 2004;291:870–879.

Malik K, Hess DC. Evaluating the comatose patient. Rapid neurologic assessment is key to appropriate management. Postgrad Med 2002;111:38–50.

Wijdicks EF. The diagnosis of brain death. N Engl J Med 2001;344:1215–1221.

Chapter 4

Corbett JJ. The bedside and office neuro-ophthalmology examination. Semin Neurol 2003;23:63–76.

Lueck CJ, Gilmour DF, McIlwaine GG. Neuro-ophthalmology: examination and investigation. J Neurol Neurosurg Psychiatry 2004;75(suppl 4):iv, 2–11.

Newman NJ. Neuro-ophthalmology and systemic disease—Part I. An annual review (1994). J Neuroophthalmol 1995;15:109–121.

Newman NJ. Neuro-ophthalmology and systemic disease—Part II. An annual review (1994). J Neuroophthalmol 1995;15:241–253.

Chapter 6

Cervero F. Spinal cord mechanisms of hyperalgesia and allodynia: role of peripheral input from nociceptors. Prog Brain Res 1996;113:413–422.

Landy S, Rice K, Lobo B. Central sensitisation and cutaneous allodynia in migraine: implications for treatment. CNS Drugs 2004;18:337–342.

Chapter 7

Baloh RW. Clinical practice. Vestibular neuritis. N Engl J Med 2003;348:1027–1032.

Furman JM, Cass SP. Benign paroxysmal positional vertigo. N Engl J Med 1999;341:1590–1596.

Grubb BP. Neurocardiogenic syncope. N Engl J Med 2005;352:1004–1010.

Hilton M, Pinder D. The Epley (canalith repositioning) manoeuvre for benign paroxysmal positional vertigo. Cochrane Database Syst Rev 2004;(2):CD003162.

Chapter 8

Albin RL. Dominant ataxias and Friedreich ataxia: an update. Curr Opin Neurol 2003;16:507–514.

Rubino FA. Gait disorders. Neurologist 2002;8:254–262.

Shams'ili S, Grefkens J, de Leeuw B, et al. Paraneoplastic cerebellar degeneration associated with antineuronal antibodies: analysis of 50 patients. Brain 2003;126:1409–1418.

Chapter 9

Agarwal P, Rosenberg ML. Neurological evaluation of urinary incontinence in the female patient. Neurologist 2003;9:110–117.

Delancey JO, Ashton-Miller JA. Pathophysiology of adult urinary incontinence. Gastroenterology 2004;126(suppl 1):S23–S32.

Payne CK. Epidemiology, pathophysiology, and evaluation of urinary incontinence and overactive bladder. Urology 1998;51(suppl 2A):3–10.

Thomas DR. Pharmacologic management of urinary incontinence. Clin Geriatr Med 2004;20:vii–viii, 511–523.

Chapter 10

Edlow JA, Caplan LR. Avoiding pitfalls in the diagnosis of subarachnoid hemorrhage. N Engl J Med 2000;342:29–36.

Headache Classification Subcommittee of the International Headache Society. The International Classification of Headache Disorders: 2nd edition. Cephalalgia 2004;24(suppl 1):9–160.

Lipton RB, Bigal ME, Goadsby PJ. Double-blind clinical trials of oral triptans vs. other classes of acute migraine medication—a review. Cephalalgia 2004;24:321–332.

Purdy RA, Kirby S. Headaches and brain tumors. Neurol Clin 2004;22:39–53.

Chapter 11

Damasio AR. Aphasia. N Engl J Med 1992;326:531–539.

Gernsbacher MA, Kaschak MP. Neuroimaging studies of language production and comprehension. Annu Rev Psychol 2003;54:91–114.

McClain M, Foundas A. Apraxia. Curr Neurol Neurosci Rep 2004;4:471–476.

Parton A, Malhotra P, Hussain M. Hemispatial neglect. J Neurol Neurosurg Psychiatry 2004;75:13–21.

Chapter 12

Cummings JL. Alzheimer disease. N Engl J Med 2004;351:56–67.

Knopman DS, Boeve BF, Petersen RC. Essentials of the proper diagnoses of mild cognitive impairment, dementia, and major subtypes of dementia. Mayo Clin Proc 2003;78:1290–1308.

Ritchie K, Lovestone S. The dementias. Lancet 2002;360:1759–1766.

Chapter 13

Malhotra A, White DP. Obstructive sleep apnoea. Lancet 2002;360:237–245.

Scammell TE. The neurobiology, diagnosis, and treatment of narcolepsy. Ann Neurol 2003;53:154–166.

Chapter 14

Alamowitch S, Eliasziw M, Algra A, et al.—the North American Symptomatic Carotid Endarterectomy Trial (NASCET) Group. Risk, causes, and prevention of ischaemic stroke in elderly patients with symptomatic internal-carotid-artery stenosis. Lancet 2001;357:1154–1160.

Mohr JP, Thompson JL, Lazar RM, et al. A comparison of warfarin and aspirin for the prevention of recurrent ischemic stroke. N Engl J Med 2001;345:1444–1451.

Sacco RL. Risk factors for TIA and TIA as a risk factor for stroke. Neurology 2004;62(suppl 6):S7–S11.

Tissue plasminogen activator for acute ischemic stroke. The National Institute of Neurological Disorders and Stroke rt-PA Stroke Study Group. N Engl J Med 1995;333:1581–1587.

Chapter 15

Chang BS, Lowenstein DH. Mechanisms of disease: epilepsy. N Engl J Med 2003;349:1257–1266.

Nguyen DK, Spencer SS. Recent advances in the treatment of epilepsy. Arch Neurol 2003;60:929–935.

Schachter SC. Seizure disorders. Primary Care 2004;31:85–94.

Chapter 16

Dalakas MC, Fujii M, Li M, et al. The clinical spectrum of antiGAD antibody-positive patients with stiff-person syndrome. Neurology 2000;55:1531–1535.

Lang A, Lees A. Management of Parkinson disease: an evidence-based review. Movement Disorders 2002;17(suppl 4):S1–S166.

The Parkinson Study Group. Levodopa and the progression of Parkinson disease. N Engl J Med 2005;351:2498–2508.

Chapter 17

Harris OA, Colford JM, Good MC, et al. The role of hypothermia in the management of severe brain injury: a metaanalysis. Arch Neurol 2002;59:1077–1083.

Shackford SR, Wald SI, Ross SE, et al. The clinical utility of computed tomographic scanning and neurologic examination in the management of patients with minor head injuries. J Trauma 1992;33:385–394.

Chapter 18

Hoitsma E, Faber CG, Drent M, et al. Neurosarcoidosis: a clinical dilemma. The Lancet Neurol 2004;3:397–407.

Martin RJ. Central pontine and extrapontine myelinolysis: the osmotic demyelination syndromes. J Neurol Neurosurg Psychiatry 2005;75(suppl 3):22–28.

McIntosh C, Chick J. Alcohol and the nervous system. J Neurol Neurosurg Psychiatry 2004;75:(suppl 3):16–21.

Moore PM, Richardson B. Neurology of the vasculitides and connective tissue diseases. J Neurol Neurosurg Psychiatry 1998;65:10–22.

Watkins PJ, Thomas PK. Diabetes mellitus and the nervous system. J Neurol Neurosurg Psychiatry 1998;65:620–632.

Chapter 19
Hentschel SJ, Lang FF. Current surgical management of glioblastoma. Cancer J 2003;9:113–125.

Soffietti R, Ruda R, Mutani R. Management of brain metastases. J Neurol 2002;249:1357–1369.

Chapter 20
Beck RW, Cleary PA, Anderson MM, et al. A randomized controlled trial of corticosteroids in the treatment of optic neuritis. The Optic Neuritis Study Group. N Engl J Med 1992;326:584–588.

Bergamaschi R, Ghezzi A. Devic's neuromyelitis optica: clinical features and prognostic factors. Neurol Sci 2004;25(suppl 4): S364–S367.

Calabresi PA. Diagnosis and management of multiple sclerosis. Am Fam Physician 2004;70:1935–1944.

Filippini G, Munari L, Incorvaia B, et al. Interferons in relapsing remitting multiple sclerosis: a systematic review. Lancet 2003; 361:545–552.

Frohman EM. Multiple sclerosis. Med Clin North Am 2003; 87:867–897.

Garg RK. Posterior leukoencephalopathy syndrome. Postgrad Med J 2001;77:24–28.

Chapter 21
Hussein AS, Shafran SD. Acute bacterial meningitis in adults. A 12-year review. Medicine 2000;79:360–368.

Schmutzhard E. Viral infections of the CNS with special emphasis on herpes simplex infections. J Neurol 2001;248: 469–477.

van de Beek D, de Gans J, McIntyre P, et al. Steroids in adults with acute bacterial meningitis: a systematic review. Lancet Infect Dis 2004;4:139–143.

Chapter 22
Bensimon G, Lacomblez L, Meininger V. A controlled trial of riluzole in amyotrophic lateral scelrosis. ALS/Riluzole Study Group. N Engl J Med 1994;330:585–591.

Lacomblez L, Bensimon G, Leigh PN, et al. Dose-ranging study of riluzole in amyotrophic lateral sclerosis. ALS/Riluzole Study Group II. Lancet 1996;347(9013):1425–1431.

Lacomblez L, Bensimon G, Leigh PN, et al. A confirmatory dose-ranging study of riluzole in ALS. ALS/Riluzole Study Group II. Neurology 1996;47(suppl 4):S242–S250.

Chapter 23
Koller HB, Kieseier C, Jander S, et al. Chronic inflammatory demyelinating polyneuropathy. N Engl J Med 2005;352: 1343–1356.

Kornberg AJ, Pestronk A. Antibody-associated polyneuropathy syndromes: principles and treatment. Semin Neurol 2003;23:181–190.

Verma S, Estanislao L, Simpson D. HIV-associated neuropathic pain: epidemiology, pathophysiology, and management. CNS Drugs 2005;19:325–334.

Chapter 24
Dalakas MC, Hohlfeld R. Polymyositis and dermatomyositis. Lancet 2003;362:971–982.

Emery AE. The muscular dystrophies. Lancet 2002;359: 687–695.

Newsom-Davis J. Therapy in myasthenia gravis and Lambert-Eaton myasthenic syndrome. Semin Neurol 2003; 23:191–198.

Sanders DB. Lambert-Eaton myasthenic syndrome: diagnosis and treatment. Ann N Y Acad Sci 2003;998:500–508.

Vincent A, Palace J, Hilton-Jones D. Myasthenia gravis. Lancet 2001;357:2122–2128.

Chapter 25
Online: Mendelian inheritance in man: http://www.ncbi. nlm.nih.gov/entrez/query.fcgi?db5OMIM

Nissenkorn A, Michelson M, Ben-Zeev B, et al. Inborn errors of metabolism: a cause of abnormal brain development. Neurology 2001;56:1265–1272.

Palmer FB. Strategies for the early diagnosis of cerebral palsy. J Pediatr 2004;145:S8–S11.

Rappley MD. Clinical practice. Attention deficit–hyperactivity disorder. N Engl J Med 2005;352:165–173.

Spence SJ, Sharifi P, Wiznitzer M. Autism spectrum disorder: screening, diagnosis, and medical evaluation. Semin Pediatr Neurol 2004;11:186–195.

Wenger DA, Coppola S, Liu SL. Insights into the diagnosis and treatment of lysosomal storage diseases. Arch Neurol 2003;60:322–328.

Index

Page numbers followed by *t* refer to tables; page numbers followed by *f* refer to figures.